KNOCKOUT

SUZANNE SOMERS

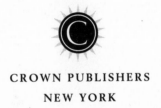

CROWN PUBLISHERS
NEW YORK

KNOCKOUT

INTERVIEWS WITH DOCTORS

WHO ARE CURING CANCER—AND HOW TO

PREVENT GETTING IT IN THE FIRST PLACE

The information presented in this work is in no way intended as medical advice or as a substitute for medical counseling. The information should be used in conjunction with the guidance and care of your physician. Your physician should be aware of all medical conditions that you may have, as well as the medications and supplements you are taking.

Copyright © 2009 by Suzanne Somers

All rights reserved.
Published in the United States by Crown Publishers, an imprint of the Crown Publishing Group, a division of Random House, Inc., New York.
www.crownpublishing.com

CROWN and the Crown colophon are registered trademarks of Random House, Inc.

Library of Congress Cataloging-in-Publication Data is available upon request.

ISBN 978-0-307-58746-6

Printed in the United States of America

10 9 8 7 6 5 4 3 2 1

First Edition

This book is dedicated to Farrah Fawcett, Ed McMahon, Fred Travalena, Merv Griffin, Eartha Kitt, Ron Silver, Dan Seals, Bea Arthur, Raul Walters, Greg Pineda, Jeannie Berzner, Jack Kemp, Wayman Tisdale, Kenny Rankin, Raymond Vloeberghs, Suzanne Pleshette, Sydney Pollack, Roy Scheider, Tony Snow, Hal Gaba, Philip Dennis, Robert Novak, Don Hewitt, Ted Kennedy, Dominick Dunne . . . all friends who died of cancer during the short time in which I have been thinking about this book.

With my love.

To live in a human body, you must have access to a certain amount of life-sustaining energy. You may either use this inherent energy in a nourishing and self-sustaining way, or in a destructive and debilitating way. In the case that you consciously or unconsciously choose negligence or self-abuse over loving attention and self-respect, your body will likely end up having to fight for its life.

—*Andreas Moritz*

ACKNOWLEDGMENTS

To Alan Hamel, my great husband and partner in life and in business for the last forty-two years; your fierce love and protection during this frightening episode was deeply moving. Knowing you wanted to go with me if I had to depart spoke volumes. Thank you for always looking out for me, loving me so much, and keeping the wolves away from the door.

To my loving and darling son, Bruce Somers, for all we've been through together; my stepson, Stephen Hamel; and my two inherited daughters, Caroline Somers, my daughter-in-law, and Leslie Hamel, my stepdaughter, whom I adore and love like my own; and to my best friend, Barry Manilow; you are the people in my life, along with my husband, who were there when I needed you most. In my valley of fear, my darkest hour, you never left my side, never let me down. This loyalty and show of love is the greatest gift in my life and I will always be grateful to all of you.

So many people are instrumental in putting together a book of this magnitude: the girls in my office; my executive assistant, Julie Turkel, making sense of an impossible schedule, tracking down and landing my interviews with these incredible professionals; and my darling other assistant Jordyn Goodman, who lights up the office, making sure I had everything I needed to pull this off; and Marsha Yanchuck, my editorial assistant of thirty-six years who singularly put together the entire resource section (which is no small feat)—all the phone calls and fact-checking. Thank you, Marsha, from the bottom of my heart.

My cool and calm editor, Heather Jackson, who in a very short period of time was able to help me pull this together and make sense of a whole lot of information. Now we can share that bottle of wine.

Marc Chamlin, my literary attorney who has been with me for the last thirteen books—I call him "the closer" and he does that so well.

To David Vigliano, my literary agent and friend—thank you for your support and loyalty and the great fun we have together.

To Sandi Mendelson, my publicist of many years and many books, and many more in the future—my deepest thanks for always being on top of it.

To Julian Whitaker for his eloquent and courageous foreword. His perspective and wisdom are evident in every word.

To Bill Faloon and the Life Extension Foundation, for giving me unwavering support and scientific backup to verify and validate the information presented in this book. Thanks to Dr. Steven Joyal, who along with Bill Faloon, sent me constant scientific backup to make these points.

Thanks to Dave Henson, my computer guy, for being available at all hours, helping me keep everything in order, finding lost pieces when I found impossible ways to file them in some way-out cyberspace.

Thanks to Cindy Gold and her great crew for the beautiful cover photo, and to Danielle Shapiro, who along with my daughter-in-law, Caroline Somers, designed the beautiful and strong cover of this book.

A huge thank-you to Dr. Stanislaw Burzynski, Dr. Nicholas Gonzalez, Dr. James Forsythe, Dr. Julie Taguchi, Dr. Jonathan Wright, Dr. Russell Blaylock, Dr. Stephen Sinatra, Dr. Michael Galitzer, Dr. Janet Hranicky, Dr. Steve Nelson, Dr. Steve Haltiwanger, Dr. Robin Smith of the NeoStem Company, Burton Goldberg, David Schmidt of LifeWave, Ralph Moss, Ph.D., and Cristiana Paul, M.S., who did so much extra work for the resource section and for her excellence.

All of you . . . made this book . . . you inspired and taught me, but most of all took away my fear of cancer. Thank you. I am deeply appreciative of all of you.

To my publisher, Jenny Frost, and her team at Crown, Tina Constable and Philip Patrick, who are not only talented but great fun to hang out with; and to all of the Crown crew who made this book possible—Christine Tanigawa, Amy Boorstein, Lenny Henderson, Linnea Knollmueller, Laura Duffy, Annsley Rosner, and Patty Berg.

To Mooney, for keeping my golden locks, indeed, golden, hip, sexy (but not desperate . . . ha-ha-ha).

And last but not least, Richard Jaffe, Esq., the renegade Texas lawyer who fights on behalf of maverick alternative doctors, for his perspective, experience, savvy, and intelligence. He went over this book page by page, word by word, making it better, protecting, suggesting, making sure I came off well and accurately. The words *thank you* do not seem enough for all you gave in this effort; inadequate though they may be, I thank you.

CONTENTS

FOREWORD BY JULIAN WHITAKER, M.D.   xv

PREFACE   xix

Part I
What Got Us Here

Chapter 1: A Cancer Story—Mine   3

Chapter 2: Meet the Doctors   18

Chapter 3: Against Our Nature: The Birth of a Big Business   28

Chapter 4: If It Could Happen to Me, What Will Happen to You?   34

Chapter 5: How Did It Get This Bad?: Conventional
          Medicine's Dark Side   40

Chapter 6: Ralph Moss, Ph.D.   43

Part II
The Doctors Who Are Curing Cancer

Chapter 7: Dr. Stanislaw Burzynski   59

Chapter 8: Dr. Nicholas Gonzalez   87

Chapter 9: Dr. James Forsythe 121

Chapter 10: Dr. Julie Taguchi 134

Part III
Preventing Cancer Before It Starts

Chapter 11: Dr. Russell Blaylock 147

Chapter 12: Burton Goldberg 163

Chapter 13: David Schmidt 173

Chapter 14: Dr. Jonathan Wright 181

Chapter 15: Dr. Stephen Sinatra 200

Chapter 16: Dr. Michael Galitzer 212

Chapter 17: Cristiana Paul, M.S. 228

Chapter 18: If You Choose Traditional Treatment, What You
Need to Know: An Interview with Bill Faloon 252

EPILOGUE 269

RESOURCES 271

BOOKS BY OR ABOUT *KNOCKOUT* DOCTORS 311

INDEX 317

FOREWORD

Suzanne Somers has written a book on cancer treatment and prevention. Suzanne is not a doctor or a scientist.

Should you pay attention?

Absolutely! And here's why.

Conventional medicine's approach to cancer prevention and treatment is a debilitating, often deadly fraud. The physicians who perpetrate this fraud must bear some responsibility, but the problem runs much deeper than individual doctors. The underlying issue is that the entire cancer treatment "industry" has been following a faulty paradigm for close to a hundred years.

A paradigm is a belief system. For instance, for centuries it was widely believed that the earth was the center of the universe. This paradigm was so firmly entrenched that it was part and parcel of church dogma of the time. When Galileo proved four hundred years ago that the earth revolved around the sun, he so threatened the existing order that he was tried by the Inquisition, threatened with torture until he recanted what he knew to be the truth, and spent the remainder of his life under house arrest. That's an example of the power of a paradigm—wrong though it may be.

The paradigm that is the basis for cancer prevention and treatment today is equally wrong. That paradigm of "purging the body of cancer cells" was initiated back in the late 1800s by William Halsted, M.D., who performed the first radical mastectomies on women with breast cancer. There was no significant follow-up with these patients to justify continuation of this procedure, but the presumption that cancerous cells must be cut out of the body was accepted without question. It just made sense.

More than a century later, this concept still holds sway, and our primary treatment modalities—surgery, chemotherapy, and radiation—are attempts to purge cancer from the body.

This approach does a lot of damage. Think of cancer and its treatment in terms of this analogy. Nations characteristically maintain a standing army to defend themselves against other nations as well as police forces to protect against nefarious elements within. If pockets of crime crop up in Chicago, Cincinnati, Philadelphia, Los Angeles, or Atlanta, you call the local police. Conventional cancer therapy, however, is like mobilizing the army, air force, and marines to invade, clear out, and bomb the enemy. It may get the bad guys, but it does obvious collateral damage—just as chemotherapy, radiation, and extensive surgery do.

Toxicity aside, it's clear that this approach doesn't work. Over the past hundred years, the death rate from cancer has hardly budged, and it will soon be the number one cause of death. Yet the trillions of dollars vested in its perpetuation have created a powerful and virulent force against change. Nevertheless, like all failed paradigms in human history, this one is coming to an end, and I expect that *Knockout* will hasten its demise.

What paradigm will replace it? It's obvious. All cancer cells, whether they're in the breast, prostate, pancreas, brain, or other organs, engage in undisciplined, rapid cell division. This is the basic defect, and this is where cancer treatment should be focused. You don't need to cut it out or otherwise purge it. All you need to do is to stop the cells from dividing, and the cancer will disappear.

The human body is capable of doing this. In fact, this is the primary discovery of Dr. Stanislaw Burzynski, who is interviewed in this book. He detected small peptides produced by the liver that control cell multiplication and found that, in the absence of sufficient amounts of these internal controls, cancer develops. Dr. Burzynski figured out how to synthesize these control peptides, which are the basis of his breakthrough cancer therapy. These peptides are like antibiotics for cancer cells. They stop cell division, and the cancer dies. Suzanne Somers has interviewed other practitioners with unique methods of treating cancer, and their successes are indicative that they too are enhancing the body's control over undisciplined cancer cell multiplication.

If you are afflicted with cancer, you will be facing a number of decisions, and it's important that you make up your mind with thought and reason, not fear. Here are some questions you should ask every physician you choose to investigate when it comes to your treatment choices for cancer.

First, is the therapy itself significantly harmful and debilitating? This is an important question. Regardless of how a therapy temporarily affects the cancer, if it weakens and debilitates the body, you become more vulnerable both to disease recurrence and to damage done by the therapy. Remember, your goal is not just to survive for two to three years but to thrive and prosper.

Second, are there indications that the therapy enhances the body's innate healing ability? Does the therapy make your internal protection against cancer stronger or weaker? Obviously, any therapy that weakens the body's ability to fight off other cancers is undesirable, as you may survive one bout only to have to deal with more virulent disease down the road.

Third, and perhaps most important, is it appropriate to seek second opinions from other cancer specialists and from practitioners who use unconventional therapies? If the physician's response is aggressive or demeaning toward other approaches, that's a red flag. No doctor should make your decisions for you. It is, after all, your life that's at stake. Physicians who care for their patients and have confidence in their abilities as physicians do not use scare tactics to coerce patients.

Knockout is a very helpful book. In it you'll find guideposts and resources for information that will empower you to make the best decisions possible. The book also contains a wealth of scientifically based advice on how through nutritional support you can reduce the risk of getting cancer or having a recurrence. Of course, there is no one treatment that can guarantee success for everyone. For many, the conventional approach feels right. If you choose this path, the interview with Bill Faloon will provide excellent advice on nutritional support while undergoing chemotherapy and radiation that can dramatically increase your survival prospects.

I do, however, believe that cancer can be cured—not improved but cured. I've seen too many patients recover from serious, even life-threatening cancers to mince words. These are people who had been told they had no chance of survival, but their doctors were wrong. Cancer can be cured. I look forward to seeing the day when that is the norm and not the exception. This book, *Knockout*, is a step in that direction.

Through my newsletter, *Health & Healing,* and my other advocacy activities, I have long been a critic of the old cancer paradigm and an avid supporter of new, more rational approaches put forth by people like Dr. Burzynski. As a warrior in this battle, it is very gratifying to me that someone like Suzanne Somers, with her stature and influence, is joining the fray. Suzanne is a courageous woman for challenging the conventional cancer treatment paradigm. You too will need courage if and when the time comes for you to face that challenge yourself. Good luck to you.

Julian Whitaker, M.D., founder, Whitaker Wellness Institute Medical Clinic (whitakerwellness.com), and editor of *Health & Healing* (dr.whitaker.com)

PREFACE

As I finished the final edits to this book, the *New York Times* featured an in-depth article about the failure of conventional medicine to cure more cancers.

According to the *New York Times*, adjusting for the size and age of the population, cancer death rates dropped only 5 percent from 1950 to 2005.

What other technology has performed so miserably over this fifty-five-year period? Would you accept a medical therapy that has not improved much since 1950?

In contrast, the death rate from heart disease dropped 64 percent in that time, and for flu and pneumonia it fell 58 percent.

The *New York Times* was especially critical of expensive conventional treatments that subject patients to much mutilation and suffering, yet yield survival improvements of only a few months.

Clearly, as the *Times* states, "we are not winning the war against cancer."

This book is written to show another side of cancer treatment and what you can do now to prevent getting this dreaded disease.

As a reader, you must know there are no guarantees. Cancer kills and continues to kill. Yet there are some who beat it. Some beat it with traditional methods, and some with alternative methods. No one can tell you what will work for sure. You need to gather as much information as you can and make your own decisions.

But there is hope, and this book offers new choices. It is important you know that there are more methods than traditional chemotherapy and radiation available, and these are what this book attempts to bring to you, my faithful readers. Although I have always leaned toward alternative medicine, the testimonials of the "cured" patients made a believer out of me.

It is a very brave choice to go against traditional medicine and embrace the alternative route. It's easier to try the traditional route and then, if it fails, go to the alternatives, but often it can be too late. My friend Farrah—would she have made it if she had gone alternative first? There is no way of knowing.

When you receive a cancer diagnosis, you're more vulnerable than at any other time in your life. I've personally had the experience twice, as you will read in this book, and my only hope for survival was alternatives. But that was my decision, what I thought best for me.

I cannot make up your mind for you. I can only offer you these incredible professionals who have chosen to go another way. Some are completely alternative, while some are more integrated, but all are having success, great success.

Does everyone survive, though? The sad answer is no. Having cancer is a lonely experience. It is the one time in your life that you cannot ask those closest to you, "What should I do?" It's too heavy a burden to place on another person. This is your life, your decision, and cancer kills.

Read this book carefully. See and feel if the information resonates. I know that for myself, after having interviewed all of these incredible doctors, scientists, professionals, and patients, my choice overwhelmingly would be to use only alternative treatments regardless of what kind of cancer I contracted.

I am not a doctor or a scientist, but merely a passionate layperson, a filter, a messenger. I spoke with so many patients who are living normal, happy, fulfilled lives, and their enthusiasm and great quality of life convinced me that indeed you can live with cancer. You can manage cancer. You don't have to be degraded by humiliating treatments and protocols. And in some cases, you can be cured of cancer.

It is with great humility I ask you to read these pages and then listen to your heart and choose what is best for you. Writing this book has taken away my fear of cancer. I hope reading it does the same for you.

PART I

What Got Us Here

By academic freedom I understand the right to search for truth and to publish and teach what one holds to be true. This right implies also a duty: one
must not conceal any part of what one has recognized to be true.

—Albert Einstein

For the great enemy of the truth is very often not the lie—deliberate, con-
trived and dishonest—but the myth, persistent, persuasive and unrealistic.
Too often we hold fast to the clichés of our forebears. We subject all facts to
a prefabricated set of interpretations. We enjoy the comfort of opinion without the discomfort of thought.

—John F. Kennedy

Chapter 1

A CANCER STORY—MINE

November 2008, 4:00 a.m. I wake up. I can't breathe. I am choking, being strangled to death; it feels like there are two hands around my neck squeezing tighter and tighter. My body is covered head to toe with welts and a horrible rash: the itching and burning is unbearable. The rash is in my ears, in my nose, in my vagina, on the bottoms of my feet, every-where—under my arms, my scalp, the back of my neck. Every single inch of my body is covered with welts except my face. I don't know why. I struggle to the telephone and call one of the doctors I trust. I start to tell him what is happening, and he stops me: "You are in danger. Go to the hospital right now." I knew it. I could feel that my breath was running out.

No time to wait for an ambulance. We race to the emergency room. I am gasping, begging for yet one more breath. I am suffocating. I am running out of time. I don't have time to think or be frightened; I can only concentrate on getting one last breath. I am dizzy . . . the world is spin-ning. Breathing is all I can think about.

We arrive. My husband has called the hospital in advance. They are waiting for me. The emergency room workers—nurses, doctors, and other professionals—are wonderful people. They have dealt with this before. They are reassuring: "Okay, we'll take care of her."

As soon as I am in the emergency room they inject me with Decadron, a powerful steroid. "Why can't you breathe?" the ER doc seems to be yelling in my ear, but I can't answer. I am unable to get words out. They inject me with Benadryl for the welts and the rash. Now I'm inside the ER, but I still can't breathe. I can't even sit up. I am bent over trying to find oxygen anywhere . . .

They put me on oxygen and albuterol to get me breathing, and slowly, slowly, life returns. I am still grabbing for each breath, and there are spasms in my lungs, like someone is turning a knob that pulls my lungs inside out, but unlike before, the breath is there . . . labored but there.

"We have to do a CAT scan," he says. I already know that there are large amounts of radiation inherent in CAT scans, and it bothers me to think of doing that to my body. This is the first time I have had any pharmaceutical drugs in me in eight years.

I always say, "I am not anti-pharmaceutical, but they should be saved as the last tool in the practitioner's back pocket." My life was just saved by pharmaceuticals. Maybe this is one of those times that radiation is justified to find out what is wrong? Because something is seriously wrong. I am healthy. I don't know anyone who does more for her health than I do on a daily basis. CAT scan . . . I don't know.

I say to the doctor, "It seems to me that I've either been poisoned or am having some kind of serious allergic reaction to something. I mean, doesn't that make sense? The rash, the strangling, the asphyxiation. Sounds classic, doesn't it?"

"We don't know. A CAT scan will tell us. I really recommend you do this," the doctor says. "Next time you might not be so lucky—you might not get here in time. You were almost out."

I know that. I could feel the life going out of me in the car ride over.

"Okay," I answer meekly. I am concerned and wary. My husband is with me, holding my hands, rubbing them. His face is twisted with fear, concern. Nothing is making sense.

A week ago, I was the picture of health. I hosted a beautiful evening at my home for all the wonderful doctors who had participated in my bestseller *Breakthrough*. It was a beautiful, warm evening, and together we all celebrated health and wellness. The stars were out that night in full force, and while the air was filled with the sounds of live musicians playing my soft jazz favorites, the forty people at the table were enthusiastically conversing about the possibilities of aging without illness; aging with bones, brain, and health intact; dying healthy at a very old age. We were all turned on. We had all realized it was attainable, and we were excited to know that we had jumped on this incredible bandwagon in time.

This was an amazing group of people. These doctors were the courageous ones who stepped out of the Western "standard of care" box to declare that the present template of medicine is not working. Drugs are not the answer. Drugs and chemicals are degrading the brains of our elders and sneaking up on the unsuspecting young ones.

I looked around at this group of healthy-looking, vibrant people and was excited to bring them all together. We were all living this new approach to wellness. And before our delicious organic meal was served, everyone pulled out their little bags of supplements. We all got a laugh over that one.

It was so exciting to talk about true health enthusiastically instead of in the hushed tones that accompany talk of a loved one in a diseased state. I felt there always seemed to be a hopelessness that accompanied so many of today's approaches to health. Even when they worked, there seemed to be an undesired reaction in the body. Somehow you weren't the same person anymore; you became slowed down, aging faster, fragile.

Socially, in most groups I tempered my conversations on my approach to health because those who entrusted their lives to allopathic, "standard of care" Western doctors might not want to entertain the idea that they might have made the wrong choice or that their way wasn't the best way. I respected that. Life and health are about choices. There is the old way and the new way, and each of us has to do what makes us most comfortable.

I chose the new way and I have never felt better, happier, more energetic, more hormonally balanced, and more sexually vibrant in my life.

So why am I *here*, in this hospital? What happened?

It's surreal, being wheeled into the CAT scan room. I'm immediately brought back to my radiation treatments for breast cancer years earlier. I know I wouldn't make that same choice today. The only health problems I've had—until tonight—have been related to radiation exposure, but thanks to the incredible doctors I had the privilege of interviewing and knowing, I was able to rectify what had been damaged—using "nature's tools," as Dr. Jonathan Wright says.

I am now dressed in a blue hospital gown, and so far I've been reinforced by three rounds of oxygen and albuterol. I'm starting to feel normal again. Drugs have been my lifesaver this time. This is what they are for. Knowing the toxicity of all chemical drugs, I've already started thinking about the supplement regime and detox treatments I'll have when I get out of here, to get all the residue of pharmaceuticals out of me. I'm hopeful this will be the one and only time I have to resort to Western drugs.

"We're going to inject you with a harmless dye," says the radiologist. "It will make you feel warm, and like you have to pee your pants, but the feeling will pass. It won't take long, maybe fifteen minutes, so just relax."

I'm already on an IV of glucose, so she injects the dye into my IV. I immediately feel the warmth, a rather uncomfortable warmth, and then indeed I feel like I will pee right on the table. *Click, click, click*, like something mechanical that's going wonky. *Click, click, click*. Again and again. I lie there still so they can get the best pictures.

"Okay, that's it," she says, then pauses. There is something in the radiologist's face, but I can't pinpoint it. It lasts only a nanosecond, but there was definitely something in her face, her tone.

"Have you had breast cancer?" she asks, seeming concerned.

"Yes," I answer.

"Right," she says.

I am wheeled back to the ER, and Alan and I wait. I want to get out of here. I want to go home.

The door opens and the doctor and the nurse come in and close the door behind them. The doctor stands and looks at me for a moment and then says, "I have brought her with me for courage because I hate what I have to say." The moment feels frozen, still.

"We have very bad news," he continued. My heart started pounding, like it was jumping out of my chest. "You have a mass in your lung; it looks like the cancer has metastasized to your liver. We don't know what is wrong with your liver, but it is so enlarged that it is filling your entire abdomen. You have so many tumors in your chest we can't count them, and they all have masses in them, and you have a blood clot, and you have pneumonia. So we are going to check you into the hospital and start treating the blood clot because that will kill you first."

The air has been sucked out of the room. I look at my husband's face and see that it is contorted with fear, pain, and confusion. My heart is pounding so hard that for the first time in my life I say, "I . . . I think you need to give me something to calm me down. I'm afraid I am going to have a heart attack."

"Absolutely," the doctor says.

My blood pressure is at 191. I am usually 110 over 80. Pounding, pounding, pounding. Disbelief! I look at Alan; there are no words. We hold hands. His eyes are liquid, as are mine. What can we even say? We've just been coldcocked.

Surreal again. I am being wheeled upstairs, checked into a hospital room. There is a flurry of activity, IVs being hooked up. I hear my weak voice asking, "What are you putting in these IVs?"

"Heparin," a nurse says, "a blood thinner for your blood clot, and in the other one is Levaquin, an antibiotic for your pneumonia, plus Ativan to calm you down." I am grateful for the Ativan. Drugs! Me, the non-drug advocate. I've had so many drugs this morning, my head is spinning. What is happening to my life? To our life?

"Call Bruce," my son, I say to Alan, trying to keep the panic from my voice. "He's shooting in Atlanta; call him on his cell phone." Then I tell him to call Leslie, Stephen, my sister Maureen, and my brother Danny. Both Alan and I are numb.

The oncologist comes into my room. He has the bedside manner of a moose: no compassion, no tenderness, no cautious approach. He sits in the chair with his arms folded defensively.

"You've got cancer. I just looked at your CAT scan and it's everywhere," he says matter-of-factly.

"Everywhere?" I ask, stunned. "Everywhere?"

"Everywhere," he states, like he's telling me he got tickets to the Lakers game. "Your lungs, your liver, tumors around your heart . . . I've never seen so much cancer."

He leaves the room and the sound of the machinery I am hooked up to fills the silence left by the shock and awe of this death sentence I've just been given. Alan lies down on the little bed with me and holds me like he'll never let go. There are no tears from either of us. We are too stunned to cry. Nurses come and go, adjusting my equipment; we just continue to hold each other for what seems like hours.

Our embrace is broken by Alan's cell phone. It's Bruce. "Ma . . ." His voice is cracking. "You are the rock of this family; you are what keeps us together."

"I know, Bruce. I'm going to figure this out. There's a doctor in Italy . . ." I trail off.

Bruce's voice is emotional. "I can't imagine being in a world without you, Ma."

I have never felt so sad. I have never felt so out of control and helpless. I am trying to be convincing, I am trying to be upbeat, but the words aren't coming out of me.

Caroline, my daughter-in-law, calls. Her mother died of breast cancer when she was thirteen, then her surrogate mother (her mother's sister) died of ovarian cancer, and then her stepmother died of ovarian cancer. Now me. This is just too much for her. I can hear it in her voice. I love her; I am her earth mother in spirit, the designate for her mother. "Bruce is flying home tonight," she says shakily, "and we will be at the hospital in the morning. I'll bring you some fresh chicken soup." That is her way, that is how she dealt with her mother's death; she takes charge, she handles things. She knows soup will comfort me. The concern in her voice is palpable. I am trying to make things okay, but they aren't, and we both know it. I don't have any spark in me. I've just been hit by an atom bomb.

One by one my children call, then the grandchildren, telling me they love me. That's when I start to cry. I will never see them grow up. Will they remember me? I love them all so much.

My stepdaughter, Leslie, doesn't call; she just gets in her car and drives to the hospital. She walks into the room, takes one look at her father, usually a take-charge kind of guy, and sees that he is not able to function. He can't talk. Leslie and I have been through a lot, and we have come out of it so unbelievably close, so loving, and such great friends. It is a parent/daughter/friend/business partnership that is sacred to me.

The oncologist is just leaving the room again as Leslie arrives, and I can tell her mood is anxious but fierce. She dislikes Dr. Oncology immediately. She says, "What an asshole. How does he know you have cancer? How can he be sure? You just had your stem cells banked in August with the NeoStem company. You had to do a complete cancer workup before they would bank your stem cells. You were clear. Your blood work was perfect." *Yes*, I think. *How could I have cancer?*

Then the lung cancer doctor enters the room. Maybe he has better news. But no—he says, "I just looked at your CAT scan, and you have lung cancer that has metastasized." He is nicer, more thoughtful. "I mean, I'm going to think about this," he says. "Maybe it's something else, but this sure doesn't look good. I'll be back tomorrow." Leslie takes out pen and paper and is making notes. She will continue to do this the entire week, writing down everything everyone is saying. Thank God, because when you are stunned and on medication, things get foggy.

Day one is almost over. The most shocking, devastating day of my life, our life! I know the facts: when you have lung cancer and it has metastasized to your liver, heart, abdomen, and all over your body, you have at most two months—maybe only two weeks or less.

I look at Alan and the sadness is overwhelming. I am in that "valley of fear" I have often heard about, and I see my death.

As night envelops the room, the nurse comes in and puts something dreamy in my IV—more drugs, but I can't resist. I want to sleep. I want this nightmare to be over. Alan climbs into my little bed under the covers and holds me tight. When I wake the next morning he is still holding me. He hasn't moved. The idea of leaving him . . . oh my God, that thought is overwhelming.

Day 2. The morning is nurses, blood pressure, routines. They've done this a thousand times before. They can't get involved, not really. It would make their job too difficult. Every patient has a story. Mine is no different. Every day, people are diagnosed with cancer, bad cancer . . . this is just another case.

I hoped in the morning we would awake to find that this is a bad dream, but reality is all around us. Bruce, Caroline, and Leslie are sitting vigil at the foot of my bed. The tone is shock and fear, coupled with Leslie's fierce insistence that this just can't be.

Bruce holds me and cries, tells me he loves me. He holds me in a way that speaks volumes. Touches my hand. Connecting. Showing that life is fleeting, and that no day should be wasted. As a teenager I gave birth to him and the connection between us has always been profound. Caroline has me dead in her head. It is all sense memory for her. Her mother's breast cancer spread to her liver and she died a month later. Caroline, hearing that I've cancer in my liver, knows the inevitable.

My stepson, Stephen, calls. He is awkward with emotions. It's because he feels it so much that he is uncomfortable with expressing it. I know that. I hear it in his voice.

The surgeon walks into my room. "I just looked at your CAT scan, and it's cancer." Again. The same doom. Each time I hear it, my soul accepts the injury. I feel deep, profound grief and disbelief that I am being forced to leave all those I love. So soon, so unfinished. It just doesn't feel possible.

Dr. Oncologist enters. "What do you want to do? We could prescribe full-body chemo."

"Excuse me," I say. Even in my drugged state I know this is not the answer for me. "Just so you know, I would rather die; I would never take any of your treatments."

Dr. Oncologist just shrugs and leaves the room.

"Asshole," Leslie says.

Caroline says, "What an arrogant prick!"

Being an oncologist involves constantly delivering bad news, very bad news. Maybe Dr. Oncologist uses his arrogance to protect himself.

Caroline says, "I looked up your symptoms and it could be something called valley fever. You get a rash, you get pneumonia. And it comes from the top two layers of soil in the desert of the Southwest. You work in your organic garden all the time, and you dig regularly in the ruins in New Mexico. It makes sense."

Dr. Lung Cancer comes in. "Could it be valley fever?" I ask him.

"Well," he says slowly, "it could possibly be, but I doubt it. But let me think about it. Most likely it's not. It really looks like it's cancer."

That night, Alan, who still hasn't shaved or showered, again climbs into my little bed with me, and the nurse puts the dreamy stuff into my IV. Alan holds me tight under the covers. The next morning, we are still entangled in each other's arms.

Caroline, Bruce, and Leslie are sitting there, Leslie with her notepad and her sleeves rolled up. Caroline is angry with all the doctors. "Idiots!" she says. "Except the internist." We all like him. He is open. He is managing all the doctors and reporting to me.

Dr. Internist says, "They want you to take Coumadin, a blood thinner, for your blood clot."

"I don't want to take Coumadin," I tell him. "I know that drug; it's got terrible side effects. I'm not going to take it. There is a natural blood thinner called nattokinase; I'll take that. But I won't take Coumadin."

Dr. Internist laughs. "Well, you know what you want."

I tell him, "Listen, I haven't taken a drug in nine years. I'm taking only lifesaving drugs for the moment, just until I can figure out what I am going to do."

The stress is unbelievable. I feel crazy—trying to figure out if I'm going to die soon, trying to avoid unnecessary pharmaceutical drugs, as I'm on so many drugs already at the moment. I realize how easy it is to become pharmaceuticalized. I am now on at least six drugs and fighting to resist more.

The nurse walks in. "I have your blood pressure medicines."

"Since when have I been on blood pressure medicine?" I ask, feeling upset.

"Oh, it's been in your IV all along," she says.

"Who ordered that?" I ask incredulously.

"Your doctor ordered it," she says flatly.

"No, I don't want blood pressure medicine." My voice is rising, "I don't have high blood pressure. I am upset. I am *very upset*! Wouldn't you be?"

Day 3. Dr. Lung Cancer and Dr. Surgeon come in, along with Dr. Oncologist. "We've been talking," says Dr. Lung Cancer, "and we think you should be biopsied. That way we can rule out anything else, and then you can decide how you want to deal with your cancer."

"What does a biopsy entail?" I ask.

Dr. Surgeon says, "Well, we will cut open your throat, put a tube down your chest, and go into your lung and take a piece of tissue. And then we will take a piece from a couple of the tumors in your chest. The complications are that we will be working around your vocal cords, and there is a possibility that we could damage them. So it's up to you."

I look at Alan. I look at Bruce, then Caroline and Leslie. Leslie says, "Do it. Then you'll know. I know you don't have cancer. You are too healthy. You do everything you are supposed to do to not get cancer. You eat organic, you take supplements, you take antioxidants, you exercise, you sleep. You are happy. You don't have cancer."

Bruce is a mess. He's so vulnerable, and Alan is shutting down. I can tell he is choosing to die with me if I am going to die.

"I'm going to have the surgery," I tell everyone later that day. We all agree that it is necessary. We need the information.

Barry Manilow walks into my hospital room. He's my best friend.

"What is going on?" he asks, very concerned.

I tell him I've been diagnosed with full-body cancer but that it just seems impossible. How could it be? He can't believe it either. He calls me several times that day.

That night, linked up to this IV, which I am now referring to as "my buddy," I am sure feeling the drugs; I get out of bed and start dancing with my rolling IV, singing, "Wherever we go, whatever we do, we're gonna go through it, together." We all crack up. It's a needed relief from all the doom.

My family around me, Barry calling, Alan never leaving my side, my sister, like Bruce, telling me she can't live in a world without me. And it hits me. Like a loudspeaker is in my head, I hear it; so real that I look around to see if anyone else hears it, but they can't. It is only for me to hear. It was an epiphany. In the face of seeing my death, while in the space of this valley of fear, the words ring through my head: **It's not who you are, it's not what you have, it's not where you live, it's not what you do, it's only, only about who you love, and who loves you. And the more you love, the better!**

A moment of complete and utter clarity. And I know that no matter what happens I will never be the same. I feel only gratitude that I have such deep and profound love in my life.

Once again Alan climbs into my little bed with me; the nurse puts the dreamy stuff in my IV. Tomorrow I will be going into surgery to find out if I am going to live or die. Most probably die, because four doctors plus the emergency room doctor and the radiologist have diagnosed me with full-body cancer. Yet I feel grateful. Even in this moment when I want more life, when I want to live with every fiber of my being, I know that I have more love in my life than many people ever experience. And I fall into my dreamy, drugged sleep holding my husband, who never lets me go.

Day 4. This morning is different. Nurses very busy, lots of tests, blood pressure, then two nurses (men) in white coats come to get me to wheel me downstairs into surgery. I hold Alan's hand and look at him with a longing that hurts my heart. My aching, pained heart. The feeling is indescribable.

"I love you," I whisper. He kisses me on my face and forehead and tells me I will be okay.

Dr. Surgeon comes up to me right before I go out. We're all wearing shower caps, which makes me laugh, but I'm nervous. "Look, Doc," I say groggily, "I'm a songbird—I have a need to sing every day of my life. Please, please be careful and save my vocal cords." And then I am in space.

Where do we go in that space? It's like time lost. How long am I there? Where is "there"? But I'm waking up. I can sort of hear that Alan is talking to me. I'm trying my best to hear, struggling. What is he saying? I'm so groggy.

"You don't have cancer. You don't have cancer," he whispers to me. He strokes my hair. I cry.

My eyes open. I can't believe it. I don't have cancer . . . I'm going to live.

I'm out of the ICU and back in my hospital room. Bruce, Leslie, and Caroline are around me. Bruce is speechless. Caroline is simultaneously happy and pissed off at what they put us all through, and Leslie keeps saying, "I knew you didn't have cancer. I knew it!"

You would think I'd be ecstatic. I want to be, but I am experiencing post-traumatic stress, I guess. Sadness gets into your cells. My body, my cells, accepted the death sentence of inoperable cancer as fact, and now they are shut down. My soul has been injured.

How do you heal an injured soul? I can't find my happiness. Yet I am relieved.

Day 5. Dr. Oncologist comes into my room. Now, you would think he'd say, "Well, sometimes it's good to be wrong." Or "Isn't it great that you don't have cancer?" But no. He walks in, doesn't sit down, just looks at me and says angrily, "Well, you should have told me you were on steroids."

I am flabbergasted. I don't know what to say to him; I am so stunned by his lack of compassion that I just stare at him. I am not on steroids. I would never take steroids. But because he is stuck in old thinking and so out of touch with new medicine, he has no clue and doesn't understand cortisol replacement as part of the menopausal experience.

I don't know where to begin with him. He's too arrogant to listen to a "stupid actress," anyway. So much of his attitude with me has been the unsaid but definite "So you think all your 'alternatives' are going to help you now, missy?"

Why steroids would have anything to do with being misdiagnosed with full-body cancer, I can't guess. But we still don't know what has gone wrong in my body. We still have to find out what caused me to end up in the ER.

I think Dr. Oncologist is embarrassed that he so horribly misdiagnosed me. That he put me and my family through a trauma no one should have to endure. (I hear later that my personal oncologist called him and said, "Don't tell her she has cancer until you do a biopsy," and he arrogantly replied, "Look, this is bad—the cancer is everywhere. You can't give this woman false hopes.") I think for all these reasons he is embarrassed . . . and mad. Would he rather I have cancer than be wrong?

A simple "I'm sorry" from any of the doctors would go a long way, and would help in healing. How hard is it to make an apology? Are doctors so concerned with lawsuits that they can't be human anymore? What hap-pened to the Hippocratic oath that all doctors take: "First do no harm"? Ego. Arrogance.

So he has to find a reason to have made such a stupid, arrogant mis-take. Man, is he searching for something, anything. What am I going to say to this guy? He isn't worth it—I just want him to go, to get out of my room. I never want to see him again. He turns abruptly and leaves.

Later that day, just as I'm beginning to see some light, hope, and a fu-ture with my loved ones, the infectious disease doctors march into my room, four of them, in white coats. One of them, whom we'll nickname "Nurse Ratched" after she leaves the room, is the head of infectious dis-eases for the hospital. She says, "Now that we've ruled out cancer, we all think you have a serious infectious disease."

Oh God, I thought. *It's beginning again!*

"Like what?" I ask, not sure I want to hear the answer.

"Well," begins Nurse Ratched, "we believe you have either tuberculosis, leprosy, or coccidiomycosis, which is valley fever, which can bring with it meningitis and brain damage."

Caroline jumped in. "That's what I thought it was, valley fever. Everything I read about it describes her symptoms."

"Well," says Nurse Ratched, dismissing Caroline, "it's most likely tuberculosis. After looking at her CAT scan, this is what *we* all believe. Now, Suzanne, I know you understand our job is to protect the community, so we are going to move you to an isolation room so your germs cannot escape into the hospital community."

I am once again in shock. TB? Leprosy? Really?

My kids and Alan pack my things up; I am covered with a blanket, a shower cap, and a face mask and wheeled upstairs to what turns out to be a closetlike room, obviously rarely used, with a huge motor that supposedly takes my germs out into cyberspace or somewhere.

All the nurses and doctors who come and go from my room are now in full protective clothing, covered head to toe in what looks like beekeeper suits. I can't tell if they are men or women, and I feel like a living human germ.

I am *contaminated*. I am a *danger to the community*.

When the door opens I see that a police guard has been placed outside my room for security reasons, but I misunderstand. I think it's to keep me from escaping. *Don't let HER out. She will harm you.*

My children are no longer allowed to be in contact with me. No visitors. They either don't care about Alan or realize that he will get crazy if they try to keep him out.

That's when I lose it. I break down in sobs. It's all been too much. So much stress and craziness. I sob and sob. Alan still does not leave my side. He still has not showered or shaved, and he climbs into my little bed in this horrible noisy room and gets under the covers with me and all my germs to go to sleep. Another day gone. What will tomorrow bring?

By now I am beginning to be able to think. I'm still stunned, but the fight is coming back. I e-mail a couple of the doctors I know from my books *Breakthrough* and *Ageless*. Each of them has suggestions for building back up, for detoxing the drugs out of me, for finding natural approaches to what is being diagnosed as either TB, valley fever, or—God of gods!—leprosy. Just crazy!

Dr. Jonathan Wright says, "You gotta get out of there."

"I know," I say. "But they won't let me go, I am evidently a threat to the community."

"Listen, I have your blood work from a month ago and it is all stellar. There is no way you could have these diseases. TB would have presented itself long before this, and leprosy is a joke. It doesn't look like that on a CAT scan."

Dr. Infectious is back in my hospital room again. "I want to go home," I say firmly.

Dr. Infectious answers, "Well, that is not possible. We have to wait for your cultures to come back."

"How long will that take?" I ask.

"At least a couple of weeks, maybe six weeks," she says matter-of-factly. It's no problem for her to have me sit idly waiting for test results.

"No, no, no!" I say loudly. I have the urge to start pounding on the bed-side table violently. "No, I am not staying here! I want to go home. *I want to go hoooome!*" I say murderously. (Shades of Shirley MacLaine in *Terms of Endearment*.) "I WANT TO GO HOME. I AM GOING HOME!"

"Well . . . ," Dr. Infectious begins anxiously. (*Good*, I thought. My fight is coming back. I think she's nervous that I'm going to make a scene, and I am. I've had it.) "I will release you, but you must sign a paper agreeing to be quarantined to your property for six weeks. You may not go to any public place. If you do not sign this paper, I will report you to the Department of Health, and you do not want that publicity. You must take the medicines for TB, leprosy, coccidiomycosis, and meningitis. We also want you to take Coumadin and the antibiotic Levaquin for your pneumonia. And by the way the leprosy medicine may make you sweat blood."

Really, truly, I am a nice person, I am always polite, but I am having thoughts of saying terrible things to her. But I don't, can't. She has the power, and until I get out of here, she is the warden. I am powerless. Patients are rendered powerless. Now I know it firsthand.

I e-mail Dr. Wright. "Sign the paper," he says. "Tell her you'll be a good girl. Tell her you will take the medicines. When you get home, send me the names of the medicines and I will research them for you."

So four hours later I am being wheeled out of the hospital, with $5,000 worth of medicines in my hand I know I am not going to take. (I just look at it as my getaway money.) I am covered from head to toe to minimize my exposure to the community, and I am put in my car.

As Alan gets into the driver's seat, I feel exhausted. I have never been through such a terrible ordeal—and I was an abused child! My childhood was spent hiding and sleeping in a closet to protect us from the violence; but never, never have I experienced anything like this.

As we drive home in the beautiful southern California sunshine, I look around the streets of Los Angeles, knowing that the world continues on, and I say to Alan, "I feel like we've both been in a terrible earthquake and a huge building fell down on us, and at the very, very last moment, just as we were running out of air, they were able to pull us out of the rubble. So I am relieved to be out from under, and I am relieved to be going home, but we were buried alive and it is going to take some time to get over the trauma."

We drive onto our property, quarantined from the outside world for diseases no one is even sure I have. Immediately I e-mail Dr. Wright with the names of the medicines I have been given. He shoots back an answer within twenty minutes.

"First of all," he says, "these drugs will kill you. Seriously, they are so toxic to the body that I don't know what this doctor is thinking. Second, it is mandated by law that these drugs not be given unless there is an absolute diagnosis, which you do not have. It is also mandated by law that you only give these drugs one at a time, to see how the patient tolerates them, because these are all so toxic to the liver. So I am not exaggerating that these drugs have the potential to kill you or seriously injure and debilitate your liver. How long did she say she wanted you to stay on these drugs?" he asks.

"Anywhere from two to six weeks," I answer.

"Good God," he says. "You have to do what feels comfortable to you, but until these cultures come back, I advise you for your health's sake not to take these drugs."

As he is talking I begin dumping thousands of dollars' worth of useless, toxic drugs into the trash can. What a waste. What trauma. What a terrible thing to thrust on me so she can "protect the community," even though she does not have a diagnosis. She would rather destroy my liver and make me sick for life so she can write in her report that she has followed protocol (wrongly, I will later find out). This is dangerous medicine. And once again, I feel sure that I am experiencing my second horrible misdiagnosis in one week. How can this be? How can this be happening to me?

While in the hospital I kept repeating to all the doctors that I felt either I had been poisoned or was experiencing a severe allergic attack. Just weeks before this episode I had had my killer cells tested to measure the strength of my immune system; I clearly remember what my doctor had said looking at my results: "Wow, your numbers are great, they are at 43." I said, "I have no frame of reference." "Well, most adults your age have immune systems at 2 or 3, you are at 43!"

So how did I go from perfect health and a very strong immune system to lying in a hospital bed, near death, diagnosed with full-body cancer? No one could answer this question and none of the professionals were all that interested in finding out. My queries were dismissed as insignificant. Something terrible had happened to me. Something I ate or something I breathed, or maybe it was foul play. Who knows? The whole thing was very disturbing. All I knew was that I did not have cancer. The biopsy confirmed this to be true. No cancer anywhere.

What if I had taken the full-body chemotherapy as suggested? I shudder to think what might have happened to my health. It would have been seriously degraded. How often is this happening to innocent, trusting patients?

I'll never know what caused the attack, but I do know that being an informed patient saved my good health. I had enough knowledge to realize that even if the diagnosis were true, that if I did indeed have cancer metastasized throughout my entire body, I had other options and chemical poison was not an option for me.

If this horrible misdiagnosis could happen to me—a known health advocate, a bestselling author of health books, and a famous person—then what is happening to the rest of the people in this country? What happens to the average Joe who trusts in the system, the average Joe who when diagnosed says, "Okay, Doc, if that's what you think, bring on the full-body chemical poisoning. We'll figure out how to pay for it somehow."

I was lucky, though, because I knew something that the average Joe doesn't: Prior to this episode I had been keeping a file on doctors who were curing cancer without drugs, surgery, or poisons. I never thought it would be something I might need to access personally. In my darkest moments, even when it all seemed hopeless, I had one little ray of light to hold on to—that "out there" was another way. It gave me hope, and is my reason for writing this book.

Now I want to introduce you to these healers, so if ever you find yourself in a similar horrifying situation, you will know there are options, choices. . . . Information is power, and being informed will always allow you to make the best choices for yourself or your loved ones.

Chapter 2

MEET THE DOCTORS

Just to say the word *cure* is apparently sacrilegious. There is no cure for cancer, we all know that. "They" have told us so. We can "shrink the tumor." We can "respond." We can be "in remission." We can grab a few extra months of life . . . except that the destruction done to the body in most cases does not warrant the extra breaths the patient is allowed. (And it is labored breath at that.)

But . . .

Dare I say it? Yes.

There are doctors out there who are curing cancer!

I am speaking of people who are getting well. People who are living long, productive lives. People diagnosed with stage IV cancers, people who chose another way and avoided the degradation of chemical poisoning and mutilation.

I had heard about these doctors at the medical conferences I attend: conferences on cutting-edge, antiaging medicines, for Western-trained medical doctors who are fed up and disillusioned with the medical system. And I've had the privilege to interview these doctors, professionals who courageously speak of their disillusionment with the present template of "standard of care" (or "cover your butt") medicine. They are concerned that our current system is not working and that people are on too many drugs and not getting well.

These are pioneers, doctors who have figured out how to knock out cancer. As a result they have been attacked, sued, called frauds, ridiculed, and ostracized for having the audacity to think outside the box. Thank God for courageous people.

With an epidemic at hand and the poor results we are observing with the use of chemotherapy, you owe it to yourself to at least be aware that other protocols exist.

There is a choice. But when you are diagnosed with cancer, you won't hear about "another way." Instead, "standard of care" is always the same: surgery, radiation, chemotherapy, and harsh aftercare drugs. You rarely hear about the logic of combining "standard of care" with alternative treatments so that they might complement each other. (I know this firsthand.)

Everyone knows the damaging consequences of chemo (what I call poison therapy) but it's rare to consider complementing it with IV nutrients or vitamin C, an area Dr. Linus Pauling so eloquently researched.

If you do suggest to your doctor that you have heard of doctors who are having success without drugs, you may be brushed aside as unrealistic and foolish. Some traditional doctors may even dismiss these other protocols as crazy and wacky. But I ask you: What is crazier than pumping a body full of poison? And then there's usually six weeks of radiation. But wait . . . isn't it radiation that *gives* us cancer?

You have a choice. A choice! Again, what you choose is not my business, but you need to know that there are those who are approaching this nasty, killer disease in a different way. My goal in writing this book is to introduce you to those who are healing, curing, building up, and replacing what is missing, as another way.

By 2010, cancer will be the leading killer in the world!

So it's likely it could be you.

If you ever find yourself in this horribly frightening position (and I hope you won't), you will be glad you know about these proud, determined, and cutting-edge Western doctors. They are having success. Not with everyone. That is the tragedy of cancer. Diet, lifestyle habits, and time of diagnosis contribute greatly to whether or not a patient will live. Not all cancer patients are lucky enough to catch it in time, but enough people are getting well for these doctors to know they are on the right track.

None of these doctors has a 100 percent success rate, so to expect a miracle would be too simplistic. Each protocol requires collaboration with the patient. In all cases, nutrition must be taken seriously, even held as sacred.

The important information to walk away with from this book is that cancer is mostly preventable, manageable, and sometimes curable, but it is up to us individually to make the effort. To continue the present poor, nonnutritious, chemicalized diets will surely put you on the other side of wellness.

I am not a doctor or a scientist; I am merely a filter for these Western-trained doctors and scientists. I am a passionate layperson; I write on behalf of us.

THE DOCTORS:
YOUR HEALTH WARRIORS

A number of the doctors interviewed for this book have experienced first-hand the horrors of what happens when you go against the mainstream medical establishment, but they've fought and won, all with one purpose in mind: to heal. They provide us with needed choice, creative medicine, and an opportunity to take care of our bodies and our health in supportive, nontoxic ways.

First, you'll read an interview I did with Ralph Moss, Ph.D., who has written extensively on our failing medical system, in particular with regard to cancer. He is the author of many books, including *Questioning Chemotherapy*. He has some horrifying insights into why the medical system is in this state.

At the forefront of treatment and at the center of this book are Dr. Stanislaw Burzynski, Dr. Nicholas Gonzalez, and Dr. James Forsythe. I've interviewed many of their patients, who all claim that unorthodox treatments by these doctors have saved their lives. Throughout this book you will hear from many of the patients of these doctors. These are people who are living with excellent health and great quality of life. Many have chosen to forgo chemical poisoning and instead take advantage of the life's work of these doctors.

> Many oncologists recommend chemotherapy for almost any type of cancer, with a faith that is unshaken by the almost constant failure.
>
> —Albert Braverman, M.D.

Dr. Stanislaw Burzynski's work consists of replacing antineoplastons, a peptide that according to him is missing in cancer patients. These small peptides produced by the liver control cell multiplication. Dr. Burzynski found that in the absence of sufficient amounts of these internal controls, cancer develops. His theory is that if this peptide is replaced, cancer is knocked out. And in many, many cases his patients have recovered. He has been treating patients for over thirty years.

Now, when they recover, when they are well, happy, healthy, and strong . . . is this "cured"? From my perspective, the word *cure* seems appropriate for those who do respond and show no evidence of cancer for years afterward. But when I interviewed Dr. Burzynski, he was reluctant to make that claim: "I don't give false hope; I don't want anyone to have any illusions. Everything we claim is right on the films." Yet when I spoke to his "cured" patients, they were eager to say they no longer had cancer.

To keep things fair, Dr. Burzynski has never done X-rays or CT scans himself. His patients undergo scans and magnetic resonance imaging (MRI) at centers near their homes and then bring the results to Houston.

Dr. Burzynski's work evokes much controversy. For years the Texas Medical Board tried to take away his medical license, and when the big guys, the Food and Drug Administration (FDA), tried to put him in jail, Dr. Burzynski had several things going for him. His patients were passionate in his defense and were absolutely devoted to him.

Dr. Burzynski's longtime advocate, Richard Jaffe, is a nationally recognized health care attorney. He has written the book *Galileo's Lawyer*, which is an insider's look into the alternative health world with Dr. Burzynski as his main inspiration:

> *The Medical Board Hearing lasted several days. The patients were powerful. They just got up and told their stories.*
>
> *All of them had terminal cancer with very short life expectancies. They all found their way to the Burzynski clinic, and they were all disease free, some for many years. A number of them were still on maintenance treatment and, as could be expected, they were very concerned about continued access to Burzynski and the medicine. Many of the patients were small children with brain tumors.*
>
> *The Kunnaris were one of the families who came to Austin to testify (read their testimony on pages 83–84). They live in upper Minnesota. They were not rich and could not afford to fly down, especially since they would have to take all four of their young children with . them. So they all piled into their big station wagon and drove twenty-*

four hours straight through to Texas, Jack and MaryAnn switching driving every few hours. They put a bunch of sleeping bags in the back for the kids because showing up for Dr. Burzynski, the doctor who had saved their son from a terminal brain tumor, was so important.

This is typical of the passion patients display for Dr. Burzynski.

The same thing occurred when the FDA tried to put Dr. Burzynski in jail.

There were two trials. At the beginning of each trial hundreds of people came out showing their support. Two-thirds of them were patients and the rest were families. They couldn't even fit all the media into the courtroom because there was so much interest. I asked Jaffe what those days were like. He told me, "In my twenty-five years of practicing as a health care attorney, I have never seen a physician who has been subjected to the unrelenting government persecution that Dr. Burzynski faced. Early on, the FDA tried and failed to obtain an injunction stopping him from treating his terminally ill cancer patients. Between 1985 and 1995, Burzynski was investigated by four federal grand juries. The first three refused to indict him; the fourth did. Fortunately, the gods were smiling on us. We won the case and Dr. Burzynski was acquitted on all charges after two federal criminal trials. . . . Congress held several hearings on FDA abuse in which the Burzynski persecution was front and center. Eventually, Congress forced the FDA to allow him to continue to treat all of his patients and begin clinical trials. Throughout those dark days the clinic's doors never closed, due largely to Burzynski's courage, the extraordinary efforts of many of his successfully treated terminally ill patients, and maybe some pretty fair legal work."

According to Jaffe and Dr. Burzynski himself, another absolutely critical factor in the success against the FDA was the support and friendship of Dr. Julian Whitaker (who has written the foreword to this book). After Dr. Burzynski was indicted, Julian visited the Burzynski clinic and became convinced that patients were being cured of terminal cancer. Julian became a tireless advocate for Dr. Burzynski. He repeatedly wrote articles and editorials about Burzynski in his massively popular newsletter.

Dr. Whitaker helped stop rumors that the clinic was out of business, and many new patients found their way to Dr. Burzynski because of him. This helped keep the clinic's doors open.

Dr. Whitaker also asked his subscribers to help pay for Dr. Burzynski's defense and did they ever! As many as ten thousand of his faithful subscribers sent in donations. Through *Health & Healing*, Dr. Julian Whitaker single-handedly raised many hundreds of thousands of dollars, in amounts of ten, twenty-five, and fifty dollars, for Dr. Burzynski's defense. Without Dr. Whitaker's efforts, the Burzynski clinic might not have survived the government attacks.

In the end, Dr. Burzynski fought the United States government and won!

Another maverick is Dr. Nicholas Gonzalez, who resides in Manhattan and treats patients with all types of cancers. He offers an aggressive nutritional program for the treatment of advanced cancer as well as for a variety of other serious illnesses ranging from chronic fatigue to multiple sclerosis, and it is working. Dr. Gonzalez's patients also have a reverence for him and his protocol, and one after another shared their stories of success with me. But the long, healthy lives they are living is the greatest testimony. His patients swear by his therapy. They are its living proof.

Whatever the underlying problem, his therapy involves three basic components: individualized diet, individualized supplementation, and intensive detoxification. The diets prescribed can range from a vegetarian raw food approach to a red-meat one; it all depends on the person's needs and type. The supplement programs are varied, and involve vitamins, minerals, and trace elements in various forms and various doses as well as glandular and enzyme products. Each of these individualized programs is chosen to meet a particular need for each patient. Much in the way that bioidentical hormones are individualized for each person, there is no "one program fits all." And this is why it works.

Dr. Gonzalez is best known for his work with advanced cancer. He believes that diet, vitamins, minerals, and trace elements help improve tissue and organ deficiencies but that it is the pancreatic enzymes that target and kill cancer cells. The detoxification routines help the body neutralize and excrete the multitude of waste products produced during routine metabolism; in the case of his cancer patients, this results in tumor lysis, meaning the cellular destruction needed to kill cancer that occurs with chemo (sometimes) and enzymes (frequently).

Dr. James Forsythe is a remarkable man. Trained as a traditional oncologist, he soon became dismayed and depressed as a result of the poor outcomes of his cancer patients on the "standard of care" treatments. Over twenty years ago, he became interested in combining conventional and alternative medicines. He was the only oncologist in his area who would treat patients who were under the care of an alternative-medicine physician. He couldn't help noticing that the patients who were integrating conventional treatments with alternative therapies were doing better.

They had fewer side effects, and their quality of life was far superior. This convinced him that conventional medicine was lacking in terms of keeping patients' immune systems stimulated.

He began to study alternative medicine, and in 1995 he received his homeopathy certificate. His protocol for cancer patients emphasizes good nutrition as a core requirement; a balanced lifestyle that includes exercise, rest, sleep, and emotional harmony; detoxification; and treatments that ensure that the organs and other body systems work efficiently. His patients are getting well, and you will read about them in *Knockout*. But you wouldn't be reading about him had the federal government succeeded in discrediting him.

It is hard to imagine that on February 16, 2005, the government tried to close his office, put him in prison, and ruin his reputation because he prescribed human growth hormone to a government shill posing as a patient. Dressed in black flak jackets and with guns drawn, several federal agents prepared to knock down the door of his home with a battering ram, demanding to know if he kept guns in the house. He was treated like a criminal rather than one of America's most respected doctors; he was ordered to kneel and a gun was pushed to his forehead. He became the first and only physician in the United States ever to be charged with prescribing HGH to patients for off-label use as an antiaging treatment. Federal agents and prosecutors trashed his pristine reputation and tried to portray him in the news media as a sleazy doctor who employed questionable techniques. After his false arrest it took fourteen months for his acquittal, but after just a few hours of deliberation, the jury reached its innocent verdict following what some Nevada journalists hailed as the "trial of the century" for the state.

In Part III, you will hear from Dr. Russell Blaylock, renowned neuroscientist and oncologist, who will open your eyes to the importance of nutrition relative to cancer protection and prevention. Every doctor in this book stresses the importance of nutrition. Dr. Blaylock claims it is the food we are eating that is killing us: processed foods, foods in bags and boxes, foods with unpronounceable names, irradiated foods, genetically modified foods, foods sprayed with pesticides, foods containing glutamates such as MSG.

Our houses are loaded with chemicals: we spray with poisons, we use products that create household toxins, and cities dump fluoride into our drinking water. What are we thinking? The human body was never meant to process this onslaught of chemicals. With this chemical and environmental attack, how can we expect to remain cancer free? But Dr. Blaylock understands much about prevention and gives us the tools to avoid getting the disease in the first place.

Burton Goldberg is a researcher and seeker of truth. He has devoted his life to finding the cause of cancer and promoting integrated protocols to wipe out cancer. His work in nutrition and alternative medicine is unmatched: in fact, he funded and oversaw the writing of the bible on alternative medicine.

Dr. Jonathan Wright is another of the pioneers you'll meet here. His understanding of the hormonal system is mind-boggling. He was the first doctor to introduce bioidentical hormones to the United States over twenty years ago.

Now, what do bioidentical hormones have to do with a book about doctors curing cancer? Just about everything. You will be blown away when you read his explanations of the cancer-protective nature of natural hormones. When you consider that most women develop cancer when they go into hormonal decline, I believe you will be more than interested to read that proper replacement in the right ratios will protect you from getting cancer.

Much like Dr. Burzynski's theories on genetic switches that you'll be reading about later, hormones are also genetic switches. Hormones work because they regulate the activity of the genes. Estrogens work because they activate certain genes and silence others. If you don't have hormonal balance, you will speed up cancer development, but regulating hormonal balance can control cancer while restoring quality of life.

Dr. Julie Taguchi, a conventional oncologist, conducted a study of fifty-five women who refused traditional chemotherapy and radiation and instead chose to treat their cancer by using bioidentical hormones and nutrition. Today all fifty-five women are five, six, seven, and nine years out. I am one of those women. You will be fascinated by what she has to say.

What if you could wear a little, inexpensive nanotechnology patch daily that constantly detoxed your body of cancer-causing free radicals? Wouldn't you like such a simple and healthy edge against toxicity? David Schmidt of LifeWave has created such a device.

Dr. Michael Galitzer has realized we can prevent getting cancer by utilizing natural strategies, energy medicine, nutrition, and nondrug therapies.

Dr. Stephen Sinatra teaches the power of the mind with regard to healing. If you believe that you can get well, that is the power. And that power of belief might just heal you from cancer or other serious disease.

Cristiana Paul, M.S., my personal nutritionist, lays out a supplementation regimen for cancer protection and discusses the importance of antioxidants in fighting free radicals in the body that can lead to cancer. Supplementation is a must in today's toxic world, and she will lead you through this mysterious and little-understood nutritional science.

If you feel more comfortable with traditional approaches to cancer treatment, you must read the interview with Bill Faloon from the Life Extension Foundation before you start treatment or have surgery. There is invaluable information there that will improve its effectiveness—and potentially your outcome.

ONE MORE THING

Each of these doctors has patients who agreed to speak with me—and their stories are incredible. Their testimony is very hopeful and inspiring.

Because these doctors are often muzzled by the FDA and the pharmaceutical companies, you most likely would not hear of them if not for this book. So I asked the doctors to explain their protocols and how they came to this thinking.

You are going to be fascinated. But most important of all, you are going to be made aware that there are doctors out there who are in this for the love of good medicine. There is very little money to be made in the world of alternative medicine. Insurance stubbornly refuses to cover the costs, and in good conscience these doctors cannot charge much. But these doctors love their work.

In my opinion, the worst job in this country is to be an oncologist. It is a job that requires delivering devastatingly bad news to patients on a daily basis. In my book *Ageless*, I recounted how my oncologist said something so very poignant to me: "I dream of the day when I no longer have to poison people." I think that says it all, yet it is precisely this disease and the exorbitant chemotherapy charges that keep our hospitals afloat and our insurance premiums high. Most hospitals require the ongoing use of toxic, conventional therapies to keep their doors open, such are the huge profits. And chemotherapy is often administered in oncologists' offices, bringing in profitable revenue.

You the patient, like me, need to know the realities, and that there are other ways to approach what is now an epidemic.

In Part III of this book we will teach you how to live your life to prevent getting cancer. It is preventable, even in this toxic soup we all live in. Each doctor interviewed verified this statement.

We can win the fight over cancer, and we can get well even if we are given this deadly diagnosis.

There is lifesaving information in this book. From the bottom of my heart, I pass it on to you in hopes that you never need the information. But if you do, remember that out there, with the real pioneers, there is another way. And you have a choice.

But let's understand how we got here in the first place. What went wrong?

Chapter 3

AGAINST OUR NATURE: THE BIRTH OF A BIG BUSINESS

Certain lapses of judgment indicate the radical failure of an entire sensibility.

—Susan Sontag, *Against Interpretation*

Nine years ago I was diagnosed with breast cancer. Being told you have breast cancer or any other cancer will bring the strongest person to his or her knees. There is a feeling of shock and disbelief, and your mortality stares you in the face. Suddenly all the things that seemed important are so trivial: that big deal you were impatiently waiting for to come through, the petty nuisances of life, or minding other people's business. It's all so . . . meaningless.

You are now looking at your life clearly. Have you lived it well? Have you loved enough? Have you been loved? Did you waste your time? You begin to review your lifestyle choices: "Why did I eat all the crap?" "Why didn't I take nutrition seriously?" "Why did I ever smoke?" Why, why, why? And now it seems too late.

We all have cancer in us. For most people the cancer stays at bay as long as we remain hormonally balanced, we give our bodies the proper nutrition, rest, and exercise, and we manage our stress. A hormonally balanced woman is a reproductive woman. Balance occurs when the body makes hormones in the correct ratio and amount every day of the month in a rhythm, the rhythm of life—our cycle.

Each day of the month is important in this cycle, and when you understand how exquisitely nature has formed us, imagine what chaos is created when we interrupt this beautiful cycle with chemicals that prevent full ovulation. Imagine the chaos when a period is manipulated to accommodate a hot date or a weekend caper. We all did that. These pills came with no warning. The doctors never told us of the dangers.

Why didn't we hear our bodies yelling (screaming) by way of bloating, weight gain, and mood swings? How else can the body talk? Symptoms of any kind are the body's language. We were deaf, we couldn't hear, we were not taught to hear, we did not know what to listen for, and now those of us who walked into this blind and trusting, taking these types of contraception, are getting breast cancer in epidemic proportions.

What puzzles me is that no one seems to be upset. No one is pointing the finger. The pharmaceutical companies are taking no responsibility. What doctor wants to put his hard-earned career on the line by talking? The pharmaceutical companies and their sidekick, the FDA, are certainly not going to say "Oops!" In fact, the pharmaceutical response is the creation of a new "miracle" birth control pill, one that gives women only four periods a year. Four periods a year! What are we thinking? Imagine what havoc that creates with the nature in us. Seems like a perfect cancer setup to me.

And maybe that's the point. Cancer is big business—approximately $200 billion a year!

When it was announced on Larry King's show that I had breast cancer, a friend set me up on a phone call with a person involved in the cancer industry, who asked for anonymity and confided in me, saying, "The truth is, we don't want to find a cure for cancer. It's too big a business." Cancer is the disease that keeps the hospitals open; it brings an extra $100,000 each year to oncologists' practices (and this is a modest estimate).

According to Bill Faloon, founder of the Life Extension Foundation, chemotherapy bonuses to oncologists are routine. There is incentive to keep cancer alive and well. The unnecessary drugs we are being given in unprecedented amounts are one culprit, and we patients are ignorant about the game plan because we have gotten used to the quick fix. It's easier to take a pill or pump ourselves full of chemicals. And as with all of us women who blindly took birth control pills, a day of reckoning arrives—the day you hear the doctor say, "You have cancer."

In this country, most often we don't even bother to do chemotherapy sensitivity tests before administering this poison to a patient. Why not? Why not find out if at least there is a shot that the chemo you are being administered will have any effect? I suspect the reason is that if this poison doesn't fit, they will lose the revenue.

My friend Farrah Fawcett, who underwent two courses of excruciating,

debilitating, immune-system-ruining chemotherapy for anal cancer—
only to have the cancer return in three months—was told upon doing a
chemosensitivity test in Germany that the chemo she had been administered in our country had been completely ineffective. A waste of time.
Useless. All it did was seriously degrade her health.

Yet we look around, trying to pinpoint anything else that might be the
source of cancer, and we march for breast cancer to bring in millions of
dollars for the drug companies to create even more drugs.

BUT WHAT CHOICE DO I HAVE?

Dr. Stanislaw Burzynski, interviewed in this book, said about pancreatic
cancer, "We in the medical world know without a doubt, that chemotherapy absolutely, positively, does nothing, nothing whatsoever and is completely ineffective for pancreatic cancer."

Dr. Nicholas Gonzalez states, "There are only three kinds of cancer
that respond to chemotherapy, if they do, in fact, respond: testicular cancer, some lymphomas, and childhood leukemias."

Dr. Ralph Moss was fired from Memorial Sloan-Kettering Cancer Center because he wouldn't disseminate the research on laetrile, a natural
drug that showed much promise.

These are opinions from people with a definite point of view but
nonetheless it behooves us laypeople to look into other options. And that
is what this book is trying to accomplish: to look at the possibility that
there is another way. With *Knockout*, I am presenting to you doctors who
are treating cancer patients in new ways.

This book was written to warn patients to think and look into alternatives first, before you blindly walk into "standard of care" surgery, radiation, chemotherapy, and harsh aftercare drugs. Again and again, we have
seen so many suffer from horrible poisons and, unfortunately, most often
live out their last months of life horribly degraded, only to die a tortured,
expensive death.

Over and over, the patient is sold the chemotherapy rap, that it will
"shrink" (not cure) the tumor. Or experts will use words like *respond*.
So, because we believe and trust that "they" know best, we agree to be
poisoned.

It has got to stop. We patients have to know the truth, learn the realities. With information there is power.

THE CHEMOTHERAPY RACKET

How often is this happening on a daily basis in our country? How cavalier is it that chemotherapy is thrown about as though it is *the* viable solution? Not a cure, not even a promise, just an antidote for what is perceived as cancer. In my case, there was no mention of a chemosensitivity test in either of my two diagnoses to find out whether I would even respond to chemotherapy.

This entire scenario got me thinking that perhaps chemotherapy is a racket. Chemosensitivity tests exist. They do them routinely in Germany. Burton Goldberg will tell you about them in his chapter. Shockingly, Dr. Robert Nagourney in Long Beach, California, and Larry Weisenthal in Huntington Beach, California, are the two lone doctors in America doing these difficult sensitivity tests. They know the benefits.

The doctors in this book all make the claim that chemotherapy is for the most part a failed protocol—in fact, a dismal failure. Our oncologists are stuck with a protocol that, with the exception of a few select cancers, doesn't work. But they have no other ideas about what does work, as this is all that is taught in American medical schools (which are compromised by funding from pharmaceutical companies).

It is in the interests of big business to teach this moneymaking protocol and from a business standpoint they have the perfect template in place: fund the students who will administer their medicines, fund the hospitals to administer their medicines, lobby in Washington, D.C., for a standard of care that revolves around their medicines, make it illegal not to use their medicines, and ostracize doctors who don't toe the company line, calling them quacks, charlatans, and frauds and running them out of town.

Pharma is not interested in anything that comes from nature. Anything from nature cannot be patented, and if it can't be patented, there is little revenue in it. This is why so often many natural alternatives to serious disease never see the light of day.

Chemotherapy is big business, and the business end has been thoroughly thought out. Our med students are taught the company line, and after years of being intensively taught how to administer poisons, they are then graduated to go out and give these lethal medicines. To question this would discourage financial grants, and no one wants to be cut loose from pharmaceutical funding: hospitals depend on it, universities depend on it, many doctors and Ph.D.'s depend on it. To admit that there might be another way could jeopardize the big hand that feeds them. And if they were to find another way, it might indicate that their schooling and the study of cancer were on the wrong track.

DO YOU STILL TRUST THE FDA?

Writing a book that challenges today's entrenched cancer establishment can expose me to intense criticism.

As you can imagine, those who financially benefit from maintaining the status quo would prefer you not read my book. One tactic they may try to discredit me with is to state that the novel therapies used by doctors I interview are not approved by the FDA.

Despite widespread publicity about the FDA's many failings, the media sometimes buy into the argument that anything not approved by the FDA is automatically suspect. There is a major fallacy in this assertion. When the FDA did an internal audit of itself, its own report stated that it lacks the scientific capability and competence to evaluate new medical technologies. What this means is that the FDA no longer has the scientific legitimacy to be the sole arbitrator of what works and what doesn't.

I have read enough horror stories about what really goes on inside the FDA to write an entire book on the subject. In order to deflect those who attack me for recommending therapies that are not yet FDA approved, I asked the Life Extension Foundation to provide a brief update about what's wrong with the FDA and why cancer patients should not base their treatment decisions on arbitrary FDA proclamations. You can find a link to that update at www.lef.org. As you will read, not only has the FDA admitted it is incapable of evaluating new medical technologies, but congressional investigative committees have uncovered shocking instances of FDA decisions based on protecting pharmaceutical company financial interests and not the public's health.

CAN'T WE DO BETTER?

I believe that every day people are being misdiagnosed with diseases they don't have and being treated with harsh medicines for conditions they don't have.

Most hospitals are no longer safe. Medical laziness, overstretched staffs, and intellectual sloppiness pervade every hospital in the country. In fact, the second-largest number of accidental deaths in this country occurs in our hospitals. Why aren't we mad as hell?

It's not important to pinpoint the hospital where my nightmare occurred. I'm not out to ruin reputations. I'm trying to tell you, my faithful
readers, that you need to have the information to protect yourself if you
are ever in a terrible situation, as I was.

I'm not trying to "get" the doctors. They are just part of a system that
follows procedure. They are just part of the sloppiness, a sloppiness that
leads to a lack of thorough investigation, bolstered by a reliance on a pre-
ceding doctor's evaluation. Other than Dr. Internist, who was listening to
me but was hamstrung by hospital protocol, and Dr. Lung Cancer, who
allowed a little room for doubt, none of my other doctors even wavered
slightly from the cancer diagnosis.

Maybe it's my forgiving nature, but what's weird is that other than Dr.
Oncologist and Dr. Infectious Disease, I liked the other doctors. I admire
doctors. And in their way, each of them was trying to do his or her best.
They are good people, but they were terribly wrong.

My life and emotional and physical health were at stake, and in today's
climate of litigation, not one has had the integrity to say "I'm sorry." That
would have helped my damaged and hurting soul, and might have
speeded up my healing from the post-traumatic stress I experienced,
which took months to get over.

I had surgery I did not need; I had an anesthetic I did not need; I had
such intense trauma that my normally low blood pressure went up to
191, which required me to be on strong medicines and sedatives. The
nervousness surrounding the surgery was clearly unnecessary; I am sure it
took years off my life. I was forced to see my death; I was forced to feel
the trauma of leaving the people I loved most in this world and the
aching pain of that loss.

How do you heal a soul? It has no marked place in the body, yet it is
who we are, the essence of each of us. It radiates out of us when we are
emotionally healthy and is palpable when a person has a damaged spirit.

And how do we heal what's wrong with health care that's so lacking
in . . . well, a good standard of care?

Chapter 4

IF IT COULD HAPPEN TO ME,
WHAT WILL HAPPEN TO YOU?

If I were to contract cancer, I would never turn to a certain
standard for the therapy of this disease. Cancer patients who
stay away from these centers have some chance to make it.

–Professor Georges Mathé, "Scientific Medicine Stymied,"
Médecines Nouvelles, 1989

The first night home, I sat on the porch of my bedroom, and as I looked
out at the calm, beautiful view below me, I was stunned by the week I
had just experienced. I was weak and unable to eat. I had lost ten pounds
in seven days, I was dehydrated, and my usually strong, confident voice
shocked those I spoke with on the telephone. "You don't sound like yourself," my sister Maureen said over and over.

I couldn't "get it up" for anyone. The sadness was overwhelming. It per-
meated my cells. Thinking that I was going to die, thinking that life was
over, had gotten into my being. I just couldn't shake the sadness. My cat,
who is an outdoor cat, somewhere between wild and domestic, and usually stays outside all night hunting, insisted on coming into our bedroom
and sleeping curled up next to me. He stayed there for days. Very strange
behavior for him. Sweet Ficus . . . I love that cat.

I couldn't watch television. Obama had been elected president, and I
had missed it. I never saw any of it. I had no energy, I had no happiness.
I didn't understand it. I wasn't going to die; they had been wrong. Yet I
couldn't shake the sadness. The diagnosis had scared me to death. I was
shaken and I had to figure out a way to recover.

The only thing they did right was to save my life in the emergency room, which was no small thing. I am grateful for that; they were wonderful. They reacted fast, they made me feel that they were in control and were going to take care of things, and they did. I needed them.

After that I should have been sent home. Instead, that was when the nightmare began.

Two weeks went by. Bruce and Caroline came over and brought yummy lamb shanks and mashed potatoes for dinner. The tastiness of Caroline's great cooking helped me begin to get my appetite back. Having my grandchildren doing their homework at the dinner table was part of my healing: normalcy, the routine of life, nothing fancy, just loving family and good nutritious food. That was what brought me back.

Ficus followed me everywhere. He didn't seem to want to go outside and hunt in the evenings. If we put him outside, he sat by the window and cried until we let him back in.

We celebrated Bruce's birthday with a cake my granddaughter made. It was so important to me to be with them, to be home, to be safe, to be normal. These things heal a traumatized heart. They knew it, and it also helped them to see me get my strength back.

"Dr. Internist is on the phone," Alan said one day at about the two-and-a-half-week mark.

My heart started pounding. "Hi," I said anxiously. I knew he had information on the cultures.

"Well, good news," he said. "You don't have TB or leprosy!"

I felt like laughing, I mean, geez . . . leprosy!

"We don't have all the cultures back," he continued. "But seeing these results, I feel real good that the rest of the cultures are going to be clear. Dr. Infectious wants you to continue taking the medicine until the cultures come back from the CDC, and that will be another four weeks." I listened to him but I had already decided not to take the medicines. I know of patients who were on them and they developed terrible side effects, including blindness, neuropathy, and jaundice. Why would I subject myself to that?

I sensed he knew I wasn't going to take medicines without a definite diagnosis. Finally, here was a doctor who, when outside of the hospital setting, was trying to be straight with me. Doctors in the hospital are muzzled by hospital protocols.

Two weeks later, Dr. Internist called again.

"Something interesting came in today from the lab. One culture, just one of the many, came back with a rare strain of valley fever."

Wow! There. We had it. It was just as Caroline had suspected and what she had questioned the doctors about repeatedly but had been brushed off.

Valley fever, coccidiomycosis. Symptoms: fever (check), chest pain due to intense constriction, shortness of breath (check), anaphylactic shock leading to death (check), chest pressure resembling heart attack (check), chills (check), night sweats (check), fatigue (check), joint aches (check), red spotty rash, painful red bumps and welts all over the body (check), residual infection as in pneumonia (check), can look like cancer on X-ray if not diagnosed properly and can lead to biopsies (check and check), can be seen as TB if not properly diagnosed (check).

In the hospital I kept saying to the doctors, "I'm having an allergic attack or I was poisoned." Dr. Oncologist repeated over and over, "This is cancer. No herb could do this."

Valley fever is a fungus prevalent in the desert Southwest, prolific among migrant workers because they work in soil. The spores in this fungus live in the top two layers of soil, and people who work in their gardens (I work in my organic garden at my desert home constantly) or those exposed to dust in the New Mexico regions (I go on archaeological digs with my friend Forrest Fenn on his property outside of Santa Fe regularly) are more likely to get it. Imagine, just a few questions could have opened up the possibility that I did not have cancer and that we were dealing with something else. Obviously, somewhere between my digs and my garden, I had breathed in this fungus. It may have been dormant in me for years, but it is clear that something had knocked out my immune system.

I went to Dr. Galitzer's office in Santa Monica to have an IV of vitamin C and glutathione. I needed to build up my body. The vitamin C would strengthen my entire system after all the trauma and physical damage that had been done, and the glutathione would start the detoxification I was going to need over the next few months. While I was there he said something that immediately stopped me in my tracks: "I used to be an ER doc and when a patient came into emergency, we automatically did a CBC blood test and we always checked for eosinophils."

"What are those?" I asked.

"If the eosinophils come back high, then we know we are dealing with a poisoning or an allergic attack," he said.

When I got home from Dr. Galitzer's that day I pulled out all the lab work I had kept in a file and looked at the blood test results I had obtained from the emergency room.

There it was—eosinophils. A normal range was 0 to 5. My level was at 16! It was right there. I had been slammed by this life-threatening reaction, and there it was, the results, right in front of me, clearly for all to see. This meant that no one, *no one*, apparently bothered to look at the blood test. Had they done so they would have realized they were dealing with a poisoning or an allergic attack, and it might have led them to realize I had valley fever. But instead all the professionals went right to the CAT scan and diagnosed me with full-body cancer, which put me and my family into severe trauma. I was horribly, frankly stupidly, misdiagnosed.

Having a true diagnosis started to relax me. Now I knew what I was dealing with and I could take the steps I was comfortable with to get this fungus out of my body. In reading about it, I realized it wasn't going to be easy. Fungus is trickier than say, a staph infection that you wipe out with heavy-duty antibiotics. A fungus needs antifungals. And it was very clear that the medical community was not very informed about how to deal with it. But I wasn't worried. I am a researcher. I would find the right antidote, hopefully herbal, and kill this thing.

I was beginning to feel better, getting my strength back. One day Ficus didn't want to come in and lie on the bed with me. I smiled and said to Alan, "I'm well. Ficus just told me so."

GETTING IT RIGHT

Most people would have gone along with the treatments involved in this wrong diagnosis. How changed my life would be today. I shudder to think how often this happens to others.

The only ray of hope I felt throughout the entire craziness of the hospital fiasco, in the darkest depths of being given my death sentence of full-body cancer, was that I knew there are doctors out there who are curing cancer without drugs.

My awful experience became the fuel for the book you hold in your hands. It led me to write *Knockout* so that, if I could help it, no one else would ever feel as stressed, frightened, and helpless as I did during that week in the hospital.

Had I been a different kind of patient, I most likely would have accepted full-body chemotherapy for what turned out to be a horrible misdiagnosis. After all, my CAT scan showed, proved, full-body cancer. And as we know, the doctor is always right; in my case it was *six* doctors confirming my demise. When I told them, "I would rather die than take your therapy," I was treated as insolent, ignorant, stupid, and smug.

A DIFFERENT PATH

There are many tragedies of cancer. And one of them is that there are many patients who walk into the present "standard of care" therapy with complete trust, not knowing the correct questions to ask. They listen to their doctors, who say things like "The tumor will respond nicely." Well, what exactly does that mean? Or the oncologist will say, "The tumor will shrink." They never say *cure*, *heal*, or *destroy*. They can't, because in most cases that is just not true.

Patients are not offered chemosensitivity tests to determine if the chemo they will be administered is even a fit. The patients do not even know to ask about such testing because for the most part they do not know it exists.

Because of my own horrendous misdiagnosis and the fact that I have a louder voice, I feel I must express my outrage at the present system and the "standard of care" protocol that is presented as the only option. This is just not so. There are other treatments.

The forward-looking, courageous doctors in this book are thinking outside of the box. "Standard of care" will always be there, but you owe it to yourself to look into alternatives before making the biggest and maybe the most drastic decision of your life.

Many doctors I have spoken with came to the realization that they could no longer live with themselves by delivering a protocol that completely degrades a person. The present protocol most often creates a quality of life both horrendous and torturous. And at its end it usually leaves behind a ruined immune system, one so devastated that it can no longer perform its intended tasks. The patient is left with a body that no longer operates in any way like a healthy person's. And the true tragedy is that most times, after all of this torture, the patient dies anyway.

The doctors you will meet in this book have stepped outside of the accepted box at great personal and professional expense, and often have taken a big financial hit as well. But rolling in money does not seem to be their driving force. What they care about is that they are making people well. What's more, the doctors in this book are excited about their practices and the successes they are having. Again, not all patients have the same degree of success, and some will die. But many patients are making it, while also preserving a good quality of life.

For me this is a better option. It's a shot, a possibility. These are the odds I want.

Take it seriously. It's your life—no one will be as sorry as you if you end up sick. No one can do this for you. It's all up to you. How badly do you want health?

I am not telling you to do anything more than open your mind to the concept that there are other options. If nothing else, writing this book has taken away my fear of cancer. Now that I have not only spoken to these incredible doctors and professionals but also heard from the cured patients themselves, I believe cancer is preventable, manageable, and curable in many cases.

With cancer soon likely to be the number one killer in our country, we have to start now to change our diets and lifestyles if we are to avoid this fate. If sadly, you are one of those who receive a cancer diagnosis, *Knockout* gives you options for nondrug healing or integrated healing, plus a means to change your life to prevent a recurrence. This is a book to teach us all how to knock out cancer.

One of the first ways to change the future is to fully understand the past. My interview with Ralph Moss (chapter 6) provides a reasoned look at how we arrived here, so that we can own the power to change our future path.

Chapter 5

HOW DID IT GET THIS BAD?: CONVENTIONAL MEDICINE'S DARK SIDE

Tragic sins become moral failures only if we should have known better from the outset.

—Jared Diamond

Known for their athleticism, postage-stamp skirts and persuasive enthusiasm, cheerleaders have many qualities the drug industry looks for in its sales force. Some keep their pompoms active, like Onya, a sculptured former college cheerleader. On Sundays she works the sidelines for the Washington Redskins. But weekdays find her urging gynecologists to prescribe a treatment for vaginal yeast infection.

—Stephanie Saul, "Gimme an Rx! Cheerleaders Pep Up Drug Sales," *New York Times*, November 28, 2005

Thirty years ago, Henry Gadsden, chief executive of Merck, told *Fortune* magazine that he was distressed that his company profits were capped because his product was limited to sick people. Instead, he said, he'd rather be like Wrigley's chewing gum. He said his dream was to make drugs for healthy people. Then, he said, he could sell product to everyone.

Unfortunately for us, Henry's dream has come true.

What used to be the normal ups and downs of everyday life have become diseases. When common complaints are transformed into frightening conditions, the result is healthy people being turned into patients.

During World War II, American GIs who captured Japanese soldiers noticed that the Japanese rations tasted a whole lot better than the food the American soldiers were eating. U.S. scientists analyzed it and found that the reason the Japanese rations tasted so much better than ours was that they were putting a whole lot of MSG in their food.

Our scientists shared this information with American food manufacturers, holding a conference with them at which they concluded that this additive used in processing would make food taste better. As a result, since 1945 food companies have been adding chemicals to our food. In 1970, 262,000 tons of MSG were added to American foods. These fake foods are bad for our health and waistlines. And because we send food all over the world, we're beginning to see people from all parts of the globe starting to have problems with obesity even in places where it was never a problem before.

So you can see clearly how things have changed in a short time. As a nation we are taking pharmaceutical drugs and chemicals in amounts unprecedented in the history of mankind. We now have a pharmaceutical drug for pretty much every single human ailment. The result is a toxic buildup that steals the minds of our young and eliminates the wisdom pool of our elders. By the time our seniors reach their golden years, they can't think from the toxicity. Where will we find our wisdom?

We are also undergoing an environmental assault unprecedented in the history of mankind. Our air is polluted; our water is bubbling with fluoride, aluminum, and other chemicals. Our houses are like chemical plants from all the toxins used to keep the house "clean." Gone are the days when women cleaned the house with lemon juice or vinegar and water, used mineral oil for furniture polish, or used Ivory soap to get rid of ant infestations. Now we spray with poisons and we "freshen" the air with chemicals. We clean with toxins, and the buildup is killing us.

Couple this with toxicity from the chemicals in our food—preservatives and artificial sweeteners, high-fructose corn syrup, animals fed with corn (making their meat high in less healthful omega-6s instead of rich in healthful omega-3s)—and it all results in cellular destruction, which is a sure route to cancer.

We consume an excess of oils high in omega-6s—sunflower, corn, safflower, canola (ever see a canola plant?), peanut, and vegetable—which are damaging to each and every cell in the body. Omega-3s (found in olive, flax, and coconut oils) in cell membranes help keep the membrane elastic, protecting the cell, allowing for oxygenation and hydration, and promoting healthy cell function. An excess of omega-6 oils, however, can produce cell malfunction, and cell malfunction can lead to cancer. It's insidious. We buy into the theory that these harmful oils are not only heart healthy but also promote general good health, when nothing could be further from the truth.

Then there are aluminum cooking utensils, and plastic bottles that leech phthalates and dioxins into our bodies. And we wonder why we are now facing an unprecedented epidemic of cancer, Alzheimer's disease, and heart disease.

Western medicine's answer to this dilemma is to poison (with chemotherapy) the enemy that was created by poisons. Now how crazy is that?

We have lost our way. We have gotten away from the nature in us and the nature given to us. We have genetically modified foods. Most people eat very little real food and do not realize it. Food, water, air . . . all are essential to life, and we have contaminated them all.

In order to get well and stay well, we have to change our ways.

I spoke with Ralph Moss, Ph.D., on how we arrived where we are today and on the state of treatment in today's Western medicine. He is not an alarmist, but he is a realist, and he is alarmed. As a science scholar, he believes that before you widely use a treatment, it must first be proven. Please read his observations on the effectiveness and the ineffectiveness of cancer treatment today in this country. They are very eye-opening and honest.

I'll say it again: Remember, information is power.

Chapter 6

RALPH MOSS, PH.D.

Ralph Moss is a highly respected science writer and critic of conventional cancer treatment. Dr. Moss obtained his doctorate in classics from Stanford in 1974. He started work in the cancer field in the public relations department of New York's Memorial Sloan-Kettering Cancer Center, one of the premier cancer centers in the world.

Over the last thirty years Dr. Moss has written many books on cancer, cancer treatment, and the cancer establishment, including *Cancer Therapy: The Independent Consumer's Guide to Non-Toxic Treatment and Prevention; Herbs Against Cancer: History and Controversy; The Cancer Industry: The Classic Exposé on the Cancer Establishment; Questioning Chemotherapy,* a powerful and intelligent critique of chemotherapy; and *Complementary Oncology* with Josef Beuth, M.D.

His books provide a wealth of information on health and healing. He probes scientific and statistical evidence to reveal the shocking truth that chemotherapy is mostly inappropriate, ineffective, and in fact dangerous for most of the people who receive it—yet up to six hundred thousand Americans every year get chemo at their doctors' recommendations.

When asked what lessons he has drawn from his thirty-plus years as a science writer, he says, "Once we start to reshape our writing about science to accommodate the wishes of doctors, patients, or institutions, rather than the facts, we are sure to end badly. We must always speak to cancer patients with a finely balanced mixture of compassion and honesty. Finally, we must always demand a fair evaluation of all treatments, conventional and alternative. Only on a level playing field can the true value of any cancer therapy be determined."

I found speaking with him to be not only fascinating but enormously enlightening. His frankness is refreshing. He is a scholar not driven by the almighty dollar. You will enjoy and be shocked by what he has to say.

SS: Thanks for speaking with me, Dr. Moss. Tell me, why do doctors keep prescribing chemotherapy? If we know it's not going to do any good in most cases and it robs the patient of all quality of life, why continue?

RM: It's good to speak with you. First of all, let me chop this answer into little pieces. I am really only interested in what works and what doesn't work. I'm especially interested in proof of effectiveness or ineffectiveness, and especially proof of the effectiveness of treatments through the gold standard of randomized controlled trials. This is what I learned from my nearly ten years of involvement with the National Institutes of Health, when I was an advisor for what was then the Office of Alternative Medicine.

The government and the medical establishment have a very high standard of proof, called "increased overall survival through randomized control trials." The problem is that this standard is rigorously upheld only for the nonconventional cancer doctors; it's bent for the conventional doctors.

SS: You mean the rules are bent for pharmaceutical-company-sponsored treatments?

RM: Yes. Because of that, you don't have a level playing field. In fact, the people who are least able to perform those trials, and least able to afford to have them done, are the ones from whom it is most often demanded.

SS: You are speaking about alternative doctors who are in the trenches and having successes with patients?

RM: Correct. By and large, the people who have the money, and the organizations that have the resources and the knowledge to do those trials, aren't required to do them.

There's a terrible injustice in the way that drug development is set up. It's an injustice to advocates. New, less toxic, and more promising treatments are never adequately researched to the point where they could be scientifically confirmed.

SS: The problem being the seeming partnership of the FDA with the pharmaceutical companies?

RM: Well, that's the way the system works. I don't think the FDA and the pharmaceutical companies are getting together and rubbing their hands and saying, "Isn't it wonderful to screw the public?" At least, I hope not.

SS: Yes. But certainly the events of the last few years have given us enough reason to be cynical, given what is happening in the country relative to pharmaceuticals as a whole. I mean, just watch TV any one night and you will end up thinking you need a drug for something.

RM: Well, what I saw at Sloan-Kettering when I was there from 1974 to 1977 was a more complicated picture. The same people who covered up positive animal experiments with laetrile, a promising nontoxic cancer drug, were the same people who a couple of years before were trying to get clinical trials done with laetrile.

SS: I don't understand.

RM: These people from Sloan-Kettering went to Washington on two occasions, in 1974 and 1975, to plead with the government and the powers that be to let them do clinical trials. They believed that laetrile had promise. The testing on their animals was coming out positive. Initially the people from Sloan-Kettering were perceived to be the "good guys." But the same people who initially tried to break the blockade against nontoxic agents in general, and against laetrile in particular, lost their nerve. The price of continuing to present this drug as a viable answer in the face of blistering opposition from the FDA, the American Cancer Society, and somewhat from the National Cancer Institute would probably have been the ruination of their careers.

SS: In other words, keep your mouth shut or you're out. That's terrible.

RM: Right. When I got up and said these things in November 1977, I was fired from Sloan-Kettering because I had broken ranks with the party line, which had declared that laetrile was completely ineffective, and had been proven so. But in fact, the reality was that laetrile had performed excellently in our animal studies, and it had been proven.

SS: But you were instructed to inform the public that the results of the test had been negative.

RM: Right. When I refused to do that, they fired me. Here's the irony: the same people who fired me would admit these things in private. This was a common conversation among the administrators.

I was a relatively low-level employee, but I was in a crowd of very powerful people and it was common knowledge that laetrile was coming up positive in our tests. But any one of them would have been easily taken out in terms of their careers, and selectively they would have been damaged as a leadership group. Eventually many of them did suffer for even having let it go as far as it did.

SS: So all this was a result of a wall of opposition from the FDA and the American Cancer Society?

RM: With a powerful assist from most of the people at the National Cancer Institute.

SS: As a layperson listening to this, I'm thinking, It's coming from the FDA. But the question is why?

RM: Everything points back to the pharmaceutical industry. But I also have never seen the pharmaceutical industry dirty its hands, as it were, by itself coming forward as the opponent of nonconventional cancer treatments. I think they are much too smart to do that.

SS: So they have FDA agents do their work?

RM: Again, I have no proof of that. All I know is that in the thirty-five years that I've been studying the situation, the FDA has never approved any nontoxic drug, herb, vitamin, or anything like that for cancer. The rule seems to be that nothing of a nonpatented, less profitable nature gets through the FDA system. The only things that get through are these synthetic patented agents that are generally very toxic and ineffective. They are so ineffective that the FDA keeps lowering the bar and allowing things to be approved on lower and lower standards of effectiveness and lower and lower standards of safety.

SS: It's very clear the FDA is a handmaiden of the pharmaceutical companies.

RM: How it all goes down, who gets what from whom, I don't know. I don't particularly care; to me it's quite enough to know that they act like the loyal enforcer for Big Pharma. And that's what they are.

SS: Well, I read the report of the internal investigation the FDA did of itself last year, where they declared themselves incompetent, unable to keep up with the science, understaffed, overwhelmed, and so on. They have declared themselves ineffective.

RM: I've had some friends, believe it or not, in the FDA—most of them maverick types—who aren't the worst people in the world, no different from the average person, really, and I didn't get the feeling that they were corrupt or taking money personally from Big Pharma. However it happens, it's a mind-set, vehemently pro big business, pro Big Pharma, and vehemently against alternative medicine.

SS: How did this happen? How did it get this way?

RM: It goes back to the founding of the FDA. Initially there was this rampant patent medicine advertising going on in the United States and the FDA was created to stop this quackery and allow for more scientific drug development. So in their own DNA they have this attitude that if something is coming from small developers whose ideas are not mainstream, who don't have deep pockets and can't easily do things the way the FDA likes things done, in a multimillion-dollar fashion, then there is a presumption of guilt rather than a presumption of innocence or interest. They are very much disposed against the individual or small company that has a bright idea in the cancer field.

SS: I think about the full-body chemo I was offered earlier this year and where I would be today healthwise had I been another kind of patient who would have gone for it.

RM: Here's the irony: you would have been considered a success story. If your fungus went away on its own, then you might have been considered to be cured of some cancer you never had.

SS: You are right. Yet my immune system and quality of life would have been degraded seriously.

RM: Probably true. Yet there is some wiggle room in chemotherapy . . . it comes down to the individual in every single case, which has to be evaluated on its own merits. I do consultations for cancer patients. Recently I spoke to a young woman, thirty-three years old, with an estrogen-receptor-negative (ER-negative) tumor, over two centimeters in size, grade III, with two positive lymph nodes, triple negative. This is a very poor prognosis. The odds of her being alive in ten years are about 50 percent. Now, all the data I've seen indicated that if she does chemotherapy like Adriamycin, Cytoxan, and Taxotere, she would increase her chance of being alive in ten years by about another 13 percent.

SS: Yes, but her quality of life would suck.

RM: It could be very bad initially, but because she's young she would probably recover. I'm not arguing for it; I'm just saying that every case has to be evaluated on its own merit. To go from a 50 to a 65 percent chance of being alive is to me quite significant.

Now, I have absolutely no doubt, Suzanne, that there are better cancer treatments than chemotherapy. But because of the bias we know relatively little about the predictable outcome of doing those other treatments. For instance, Dr. Gonzalez is doing important work, but there are no studies really to tell us what the likely outcome of his treatment is.

SS: Speaking to his cured patients is more than I would need to convince me of what choice I would make were I ever to be in that situation again. Last year my oncologist told me that the cancer chemotherapy drug that I turned down, Adriamycin, has been proven to be ineffective.

RM: That is correct. A study done at the University of California, Los Angeles (UCLA), and now confirmed in the *Journal of the National Cancer Institute*, has proven that Adriamycin is ineffective in up to 92 percent of women to whom it was given, which is shocking.

SS: Because . . . ?

RM: Because in the most common kind of cancers, which are ER-positive cancers, it doesn't work. There's no need for it, yet it has potentially very serious cardiac side effects. Dennis Slamon, M.D., who is a very brave and brilliant scientist heading the Revlon Center at UCLA, took on the whole breast cancer oncology community with a speech at ASCO [American Society of Clinical Oncology] a couple of years ago in which he basically challenged them and said that most of the time they are giving Adriamycin for no good reason. Now, admittedly, he invented the drug Herceptin, which he said could be given instead of Adriamycin.

SS: Herceptin is for the HER2/neu type of cancer, right?

RM: Yes, it is primarily for HER2/neu-positive tumors.

SS: I have to say, I'm really not interested in Herceptin or Adriamycin. I'm interested in why we can't treat cancer or manage cancer naturally if we desire. Why not be offered a choice? Why put the body through such a grueling chemical invasion? Why, when the doctors in this book are having success without chemicals, do we have to keep going over and over the same crap about drugs? Isn't there a better way? I really think there is. At the very least, why aren't they giving chemosensitivity tests?

RM: The medical community doesn't believe in it. And that's a scandal of the first order.

SS: Walk me through that scandal.

RM: Sensitivity testing is done for antibiotics. For instance, if you have a really bad infection, they'll test the bugs against the different antibiotics to see which one works. You can do the same thing with cancer. An early version came out in the 1970s that was endorsed by the National Cancer Institute. That test relied basically upon inhibiting the growth of colonies of cancer cells. It turned out to be ineffective, so the bottom fell out. One of the people involved with the NCI sensitivity testing program, Dr. Larry Weisenthal, figured out a much better way to do the testing, which was to look for signs of programmed cell death (apoptosis) in the cancer cells.

So if you take the cancer cells and put them in little plates with all the different cancer drugs and combinations of the drugs, then you can easily measure the amount of apoptosis, or programmed cell death, in each of the wells, and that gives you a comparative number for which is working. In other words, you are not trying to just murder the cancer cells, you are trying to induce the best type of destruction of the cancer cells, which is programmed cell death.

But because of earlier failure of the test, the medical community didn't want to hear about it. It's like the crowd had moved on to something else, the fashion had changed, and that was the end of that.

SS: What a shame. So now chemo is "one size fits all." They just throw it at the patient and hope it works. I have just buried too many friends due to death by chemo.

RM: Well, there is light—there are Dr. Robert Nagourney and Dr. Weisenthal and a few other people who recognize the need for this and are doing these tests. But these people have been pushed aside by the mainstream oncologists. The harder these doctors pushed for this testing, the more there was pushback against them by the leaders of the cancer field.

SS: It's pretty shocking.

RM: At ASCO a few years ago they put the final nail in the coffin. They declared that these tests were ineffective. The amazing thing is that they evaluated it on the original older techniques, which Weisenthal and Nagourney do not use and haven't used for over twenty years.

SS: This is astonishing.

RM: You are right about that. Nagourney was beside himself with rage when this happened. I understand and I agree with him. I think there is very good preliminary evidence that sensitivity testing works. I think what this is really about is whether or not medicine is going to be individual or cookie-cutter, and the economics favors the cookie-cutter approach. But the science trends toward individualization; the science is screaming out on this point. We have to take each person's cancer, each person's tumor cells, and treat that particular person's cancer. That's what the science is saying.

SS: You are talking about economics, right?

RM: Yes, the economics are "Let's keep that assembly line running and push through as many patients as possible, so we can maximize our profits."

SS: I have come to that same place. . . . Maybe they don't want to know if this particular chemotherapy is going to work. I mean after all, the profits are so huge, what if the tests come back and say it's not going to work? They just lost all that revenue.

RM: It's a matter of pushing through a million patients a year. At least six hundred thousand a year are getting chemo. How are you going to do that and simultaneously analyze every patient and come up with a unique combination of drugs that can't be written up in a textbook and prescribed? You just can't hand it to a nurse and give her the recipe for a particular kind of cancer.

Everybody's different, everybody's going to respond differently; we have to titrate this, we have to give different amounts for each patient. Then, of course, it gets into other kinds of individualization: vaccines and other things that we know are beneficial to cancer patients; chronomodulation of drugs, which means giving drugs at particular times of day and night when they are the most effective. This leads to a boutique type of treatment. But as I say, the push relative to the level of profitability is toward mass production.

SS: If there was individualized treatment, everyone would want it.

RM: Right, and they are not prepared to give it to everybody, although I think it will be cost-effective in the long run.

SS: Why? Because people would have better outcomes and fewer side effects? I don't know why this can't be seen as the bigger picture.

RM: They are focused on how many patients they can see today.

SS: But if I were an oncologist and I took the oath to do no harm, I would think from a place of morality I would investigate every possible approach. It is arrogant to think the present template is the only way, especially when the outcomes at present are so dismal.

RM: I agree it's outrageous and at the point where none of us wants to be treated. When doctors become sick themselves, then they sing a different tune. There was a study done in Canada relative to lung cancer and chemotherapy. When asked, 75 percent of the doctors said they would not take platinum-containing chemotherapy themselves.

SS: That should tell you something.

RM: Right, but still, they give it. A very eminent neurologist once stood in my living room and told me that if he were to get brain cancer he wouldn't take radiation. I said, "Well, then, how do you treat for brain cancer?" He answered, "Radiation." There was no irony in his voice, no recognition of the fact that on one hand he's telling me that both he and his department chief had decided they wouldn't take radiation, but every day they send people with brain cancer for radiation.

SS: In the chemotherapy world, what is considered success? Months? Is that how it works?

RM: I just like to state what the facts state. For instance, with Avastin, which will cost the average person about $100,000 a year, it may, when given with chemo, increase survival for four or five months within the confines of a clinical trial. On the other hand, for breast cancer it has not been proven to extend survival. The advisory council of the FDA just approved it or recommended approval for brain cancer, with no evidence of increased survival. They couldn't even prove that it shrank the tumor. There was a 25 percent shrinkage of the size of the growth on an X-ray for a couple of weeks, but that shrinkage was not proven to be of cancer cells. It probably was the swelling around the tumor. Despite that, they approved this. According to press reports, it's going to generate an extra $200 million a year in sales for the parent company of Avastin, with no evidence, really nothing. If we came to the FDA with an alternative treatment with that level of evidence, they would laugh us out of the room.

SS: Again, I hate to be a broken record, but this is shocking. What was the criterion for approval?

RM: Aside from the meager clinical trial data, it was based on a few anecdotes of patients who said, "We feel we benefited by this." They were tearful and their relatives were tearful and people stood up and literally cheered when the advisory board committee agreed to approve this usage. I respect the experiences of patients, regardless of what kind of treatment they opt for. But what disturbs me is that drug companies have actually helped create some of these patient advocacy groups and they certainly fund many of the others. It's no coincidence that Breast Cancer Action, headed by Barbara Brenner in San Francisco, is the only group to my knowledge that refuses to take pharmaceutical money. And this group is the one that opposed the approval of Avastin for breast cancer last December. They get labeled militant because they insist on the science rather than just the PR.

SS: What about the drug Gemzar?

RM: Gemzar [gemcitabine] was originally approved by the FDA based on a very small quality-of-life improvement in pancreatic cancer patients. The effect in the community setting was that 20 percent had improved quality of life. Once the company got approval, they could start using it off-label for everything under the sun. But this is a drug that is relatively benign, and also has minimal effects. You rarely hear about people having major side effects with Gemzar.

SS: But this is chemotherapy, right?

RM: Yes. These are chemotherapy drugs, but they are mild forms of chemotherapy. They are given as a kind of placebo, meaning when they have nothing else to give and they don't want to burden the patient with a lot of side effects, they give this drug and everybody is happy. The patients feel that something is being done for them, and the doctor gets paid for administering or prescribing something. Then the patients expire and the families feel that at least they tried.

SS: This is the part I don't understand—the patient is given drugs that don't do much and at the end the family is grateful. Recently a young friend of mine died of pancreatic cancer, stage IV. I have never seen such destruction to a human body as I watched him disintegrate and die in four months. Then a few weeks after the death, his wife called and asked if I would come perform for a fund-raiser for his doctor. And I thought, They just killed your husband.

RM: Right, and you're going to do a fund-raiser for him!

SS: How much money does a doctor make per patient on chemotherapy?

RM: Of course, it varies; I don't know exactly because it would vary from drug to drug. It would even vary from month to month. I'll give you two sets of facts. One is that the cost of treating stage IV colon cancer ten years ago was $500. The drugs they were giving at Sloan-Kettering at that time were 5-fluorouracil and leucovorin. These are inexpensive drugs to buy and administer. But ten years later the cost of treating colon cancer is around $250,000, and that's only, as they say, for parts, not labor.

SS: You mean that is only for the cost of the drugs, and not counting all the costs of the doctor administering it?

RM: The doctor, the oncologist, in private practice can make money three ways off the drug, maybe four ways. First of all, they get paid by the patient or his or her insurance for the office visit. Second, they have the chemotherapy concession, which means, alone among all doctors in the United States and probably any other industrialized country, they get to sell the drug at retail—buy it at wholesale and sell it retail.

SS: Basically they are the pharmacy for the drug.

RM: Correct. So when the mainstream doctors criticize the CAM [complementary and alternative medicine] doctors for selling vitamins out of their offices, oncologists are doing it in spades because they are selling chemotherapy out of their offices. It's called the chemotherapy concession. There have been front-page articles in the *New York Times* business section about this.

The third way they get money—and this was also exposed in the *New York Times*—is by getting kickbacks from particular drug companies for volume prescribing. So if this month a special premium for drug X is being given, the doctor would benefit financially by prescribing that drug. There's also a lot of wiggle room in what is prescribed. It's not so cut-and-dried, so that a doctor could decide that this month all his or her patients need to take a particular drug. You get the picture. Prescribing drugs that are tied into the promotional discounts could determine a much greater profit for the doctor.

SS: And what is the fourth way?

RM: The fourth way is to become a so-called marquee professor, where you get to promote the drug in question and they pay you an honorarium or a fee from a speaker's bureau or so forth. Sometimes when you go to ASCO, particular professors are basically doing blurbs, you know, infomercials for particular anticancer drugs. I remember one who shall remain nameless who said, "It brings tears to my eyes when I think about the beneficiaries of this treatment." Now of course, he's on the payroll of the company making that particular drug. So there are a lot of ways for doctors to make money off the administration and sales of the drugs.

SS: What I'm hearing is incentive to prescribe, not only for the oncologists, but also for the hospitals to make sure that there's enough chemotherapy administered. And it feels . . . well, a little evil.

RM: It just tips the scale even further toward the use of these expensive, patented, toxic, and relatively ineffective drugs, and that much further away from the so-called enemy, which is inexpensive: natural, nutritional, usually nonconventional treatment. It gives them another reason to resist and I would say to hate the natural treatments, and they do.

SS: The people have to know this. The patients are so vulnerable, and to think that this is going on. It's all a big mess. I also hear that hospitals could not afford to stay open without the revenue from chemotherapy.

RM: A lot of things need to be restructured in many ways. It goes back again to "Are we going to have individualized care or cookie-cutter care?" Of course we all want the individualized care, but we are not offered that. Part of the reason there are alternative treatments is that they cannot fit into the dominant kind of treatment that's being given.

I've looked at the cases of Drs. Gonzalez and Burzynski, and I personally know some of their cases. I am in agreement with you that these men are doing exciting work, but we don't know the sum total of what happens to people who go to them for treatment. We don't know all the factors that lead them to having success. So I'm not arguing with you, just telling you how I deal with the question. To me it's enough to expose the fact that these treatments exist, and to expose the realities of the drugs being administered in orthodox medicine. The alternative guys have had some success and they are not being given a fair shake.

Just saying this is an extremely revolutionary position. Burzynski and Gonzalez are innovative doctors, and they have made advances in cancer and they've helped a lot of people. But their successes are not 100 percent.

SS: No one could say that. That would be Nobel Prize time. I am presenting all the doctors and protocols in this book as a choice. I present to my reader the realities of the orthodox cancer world and the realities of the alternative world. Perhaps someone will read this book and decide they want to roll the dice and go the chemotherapy route. It's not for me to decide; it's all about choice.

Tell me, will alternative medicine ever grow enough to have an equal voice or even overtake this other force that owns America, owns our government? Can little voices like ours see the light of day?

RM: I have to believe we will. To maintain my own sanity and to get me going every day for thirty-five years, I must believe it. But then again, none of us ever believes we're going to die, either, but the evidence seems to speak to the contrary.

I don't see a clear path to it, but I do see that the system is crumbling, so that might be the opening. I do see a little bit of sunlight. You, Suzanne, have a tremendous opportunity to reach the masses of people. It's unprecedented. I can't think of anybody in the country who has the ear of more people on this issue than you do. I'm not that popular a person, I'm a scholar, but I am an independent scholar. So I try to document things as best I can. Somehow I feel that if I continue to do that, eventually someone will listen. At least I'm laying down a standard of scholarship in this area that is higher than what it was before. And I think you need both.

I like to make arguments that are difficult to refute, where somebody will read what I've written and can't argue effectively against it. I've had that reaction from many scientists and doctors over the years. Most of them started out hostile but in the end were won over because I was quietly pulling up facts, and it's hard to argue with facts. I try not to go overboard with my enthusiasm or endorsement of alternative treatments because I've been burned too often. But I try to keep it all in balance, in perspective, and that's my basis or philosophy.

SS: As I have been working on this project your name has come up over and over, and always with great respect. You need to know that you are making an impact. You are very highly regarded, and I am honored to have you be part of this project.

Now that we know how we got here, just what can we do about it? Read on to see what some brilliant, cutting-edge doctors have to say.

PART II

The Doctors Who Are Curing Cancer

On some positions, cowardice asks the question, is it expedient? And then expedience comes along and asks the question—is it politic?

Vanity asks the question—is it popular? Conscience asks the question—is it right?

There comes a time when one must take the position that is neither safe nor politic nor popular, but he must do it because conscience tells him it is right.

—Martin Luther King Jr., "Remaining Awake Through a Great Revolution,"
March 31, 1968

Chapter 7

DR. STANISLAW BURZYNSKI

> The clearest example of where government overprotects people
> is its irrational insistence that terminally ill cancer patients should
> only use FDA-approved drugs or standard remedies, and can
> only use experimental drugs after the so-called "proven remedies"
> have failed. Everyone in the conventional medical community
> knows that there are certain kinds of cancer for which there are
> no curative treatments. . . . Dying patients should have the ultimate
> say as to what treatments they should be able to take, and their
> choices should include any experimental or unconventional treat-
> ment the patients can get their hands on.
>
> –Richard Jaffe, *Galileo's Lawyer*

Stanislaw Burzynski, M.D., was born in Lublin, Poland, in 1943 and is
an internationally recognized physician and scientist who has pioneered
the development and use of biologically active peptides (antineoplastons)
in diagnosing, preventing, and treating cancer and other diseases since
1967.

The Burzynski clinic has effectively treated more than fifty types of
cancer but has the most consistent successes with cancers of the brain,
breast, head and neck, prostate, colon, lungs, and ovaries, as well as non-
Hodgkin's lymphoma. Patients with aggressive brain tumors often qualify
for FDA-controlled clinical trials and can receive antineoplastons. Others
may be treated with personalized combinations of gene-targeted medications, some of them from the antineoplaston family with comparable
results.

I met Dr. Burzynski at the American College for Advancement in Medicine (ACAM) awards dinner in Las Vegas in November 2008—ironically,
one week before the events I describe in the opening chapter of this book,

when I was misdiagnosed with full-body cancer. There was a buzz about him, and I was told several times that evening, "You must meet Dr. Burzynski. He's the doctor who's curing cancer."

Dr. Burzynski is to be celebrated for his accomplishments as a brave and courageous pioneer. No one has worked harder and no one has been more persecuted for his maverick approach. The proofs of his accomplishments are the successful treatments of so many patients. The government tried to take him down but he bounced back up and landed on his feet. His successes are a threat to the orthodox cancer protocols. His approach with targeted gene therapy and antineoplastons for so many kinds of cancer is working where traditional chemotherapy rarely does.

Those who want to discredit him ask the obvious question: "If this treatment is so good, why don't other oncologists jump on board?" According to Dr. Julian Whitaker:

> Here's where it gets ugly. The paradigm that governs all conventional cancer treatment is that one must "purge the body of cancer cells." Conventional cancer treatment is a search-and-destroy mission: find a tumor, cut it out, poison it with chemotherapy, or obliterate it with radiation.
>
> If there is an approach to cancer that obviously isn't working, this is it. In spite of dramatic advances in these invasive procedures (if one could call them advances), the death rate for cancer has not budged over the last fifty years. In fact, it has increased. Yes, you may hear about cancer patients surviving longer today, but the reality is that we're talking months, not years, for most of the common types of fatal cancer.
>
> Despite the fact that this approach doesn't work, it is nevertheless firmly entrenched and almost universally accepted. One reason is because physicians are notoriously resistant to change. It is understandable. Oncologists spend three to five years in intensive training to ply their trade. Acceptance of Burzynski's discovery would nullify those efforts.

One day, I believe, Dr. Burzynski will be a historic figure. But right now he is, as in the famous Schopenhauer quote about the three stages of truth, in "violent opposition." Were there to be a cure, it would put an end to all the marches and the research dollars, and most of all a big huge chemotherapy business to the tune of $200 billion a year.

A cure would force all present protocols to halt, and those in the field would have to learn a whole new way to approach the management of cancer. And maybe that's what we are talking about here. Some cancers, from my interviews in this book, appear to be "manageable," just as diabetes is "manageable." Dr. Burzynski's patients do not see their cancer as terminal. They are living with it, managing it. Maybe that will make some more comfortable than saying the word *cure*. Semantics.

Dr. Burzynski has identified missing peptides in the blood and urine of people who have cancer. These peptides are just not there. Those without cancer have these peptides in their blood. This makes sense to me; as with bioidentical hormones: if it's missing, put it back, and then everything normalizes again. I like simplicity. Because of politics, it's not that simple. There are FDA requirements.

Dr. Burzynski fled the Iron Curtain in Poland, arrived in America with $15 in his pocket, and managed to create a life that dreams are made of—doing the work he loves and living free. With that freedom, Dr. Burzynski has devoted his life to solving what he believes is the riddle to cancer, and his answer is antineoplastons. But our government interfered and initially tried to put him in jail. Now they interfere once again and force him to alter his approach.

Dr. Burzynski is a biochemist who has invented drugs and maybe the most important and successful non-FDA-approved alternative cancer drug therapy ever in this country: antineoplastons. Unfortunately, he does not have a free hand to use antineoplastons because he is still limited by the FDA to clinical trials.

Nonetheless, he has worked around these limitations, and his patients speak about him with a kind of exuberant reverence. Even though there are some instances where he must now use low-dose, weak chemotherapy to perform clinical trials, his patients do not experience the horrible side effects normally associated with high-dose chemotherapy and many of them are living long, healthy, and productive lives.

We should be grateful for people like Dr. Burzynski with his tenacious nature. Without his passion he might have given up long ago. But passion is indefinable. In spite of everything, he has carried on, and the measure of the man is clear when you read his interview. The information that follows may one day save your life.

SS: Good evening, Dr. Burzynski. It is a pleasure and an honor to speak with you. Tell me, is this what you had planned for your life?

SB: Not exactly. Initially I thought I would study the aging process, but in Poland there were limited possibilities to do research in this area.

A few years into my studies I started working with peptides and amino acids in blood, relative to various illnesses, and I noticed substantial changes in the composition in the blood of patients who have cancer. In fact, there were several peptides which were deficient in patients who had cancer, and I thought that this could be important.

I am a curious person, and in spite of the fact that this was not what I had planned to pursue, I found myself studying cancer. Since I was about to finish I decided to do my doctoral thesis on peptides.

After graduation I really concentrated on cancer. I isolated the peptides that I found were deficient in cancer patients. But Poland was a very difficult country in which to live at that time.

SS: What do you mean by difficult? The politics? The war?

SB: Yes, politics and the war. When I was a kid, my father was arrested by the Nazis because he objected to the fact that Polish and Jewish children were forbidden to go to school. In the late forties the Iron Curtain descended over Poland and suddenly our home was no longer family property. It now belonged to the state, and the state divided our home into apartments and turned them over to workers left homeless by the war. Our family was allowed to remain in a small apartment of what was our former home, but now we were forced to share our bathroom and kitchen with all these strangers who were living with us. We also learned that one woman living in our house was a government spy. It all became very dangerous because my brother was in the anticommunist underground and already many of his friends had been killed in prison.

SS: Did your father ever get out of prison?

SB: Yes, eventually my father was released from prison, but he could never again get a proper teaching job. So when I realized I had few opportunities in Poland, I decided to come to the United States.

SS: Were you worried that you wouldn't be allowed to leave Poland?

SB: Well, I didn't know. I did know that the government was trying to suppress Polish science if research in any way threatened Communist principles. They wanted a completely docile population, where no one had an independent thought. Ultimately they wiped out the middle and upper classes, but the irony was that at the same time they wanted to keep the "thinkers" inside Poland, so they made it very difficult to get a passport.

I was not allowed to bring anything with me. When I left I had fifteen bucks in my pocket and chromatographic documentation of the thirty-nine peptides I had singled out. I had an uncle in the Bronx who said I could stay with him. A few weeks after I arrived, I got a message from the Lublin medical school that I was fired from my position as a researcher and that I could no longer have any position at any other Polish medical school. I now realized that I could not go back, so I started to look for a job here.

I was grateful to receive a faculty position at Baylor College of Medicine in Houston, which was my first job interview. At that time there was a scientist named George Ungar working on brain peptides at the university's department of anesthesiology; this department had large grants. George Ungar thought peptides might be important and agreed to allow me to have space in their laboratory to continue my research.

SS: What came out of your research?

SB: That there is a system of peptides which are deficient in cancer patients which can inhibit the growth of cancer cells, and that replacing these peptides kills the cancer cells without killing the normal cells.

In 1976, I presented this information at a conference attended by doctors from all over the world. It caught the attention of the news media, and the next day it was reported internationally by the Associated Press that a researcher at Baylor found peptides that are produced in humans which can kill cancer cells without killing normal cells. Since then my main effort has been to further study these peptides.

SS: How did you test, through animal studies?

SB: First we did animal testing, then, finally, our goal was to do phase I and phase II studies. We did that after I left Baylor. Now we are entering phase III studies and we hope to have FDA approval for marketing soon.

SS: You must feel very pleased with this progress.

SB: I feel lucky that Baylor gave me a job and allowed me to continue my research. We are also working on seeing what role peptides play in memory and what we can do to slow down the progress of Alzheimer's disease.

SS: Tell me, what exactly is a peptide?

SB: A peptide is a molecule which is composed of two or more amino acids. If you combine two amino acids through a special chemical bond called a peptide bond, you have a peptide. Protein is simply a large peptide.

SS: Okay, let's break it down even more. What is a protein?

SB: When you have more than fifty amino acids in a molecule, scientists call it a protein. A molecule with fifty or fewer amino acids is called a peptide. So peptides are up to fifty amino acids connected by peptide bonds.

SS: I'm piecing together here. Is insulin a protein?

SB: Historically, yes. Insulin has fifty-one amino acids. After the structure of insulin was discovered and insulin was obtained synthetically, everybody jumped on it and cheered because this was the first synthesized protein.

SS: I ask because I have written so many books on insulin, which I know is a protein, so I'm trying to understand. In breaking down the essence of what a peptide is, I am trying to find why you deemed them so important.

SB: Yes, well, we can't live without amino acids. Eight of our amino acids are essential, and you'll die if you don't have them supplied from the outside. For instance, you need animal proteins to supply these amino acids, and then these amino acids are used as the building blocks of peptides and proteins. We know that proteins are the building blocks of life. Without proteins you don't have any life except for some viruses, which are composed of nucleic acids and peptides.

SS: What do peptides do?

SB: We have found that peptides are extremely important molecules, in fact, very active in transferring information. By assembling various chains of amino acids you can encode practically any information which is necessary for the function of the human body. My thinking is that cancer is a disease of information processing. If you have the wrong information transfer, as in if you turn on a bad or wrong genetic switch, you activate something which would lead to cancer. But by the same token if you use the right molecular switch, the right peptide, you can turn off the cancer process and you will get rid of the disease.

SS: Kind of like pressing the wrong button on your computer and you mess things up, but if you know the right buttons to push you can correct it.

SB: Yes. Peptides also work as memory tags.

SS: Please explain.

SB: Let's assume that memory is a circuit of neurons like a special CD in the brain. These molecular CDs have peptide tags and the brain can pull them out as a memory item and that information is further processed in the brain.

SS: Why do we care about this?

SB: Because peptides play an important part in information processing. The body has a defense system, which I call the biochemical defense system which is parallel to the immune system. The immune system consists of proteins and various types of cells, and it protects us against invasion from microorganisms and abnormal cells. The peptide system corrects the information inside the cancer cell. Simply by turning off what is wrong and turning on what is good inside cancer cells, those molecular switches can get rid of cancer cells.

SS: I understand, but I still do not get why peptides could kill cancer cells.

SB: The immune system works by releasing antibodies which attach to wrong proteins on the surface of the cells and they kill them, but the peptide system works through correction of the genetic information, so it is like a second immune system.

If you use the peptide system correctly by identifying the proper molecular switches, then you can work on the genes that cause cancer, and kill cancer cells without killing normal cells.

SS: And you do this through antineoplastons?

SB: Yes, this is the name I gave to these particular peptides that kill cancer cells. The components of the immune system are called antibodies, and antineoplastons are peptides that are the components of this parallel immune system in the body.

SS: So antineoplastons kill malignant cells or eliminate malignant cells and don't harm normal cells. How do you test? I mean, if a patient has cancer, how do you know if your antineoplastons will be effective?

SB: Well, we used to test for the levels of antineoplastons in the blood. Then we found that all cancer patients are highly deficient in antineoplastons, so we abandoned this test and opted to devote our time and money on more efficient tests. Now we test for genetic compatibility. We know that antineoplastons work on human genes, and people and cancers differ genetically. So genetic compatibility helps us determine which genes antineoplastons work on and which genes they don't.

SS: You mean which genes turn on the cancer and which genes turn off the cancer?

SB: Yes, the antineoplastons that we use now work on close to one hundred different genes, which cover a broad spectrum of cancers. This means they help numerous patients. For example, there are currently twenty-four FDA-approved gene-targeted drugs, and most of them work on a single gene. That is why these drugs have very little chance to really cure patients, because in the average cancer you have typically more than two thousand genes which are involved. So how can you really bring this under control if you work on a single gene? One of the bestselling cancer drugs, Avastin, works on a single gene, so really it has very little chance to bring the process under complete control, but it can decrease tumors.

SS: Well, that's when everyone gets excited because "the tumor has shrunk," but that doesn't mean "cure," and it most often comes back, and when it does it ravages the body.

SB: Right, shrinking a tumor is temporary. Antineoplastons work on about one hundred different genes, not just one single gene, which means that patients have a very good chance to be helped, but unfortunately not everybody. It depends on which combination of genes each patient has.

SS: So you know the genes your antineoplastons work on, and is that how you select patients?

SB: Yes, we select the patients who have the best chance to respond to our treatment based on genetic analysis. Also, from our research with numerous other patients we can determine who the best candidates for antineoplastons will be.

SS: If you encounter a patient with a different type of cancer, one in which you have not had good results with antineoplastons, what do you do?

SB: We treat them a different way. We treat them with a personalized cancer treatment using combinations of gene-targeted medications.

SS: What about Ashkenazi Jews? Many of them carry the BRCA gene [BRCA1 or BRCA2].

SB: They don't have a treatment for this gene in traditional medicine, but antineoplastons [ANP] may work on such patients because BRCA may be one of the genes which can be affected with ANP.

SS: What about breast cancer?

SB: At the moment we use a different approach. We study which genes in individual patients are abnormal, trying to determine the genetic signature of cancer in these patients. With our methods, we can have answers for the patient in about three days based on blood tests. Once we identify the most important oncogenes involved in cancer for that individual, we select a group of four to six medications from those twenty-four which are now approved by the FDA, and use them to hit those genes which are causing the cancer to progress. This is like "boutique treatment" because for every patient we design a treatment plan. When we do this we have a very good chance to have positive results in most patients.

SS: How many respond?

SB: About 85 percent for whom we have the proper gene signature; about 15 percent do not respond. In our responders many of them have tumors which disappear completely and in others the tumors remain small. The problem is finding the genetic signature because for many of these different genetic signatures we don't have the blood tests . . . yet.

SS: I like the "yet" part.

SB: We learn something new every day. We have a modern clinic and a workforce that includes more than two dozen people who have doctoral degrees. At present we also use a broad spectrum approach, using medications which work on numerous genes and the patients may respond. With antineoplastons, we have a broad spectrum of activity which work on close to one hundred genes, so we select patients often with the worst types of cancers, like brain tumors, and treat them with antineoplastons. And for others we use a combination of gene-targeted therapy, plus one member of the antineoplaston family which is given orally.

> For the majority of Dr. Burzynski's patients he does not use any chemotherapy, but for some patients the chemotherapy is used in lower dosages, which are below the threshold of significant side effects. Dr. Burzynski takes advantage of the synergistic effect of such combinations that have at least three advantages:
> 1. Quick reduction of the tumor bulk
> 2. A small chance of significant side effects
> 3. Reduced cost due to the fact that he uses substantially lower dosages of medicines

SS: When you talk about gene-targeted therapy, is that chemotherapy?

SB: No, this is not chemotherapy. Most of my patients have already had chemotherapy and it has not been effective for them. The beauty of antineoplastons is that they are natural compounds. They exist in our blood and form a protective system against cancer. You don't expect to have toxic side effects from chemicals which are normal in your blood. And they cover a broad spectrum of genes, which means from the very beginning we have a much better chance to help this patient.

We use this on children who have the most common type of brain tumor, which is called astrocytoma, and around 93 percent to 95 percent respond favorably to the treatment. Of course, other malignancies might not have such good results because we don't have sufficient activity against such malignancies. This requires different antineoplastons, and we know they exist, but obviously we can't do everything at once.

SS: But you'll get there, and that is the important thing. I admire the work you are doing and your dedication, and I guess I'm supposed to say that at the end of this interview, but I am compelled to say it right now.

But let me make this simple. If I am missing, in my blood and urine, these antineoplastons, these peptides, is this an indicator that I most likely have cancer? And if that is so, then why wouldn't we test everyone for antineoplastons?

SB: Well, that's a possibility. One obstacle is that the tests are quite cumbersome. We are developing an instrument that can give you proper answers very quickly. This instrument will tell us what we want to know.

SS: What are you trying to know?

SB: We want to know which genes are silent, and silent means which genes are switched off, because these are the genes that protect us against cancer. From a single drop of blood we will be able to find out which genes are switched off. Maybe this individual has twenty tumor suppressor genes which are not active, and this would mean that this person is highly vulnerable to developing cancer or perhaps he has cancer already.

SS: What causes genes to be switched off?

SB: Just by getting older many genes switch off. They become silent and these are the genes that used to protect you from cancer but now they are off. Once silent they don't protect. We are also working on a chip which we would insert into the instrument to screen for Alzheimer's and so on, in fact, any changes leading to disease. We want to find out genetic signals in patients who have cancer and select the proper treatment. In the future, we will find out the signature of the genes which are silent and then use proper prevention.

SS: What is prevention by your standards?

SB: Prevention could simply mean use the right supplements to activate the genes which are silent and then turn the switch on. In other words, activate the genes that protect you from cancer.

SS: Sounds so simple, but I know it's not. What are the supplements?

SB: There are numerous supplements. We sell Aminocare supplements, which work on a large number of genes. Among others, the chemicals in green tea are also molecular switches which can activate some of the genes and can switch off oncogenes. These are natural ingredients which work on the genes as molecular switches.

Of course, when you have advanced cancer these supplements do not contribute very much. But at the beginning of the cancer process, using supplements and diet modification can help a great deal.

For instance, curcumin [turmeric] is a very good example. This natural substance works on some genes but not on others. If you can identify the genes that are involved, then logically you can regulate the activity of these genes and recheck again in about two months to see if the job was accomplished.

SS: I have written a lot about the benefits of turmeric. It is an amazing spice and it makes food taste wonderful, and it costs about a dollar. I use it in so many dishes. Nature has provided all these wonderful health benefits, but most Americans prefer a diet of chemicals. Sometimes, when I look at the cancer rates that are now out of control, I think, Well, what did we expect? We were never meant to ingest all these toxins. But I digress.

It seems to me that if we were able to test for these peptides and amino acids, and if we found ourselves deficient, that from a preventive standpoint we could change our diets, take nutrition seriously, and replace amino acids. Is it that simple?

SB: When dealing with patients with cancer, diet and supplements are extremely important because such people don't have much time to lose from a nutritional point of view. With horrible cancers such as pancreatic or liver cancer, if you use the right regimen, if you select the right combination—and I'm not talking about chemotherapy; I'm talking about genetic medicine—we see tumors decreasing or disappearing even within two months. But very few doctors are doing this because they are concerned that if they use a combination of three or four medications, they may have side effects, and most of the doctors don't really know how these medicines work. You need to have profound knowledge in the genomics of cancer and profound knowledge of these various medicines to make sure that the combination which you use will first of all not cause some adverse reactions and that the medicines will support rather than fight each other.

SS: And you have this profound knowledge?

SB: Well, this is my life's work. But we don't know everything.

SS: I find the present template of treating cancer barbaric. Because of the books I write, I get calls from people with cancer who have been through chemotherapy and radiation and now want to try alternatives. If a patient comes to you who has been ravaged by chemotherapy and radiation, does that make your job harder or is it hopeless?

SB: The majority of patients whom we see come to us after being told that there is nothing that can be done for them. These poor people have tried everything and we hear horror stories, where half the body is amputated by a surgeon and the cancer is still progressing throughout the body. For such people it is a very special art to treat them because you not only have to treat the cancer but also address the problems from the prior treatment. This makes the task extremely difficult. But that is our typical patient. What we try to do first is predetermine if the patient is a good candidate. Sometimes after we run our testing we find out that we cannot help. It's not going to work. But other times after the results come back we say we think we can help. What we do know is to do things as quickly as possible. These people don't have time to wait. Then we start treatment, which is a combination of gene-targeted therapies. We usually don't see adverse reactions because by proper combinations we can substantially reduce the dosages of the medicines five, sometimes ten, times lower. This can be accomplished because we use medicines which increase the activity of each other and it helps balance their side effects.

SS: Are these medicines intravenous or are they in tablet form?

SB: By giving a tablet daily and a tablet every other day we don't get the side effects. It is also substantially less expensive than if we used heavy dosages of all the medicines. We use a combination because it is easier for the patient.

SS: How long does the patient stay in Houston near your clinic?

SB: Usually a couple of weeks until he or she gets strong. We usually get answers about a patient's response within one or two months. If we find the tumors are decreasing, which happens to most of the patients, we continue the treatment until the tumors are gone.

SS: Are you saying *gone*? As in the tumors haven't shrunk, they are gone?

SB: Yes. The average time for tumors to be eliminated is three to four months. Then we switch the patient to maintenance treatment, which continues for about eight months to a year, and that's about all. Of course we follow up with the patient to make sure the cancer has not come back.

SS: I have to ask again: You are saying the cancer doesn't just shrink, it goes away?

SB: Yes, in many cases the tumors go away completely. That is, the tumor has completely disappeared. The average time for this phenomenon is about three months.

SS: How many patients would you say have had a complete response?

SB: Well, it depends on the type of cancer. For instance, for certain types of brain tumors we have had a 50 to 60 percent response. This is very high. If you are talking about other cancers, it varies.

An objective response means a complete disappearance of the tumor or substantial decrease of the tumor size.

SS: You told me earlier that 58 percent of breast cancer patients are showing substantial decreases in the size of the tumors or a disappearance of the tumor?

SB: Yes. If the disappearance of the tumor lasts more than five years, it is called a cure. This is the definition of a cure. Now, with pancreatic cancer, we don't do so well. We see less objective response, probably around 50 percent, which is still better than traditional treatment. But this is a very difficult cancer to treat.

SS: What about melanoma?

SB: With melanoma we see somewhere around 30 percent objective response, which means substantial decrease of tumor size. If we see that tumors are growing, we try to change our treatment plan. We run our gene test again, find out what is going on, maybe remove some of the medicines and add some others, and again try for another month and see what happens.

SS: Now if a patient came to you with, let's say, pancreatic cancer but had not had chemotherapy or radiation or any traditional treatment, should you expect a good response?

SB: Definitely. We have such patients and in about three weeks we will be presenting a series of such cases at a large congress in Paris. This is a conference organized by M. D. Anderson Cancer Center and the French government, and we will be showing patients who had pancreatic cancer and liver cancer who responded. These are horrible types of cancer where mortality rates are usually 100 percent. Amazingly, we have patients whose tumors have disappeared in two months—completely—with both pancreatic cancer and advanced liver cancer.

SS: Do you find Europeans are open to new treatment other than chemotherapy? In this country we don't seem to want to know about anything other than chemotherapy.

SB: I must say, for pancreatic cancer, chemotherapy is doing practically nothing. Patients have horrible side effects, and in the best-case scenario it can extend life for one month!

SS: It is clear to me, having buried two friends last month with pancreatic cancer whose bodies were ravaged and degraded to looking like Holocaust survivors, that it most certainly doesn't work. But it boggles the mind. Why are doctors still prescribing it?

SB: They are brainwashed. They have been successfully brainwashed in medical schools and their residency programs. Doctors in residency work tremendously long hours. My son is in a medical school residency program and he works like hell. By the time they come out of medical school, they just use whatever they have learned, which are old treatments. They just use chemotherapy. It is very well known that chemotherapy will do very little or nothing for pancreatic cancer.

SS: What if a patient came to you with stage IV pancreatic cancer who doesn't want chemotherapy because they know it is not going to do them any good? What can you do for them?

SB: We treat them and even if they have tumors in different areas, they may be gone in two to three months.

SS: What about liver cancer?

SB: We now know that chemotherapy will speed up the progress of liver cancer! There is no reason to use it. Scientific works have proven beyond any doubt that chemo is completely ineffective, yet doctors are using chemotherapy for liver cancer over and over again. Practically all patients with advanced liver cancer will die. But with our treatment these liver tumors have disappeared in a matter of a couple of months, if you use the right combination of targeted therapy.

SS: If you are able to prescribe the right selection of medicines, these terminal patients have a chance even with horrible cancers like pancreatic, brain, or liver cancer? I mean this is pretty remarkable.

SB: Yes, but you have to know there are no miracles. Just because a cancer doesn't respond to chemotherapy doesn't mean it's going to respond to the treatment which works on the gene. You have to find the right switch and then everything comes into place. What we need to do is get rid of the cancer stem cells. If we do that, the patient is cured. That's the route to success.

SS: And getting rid of the cancerous stem cells by using proper medicines like antineoplastons will work on the genes that get rid of cancer?

SB: Yes.

SS: You mentioned the other day when we were speaking that liver cancer would be the next epidemic. Why is that?

SB: Right now, lung cancer is the main killer cancer. Last year there were about 1.3 million deaths worldwide from lung cancer, but about 600,000 deaths from liver cancer. This year we are expecting about 700,000 deaths from liver cancer. The main cause of liver cancer is hepatitis B. The virus of hepatitis B was discovered about thirty-six years ago. Right now it is estimated that about 2 billion people, about one-third of humanity, is infected with the hepatitis B virus. Now, most of these people live in underdeveloped countries, and out of these people, half a million will develop chronic disease. Right now in China, about 400 million people have chronic hepatitis.

SS: Where is it coming from? What are we doing wrong?

SB: The hepatitis B virus particle is one of the smallest of viruses and when it enters the body it embeds into the DNA and becomes like a gene in the body which may lie dormant for a long period of time.

In some patients the hepatitis virus is able to silence the genes which protect them against cancer. This virus can switch off as many as 150 genes that are protective. This is a huge number of genes. In the current population of people who are infected with chronic hepatitis B, 10 percent of them—50 million people—will develop liver cancer. That is a scientific estimate and there is very little we can do about it. The mortality of liver cancer is about 97 percent, which means you will see in the near future a huge segment of the population dying of liver cancer, the majority of them in Southeast Asian countries.

SS: Roll back for me a little bit. Where are we getting the hepatitis B?

SB: Infections. For instance, like HIV infection, it can be transmitted through sex, from mother to child, or simply from contaminated needles and blood products. Hepatitis B is more resistant than HIV. It can survive for a week in a drop of blood, whereas HIV will die very quickly.

So this means, for instance, if a woman goes for a manicure and pedicure and the tools used were not properly sanitized [sterilized], and a customer ahead of her had a hepatitis B infection, then she could get it through her manicure or pedicure.

A large segment of European women have contracted hepatitis B in this way.

Liver cancer can also be contracted by ingesting food contaminated with aflatoxins.

SS: What are aflatoxins?

SB: Aflatoxins are chemical toxins produced by fungi which like to grow on foods such as rice, peanuts, barley, and some meats. Aflatoxins can also be found in beer and water. They enter the liver and block a very important tumor-suppressor gene, p53. Many patients who have ingested aflatoxins will develop liver cancer. Worldwide, this is estimated to be about 10 million people.

SS: Is there any way to prevent this? Prevent hepatitis B?

SB: Well, the simplest prevention is through vaccination. When vaccination was introduced in countries like Taiwan it resulted in substantial protection of the population. Our institute studied animals that were given aflatoxins and later developed liver cancer. Another group of animals were given aflatoxins plus one of the supplements which we introduced, and they proved to be resistant to preventing liver cancer by using the proper supplements. Now, if liver cancer develops, it can be treated, but not with chemotherapy, which we know doesn't work.

SS: So regarding hepatitis B, if we are fanatical about cleanliness, if we make sure when we have manicures and pedicures that the tools are properly sanitized, if we are conscious of washing our hands, and if we are all automatically vaccinated for hepatitis at childbirth, we can be protected?

SB: Certainly what you describe can help a great deal, and using some precautions can give you good protection. Now we have mandatory vaccinations for hepatitis B for children. Our dilemma is what do we do for the millions of people who already have hepatitis and are slowly developing cancer? The big problem is they need treatment which can be easily administered.

SS: And you are having success with treating liver cancer with supplements, with targeted gene therapy? It sounds too good to be true. We are accustomed to cancer treatment being torturous.

SB: We are achieving success, but we have only treated seven patients. In this country we don't yet have a large number of patients suffering from liver cancer, but the numbers are increasing very rapidly. This year about twenty thousand deaths from liver cancer are expected, and in five years or so this may increase to fifty thousand people per year.

In another eight to ten years it will become the second killer after lung cancer. At our clinic we have treated seven patients, and two of them obtained responses very rapidly and they continue to do well. Three out of the seven did not respond. We are watching the other two. It's a very difficult cancer.

SS: What do you tell your patients who are now achieving success through your treatment about prevention and preventing cancer recurrences?

SB: This is a very important part of our program. These patients have to take it seriously. First we need to get the cancer under control. Every patient has a dietary consultation, and every patient has a consultation regarding supplements—not only the supplements we want them to take but also about other supplements they are already taking, because some supplements may work against them. Some supplements can promote cancer. We can help them design what is best for their situation. We also talk with the family because most patients come with the entire family, and we give family consultations twice a week. We talk to them about the treatment itself and the proper use of the supplements.

SS: And how long does the patient stay on this regimen?

SB: The average patient takes treatment for about a year to a year and a half. Then obviously there is need for continued surveillance and the use of proper supplements, proper diet, proper lifestyle to make sure they don't develop cancer again.

SS: Where is the weak spot? Or is there a weak spot?

SB: If the patient has had chemotherapy, they are at risk to develop another form of cancer, so following the regimen is very important.

SS: As someone who once had cancer, I'd like to know: What supplements should people take to prevent cancer or a recurrence?

SB: The basic supplements that will keep your genome in pristine shape.

SS: That is out of my realm of comprehension. I don't understand the genome and its needs.

SB: The genome consists of about twenty-two thousand genes, and these genes are like books in a library. We use about 10 percent of our genes when we are young. The rest of the genes which were important for developing organs are placed, so to speak, in the "body library." By the time we reach the age of twenty-five our bodies operate on 10 percent of our genome and the rest of the genes become silent, as though these pieces of DNA are covered with plastic shields, covering books—genes— which have never been read.

SS: I'm following you.

SB: When you age, you silence additional numbers of genes. When women go through menopause another number of genes are silenced, again like we put a piece of plastic over the genes and put them back on the library shelf. These genes are no longer active. For example, when people lose hair, they are getting bald because the genes that are necessary to replace the hair are silent. Ultimately you silence the genes which are there to protect you against cancer.

SS: Oh, so that is why aging is part of why we get cancer. Those genes are silenced.

SB: Yes. Like in liver cancer. There are about 150 genes that have been silenced which would have protected you against cancer.

SS: So back to my original question. How do we prevent cancer or a cancer recurrence?

SB: What you need to do is to keep the genes which are vitally important for you, like the genes protecting against cancer, turned on, and you accomplish this with supplements.

SS: So supplements will prevent silencing the genes in the body. We want to keep these genes turned on. Now, are you talking supplements that we take only if we have cancer? And can these supplements that you design and individualize for each person turn the switches back on?

SB: Right. This is for someone with cancer. We use antineoplastons to accomplish the task. We get rid of the cancer stem cells, which are leading to cancer. We activate the genes that protect you against deadly diseases.

SS: Let's get to the nitty-gritty. What supplements?

SB: Okay, for example, curcumin and genistein may play a role for some people, and also products which are the active ingredients of green tea. There are numerous natural products which can do the task, and once you know what genes are silent you can design the program to make sure to keep these genes in good shape.

SS: Can a healthy person keep their genes in good shape?

SB: By using natural products to prevent this silencing—for instance, taking curcumin supplements or cooking with turmeric and genistein, which is a substance available in soy.

We're doing everything wrong. We are silencing genes through various mechanisms. One of them is the wrong diet. Chemicals and stress play a big role, as well as lack of proper sleep, imbalance of the body clock—activity during the night and sleep during the day—all will silence genes in the body. And then there are viruses, carcinogens, and pollution. All these factors are leading to silencing the genes which protect against cancer. And when a gene is silenced for a long period of time—and I'm talking about tumor suppressor genes—this leads to mutations, which are more permanent changes, and then cancer will progress further. These factors are created by us.

SS: The average American diet consists of processed foods, foods in bags and boxes, foods with unpronounceable chemicals in them, diet soda, fast foods, fake food . . . is that what you are talking about?

SB: Certainly. Coke can silence a good number of genes, as can being on an unhealthy diet. Cigarette smoking can silence genes, and lack of exercise. Most of these things are quite well known to people, and finally they lead to gene silencing. You will speed up gene silencing if you continue to do the wrong things.

As I told you earlier, we've introduced a line of supplements called

Aminocare that work on the mechanisms which are involved in the silencing of the genes in aging. We already have tests that prove we can extend the life of animals with these supplements by influencing the activity of the genes. These chemicals already exist in our bodies, in dairy products, and they also exist in royal jelly—which is the food fed to the queen honeybee. The queen honeybee lives sixty times longer than the worker bees because she is eating royal jelly every day. We isolated what was in the royal jelly which extends the life of animals, and we put these ingredients, as well as others, in our supplements.

SS: How important is hormone balance relative to cancer?

SB: It's very important. Hormones are also genetic switches. Hormones work because they regulate the activity of the genes. For instance, estrogens work because they activate certain genes and silence others.

> *If you don't have the right hormonal balance, then you will speed up cancer development.*

You need to regulate hormonal balance if you want to control cancer. Antineoplastons are similar to hormones, as both are genetic switches. Some of them are peptides. Hormones are carried by blood, and they enter the cells and regulate gene expression.

SS: I can't tell you how happy I am to hear you say this because I have been saying this in my books for some time. Hormonal balance is cancer protective.

SB: That's a very important message. Most doctors don't know what molecular mechanisms are or how they work. Inside the cell most of these hormones go into the nucleus and will work as molecular switches. They will activate some genes and silence others. Antineoplastons work in a similar fashion except that the molecular mechanism can be somewhat different depending on which hormone you are talking about.

SS: It seems to me as men decline in testosterone their PSA numbers go up. From a layperson's perspective it seems that putting back the missing testosterone to optimal ranges would be protective, and I have had this confirmed by many doctors.

SB: Right. But it's not the testosterone itself, but a derivative of the testosterone, DHT. You see, testosterone is metabolized in the body and it creates a much more active chemical which is causing prostate cancer. Until recently it was believed that testosterone was causing the rapid progression of prostate cancer, but a publication just last week proved the value of testosterone for patients who have prostate cancer.

SS: This must be the Abraham Morgentaler report. I read that. I think this is great news for men. For so long men have been deprived of testosterone because of an unproven fear that it causes prostate cancer.

SB: Yes, it's the derivative, the chemical which is created from testosterone, that is stimulating prostate cancer. Certainly too much testosterone will cause progression of cancer, not directly, but after it is transformed into another chemical inside the body.

SS: So do you, Dr. Burzynski, have the cure to cancer?

SB: Well, we certainly have a number of patients who are cured from cancer. If we have patients, for instance, who are twenty or thirty years free of advanced cancer, I would say these patients are cured. We have a number of such patients, so we can cure cancer . . . but not in everybody because cancer is not a single disease. Cancer is like a combination of numerous different types of illnesses, and each of these different types of cancer has numerous genetic signatures, so one cancer patient is not the same as the other.

It's difficult to say I have the cure for cancer, but I have cured some patients with cancer. In fact, a good number of them. Sadly, there will always be some cases for which I do not have the answer . . . yet. But we are always learning, and one day . . .

SS: You must feel fulfilled and satisfied with the great work you are doing.

SB: There's no doubt about it. It's a great feeling to see these people in good shape, leading normal lives. Among our patients are those who came to us as children, around twelve or so, and we got rid of their cancer. Now they have children of their own. Because of the way we treat cancer, our patients have had no problem with fertility and we don't see any problems in the children. That's very good news. They are living fully active, normal lives. That is a great feeling.

SS: I am sure it is. Thank you so much. As I said in the beginning, this has been an honor.

DR. BURZYNSKI'S PATIENTS
IN THEIR OWN WORDS

I was diagnosed in 1989 with low-grade non-Hodgkin's lymphoma. Low-grade is almost always incurable with conventional treatment. Before being diagnosed I was sick for over a year. I was having horrible stomachaches. I went to the emergency room three times, and the third time I said to my husband, "I'm going to die," because I had diarrhea so bad and for so long and I was throwing up and had lost ten pounds. I just knew something was terribly wrong, but they kept treating me for an ulcer. Finally a doctor suggested I get a CAT scan while I was in pain, and that is when they found the tumor.

They hadn't seen it with a CAT scan previously because I had a condition where my intestine folds over itself and only during pain was it visible. I had been to so many doctors and everyone had been telling me it was all in my mind or it was my diet. But now I had a fatal cancer.

They said I might live for three, maybe five, years with chemotherapy and radiation. My doctor at UCLA suggested I go to Boston for a bone marrow transplant. When my husband and I did the research, we found that one out of ten people die of this transplant treatment. I was forty years old. I had three young children, teenagers. Reluctantly I went to Boston. The specialist doing bone marrow transplants was quite interested in speaking with me because I had not done chemo or radiation yet, and they wanted to try this treatment on people who were clean, so to speak . . . and I had stage IV cancer, so I was an interesting study.

Boston depressed me. We went to the Cheers bar and I was trying to have a nice time with my husband, but the realities of what we were about to undertake were overwhelming. I didn't want to die, and I didn't want to miss raising my children, so this was what I had to do.

In our research we had read about Dr. Burzynski, and two days before I was to do the bone marrow treatment, I suddenly changed my mind and said to my husband, "Let's leave Boston and go to see this Dr. Burzynski . . ." which, I must say was the best decision of my life.

Dr. Burzynski's treatment was nontoxic, and I figured that I could always do the bone marrow treatment later if this didn't work.

As soon as I walked into Dr. Burzynski's clinic, I knew I was in the right place. It was just such a warm, caring environment; and it was then I felt there was hope, true hope. He was using only antineoplastons then, and I was offered the pump or capsules and I chose capsules. I felt it would be a lot easier. Having a catheter in my chest scared me a little.

I was on the capsules for three months when I started to notice that the tumor on my neck, that I could see, was actually getting bigger. I called Dr. Burzynski, panicked, and he said, "This means one of two things: either the cancer is indeed growing, or the cancer cells are dying and sometimes when they die it causes the tumor to get a little bigger."

All along the way Dr. Burzynski was available to explain things to me, and he was such a blessing. I flew back to Houston and this time he implanted a catheter in my chest and I am telling you—this is the amazing part—in three weeks, with the medicine going directly into my bloodstream, the tumor on the side of my neck disappeared in one night. I had been on it for three weeks, but in just one night it disappeared.

I showed my husband and we both screamed. I couldn't believe it. The next day we called Dr. Burzynski and he said I would still be on the treatment for another nine months before they could absolutely pronounce me in remission.

My doctor at UCLA was not supportive of Dr. Burzynski and called him a charlatan and a fraud, and that he only wanted to take my money, but I didn't care. I kept going for my treatments.

Nine months later I was pronounced in remission by UCLA! Right, UCLA! I stayed on the antineoplastons for another three months; I was just afraid to go off. I would still be on the capsules if I could.

All of this was without side effects. My hair didn't fall out, I wasn't sick, and while I was on Dr. Burzynski's treatments I led a totally normal life— I carpooled, cleaned my house, I could do whatever I wanted. I even went waterskiing!

When they indicted Dr. Burzynski and wanted to put him in jail, I was incensed. My husband took off work for about two months and we went to Houston during the trial. We marched every day with all the other cured patients. We had the radio station come down; the construction workers marched. And after the acquittal, we had this party with some of the jurors, and several of them said that we cancer patients looked better than they did.

I had been fighting, literally, for my life, as were so many of the others. I was in the middle of my treatment, and if they had put Dr. Burzynski under, I would have gone under too if I couldn't get his medicine.

I've thought a lot about why they did this to him, and it's because they were afraid of him. He is the discoverer, and he's a great man, and in time I believe he will be known as the greatest scientist of our time.

I have been cancer free now for seventeen wonderful years.

Dr. Burzynski means everything to me. There was a time in my life when I didn't think I would see my children graduate from high school. Now I've seen them all graduate from college and I'm a grandma. I am so happy every day that I get up and thank God, and I thank Dr. Burzynski. He is in my heart every day, and I talk to people on the phone each day who are sick and I try to make the connection with them to try Dr. Burzynski's treatment.

The other day a friend called me and told me his cousin had a brain tumor, and I said, "You know, don't be devastated by this. Just tell him to go to Dr. Burzynski."

—Mary Jo Siegel, non-Hodgkin's lymphoma, cancer free for seventeen years

I don't feel that my daughter, Sophia, would have lived if I hadn't found Dr. Burzynski. She had a deadly childhood brain tumor called pineoblastoma at ten and a half months of age. She was offered "standard of care" chemotherapy and radiation, but I looked at my little baby and couldn't put her through that. It was a terrible time in our lives.

It was my husband who heard about Dr. Burzynski, but I didn't want to go. I had been warned about him, that he was a quack and a charlatan. But my husband insisted, and it was against my instincts. Then I met Dr. Burzynski and he made a believer out of me. He said to me, "You have a very sick child. I can try to help her, but I can't promise anything, because this type of tumor pretty much has a zero survival rate."

She had an infection in her brain as a result of the surgery in our hometown, and at the time we weren't even aware of that. The doctors in our hometown just kind of kept pushing her off, as in if we weren't going to pursue orthodox treatment, they didn't see any reason to check her out. It was a raging infection that very well could have killed her. So when we got to Dr. Burzynski's clinic we had to spend three weeks in the children's hospital to clear the infection before we could deal with her cancer.

Dr. Burzynski told us the tumor was killing her fast. We felt so helpless. The fluid in her ventricles was backed up from the infection, and the doctors in my hometown scoffed at the idea of going to Dr. Burzynski.

But we decided to use Dr. Burzynski's protocol in spite of the cynicism of our doctors. He put an IV port in my little baby and she was on the treatment for several years. We had to get real creative because as Sophia became a toddler it became more difficult to keep the port attached. She was a baby and wanted to pull it out. But she handled it well.

You know, when it's a matter of life or death you figure it out. She had to stay on the antineoplastons longer than most people because she was so little and they couldn't give her huge doses of it. They just raised the amounts slowly and safely as she grew.

Today she is thirteen years old and living a normal life. It is a huge milestone. Every time I look at her, I have flashbacks. I wish so much I had kept a journal of all those dark and terrible times. I'll never forget it. But as

I look back and try to think of details I just realize how lucky we were to find this treatment.

She understands today how lucky she is, and that her life was saved. In fact she was asked to do a research paper at school this year on somebody she really admires or respects or is a hero; of course, she did it on Dr. B. It's a heartbreaker.

We get calls from all over the world about Dr. Burzynski, and I always recommend they go and just have a consultation at least. It takes a big leap of faith to go this way, but then I look at Sophia and realize it was her only hope, and now she is alive and normal and happy and growing normally. I made the right choice. Dr. Burzynski saved her life, and somebody led us there, I know it, and it worked out. Dr. Burzynski is a wonderful man and a great healer. They treat Sophia like their little princess. Our job as parents is to protect our children and keep them safe. I am thankful every day that we made the right choice.

—Jenny Gettino, mother of Sophia Gettino, who had a brain tumor
at ten and a half months of age; Sophia has been cancer free for
thirteen years

When I was ten and a half months old I was diagnosed with a rare disease called a cancerous brain tumor. My parents were very scared. My friends and family were very optimistic. It was not very easy for them. I give them a lot of credit.

What optimism means to me is to expect the best possible outcome.

What being optimistic means to me is for people to stay positive. Everyone should stay optimistic all the time. If you don't stay optimistic all the time, you will be negative, and you should never be negative.

When I was a baby, not only me, but everyone around me had to be very optimistic. Friends of mine had to be very optimistic for the same reasons. Those reasons were for me to get better and be my old self again and eventually I did. I can tell you pretty much anything you want to know about my disease. I am so lucky to be alive, and it is all thanks to my doctor. That amazing gentleman is Dr. Burzynski. He is the best doctor in the world. I love him. I wish I could see him more often, but he lives all the way in Houston, Texas. I am very happy to be alive.

When Dr. Burzynski received the call to action that he was getting a new patient, he was very happy to help. So he got to work right away researching what type of disease I had, and he found out I had cancer. Then he was trying to figure out what type of cancer I had. Then he finally told my parents the dreadful news. "Your daughter has pineoblastoma." Then he prescribed one of his many treatments for me and it worked fabulously. Before I went to Dr. B. the hospital wanted to do chemo and radiation on me. But thankfully they didn't, because I was too young for that stuff. Also, I had friends that did different treatments before they came to Dr. B.'s office, but unfortunately it was too late for them and they didn't make it. But I have my own special ways of remembering them. Some of those ways are praying and wearing things like jewelry to remember them. Sometimes my family and I go to visit their families. My parents and friends believed that I could be cured and I was. I have exceptional memory when it comes to stuff like that. I am happy, healthy, and cured. I have awesome friends and making more.

Everyone can get through the bad times if they stay very optimistic. If you have a disease or if you know someone who is sick, stay very optimistic. Talk to people and encourage them that everything will be all right. If you make it look like you are happy, it makes them happier.

If you keep a positive attitude you will be much better off. You will get through life much easier. Always stay optimistic. For me optimism is to expect the best possible outcome. That is how optimism helped defeat my disease.

—Sophia Gettino, thirteen years old, cancer survivor, from her entry in the Optimist Speech Contest

When Dustin was diagnosed with medulloblastoma, a highly aggressive form of brain cancer, it was a terrible time for our family. He was just a baby and they wanted to put him on chemo and then radiation, which would have caused mental retardation and was not recommended for his age but would have to be done if chemotherapy failed. The chemo he was offered was an experimental type that a computer would randomly pick, and among the risks were hearing loss, stunted growth, learning disabilities, bladder and kidney damage, sterility, and leukemia. There was a 20 to 40 percent chance the treatment would work. Neither of these treatments offered any hope at all, so we started looking for alternatives, and that's when we found Dr. Burzynski. We had a calling list from the Cancer Control Society in California and one of the names on the list was Dr. Burzynski. They told us about a child who had been in treatment with a brain tumor and the child had done well. Then we talked to other patients and were impressed, so we decided to look into it, and the outcome seemed to be so much better than any other alternatives.

When we met with Dr. Burzynski his optimism and his treatment made a lot of sense, so we decided to take a chance with him. He said there was a *very good chance that Dustin would respond to his treatment initially, and at that time we hadn't even been thinking long-term; we just wanted him to live a couple more years or maybe five years. Even that would have made us happy.*

In April of 1994, we took Dustin to Houston, Texas, to the Burzynski Clinic. Dustin was too young to be a part of Dr. Burzynski's study, but in response to our pleas, Dr. Burzynski agreed to treat him. Dustin was equipped with an IV pump that he carried around in a backpack so he could receive antineoplastons intravenously. We were taught how to program the pump for specific treatment times and dosages. We learned sterile techniques in case the IV tubing got pulled out or damaged, and we learned how to deal with emergencies.

Dr. Burzynski told us that he would stop treatment if there were no positive results on his first MRI, but to our great joy, the six-week MRI showed no evidence of a tumor. Every three months we made the trip to Houston for Dustin's checkup and to get more medication. After one year on antineoplaston therapy a tumor once again was seen on a follow-up MRI, showing the aggressiveness of medulloblastomas. It was heartbreaking. So they increased his dosage and he continued to have periodic lab tests and MRIs done. Eventually that tumor disappeared.

Today he is well. He's a normal teenager. He's got a certified nursing assistant license and is working as a certified nurse, while he is going to college to become a registered nurse.

He is very aware more and more as he gets older that he had a second chance at life. This year he thanked us for all we had done for him, and he realizes that it was a big thing he went through, and he is also very grateful to Dr. Burzynski.

I believe he's cured. Definitely. He has outlived the original prognosis by years and years.

I think Dr. Burzynski is the greatest doctor in the world. He's very brilliant, and as far as I am concerned he's a genius. He's also a very caring person, and he doesn't want to do harm to anybody; he just wants to help. I think he's a great man. He saved my son's life and we couldn't have asked for anything better.

I tell people who call for information on Dr. Burzynski, what is it going to hurt? The treatments are very safe, there are no harsh side effects, and it's not going to hurt you. We really feel that God led us to Dr. Burzynski in the first place . . . right from the start.

      —MaryAnn Kunnari, mother of Dustin, who had medulloblastoma, a highly aggressive form of brain cancer, at the age of two and a half; now cancer free for fifteen years

*I'm fifty-eight years old and today I am healthy, but I have had breast cancer
five times. It started in 1993. I was forty-three years old when I found a
lump. After an excisional biopsy, they determined it to be breast cancer. My
treatment was thirty-one rounds of radiation. Then in November of 1995
I found another little lump around my bra line, and that also turned out to
be breast cancer, but very small. It was in the same breast, about an inch
away. If you had to have breast cancer, it was a darned good scenario.*

*In 1995, I opted to get a mastectomy with immediate reconstruction
because I just didn't want to deal with this anymore. Since I already had
implants I knew what to expect and felt it would look pretty much the same.
But in December, my breast started popping open and fluid started to leak
out, so it would have to be drained. It did that for quite a while, so the plastic
surgeon stitched it up, but it kept popping open again. Shortly after that I had
a mammogram and they found carcinoma in situ [DCIS] on the other
breast, so I had surgery and immediate reconstruction in that breast, and
then I started having this same problem with this implant. My body just
doesn't like foreign objects. Once again, six months later I had an MRI and
they found a little uptake in the sternum area, which turned out to be
another small breast cancer, the same type I had before, that probably
stemmed from an internal mammary lymph node pressing onto the sternum.
So I had more radiation. In June of 2003, I started getting my tumor marker
numbers checked, and in November of '04 my numbers went up a little bit.
Normal is from 0 to 32 and mine was at 34. Then in February it went up to
37. I talked to my doctor and I was pretty freaked out. They started talking
chemo. And I thought, No—this time I'm doing it a different way.*

*I read about Dr. Burzynski in Dr. Julian Whitaker's newsletter, so my
husband and I decided to go to Houston to meet with him. I had a CAT scan
and another MRI on my brain, and thank God the brain was fine. But they
found a little tumor in the bone in my left shoulder area. I had had some
pain in that shoulder, but I figured it was like a rotator cuff injury because
I exercise a lot.*

*Dr. Burzynski put me on sodium phenylbutyrate and antineoplastons.
I started with thirty-six pills a day. He took my tumor markers and also
started me on Xeloda, which is an oral chemotherapy with very few side
effects. It allows you to have a better quality of life while the medicine is
doing its work.*

*Now my tumor markers are in the normal ranges. I feel fine and healthy. I
continue on Dr. Burzynski's medicines because I'm too chicken to stop them. I
feel like they are really helping me, and I don't think they are toxic. Every
time I have my tumor markers checked I get very anxious, but my numbers*

have been good and I just feel so healthy. This whole experience has taught me I am loved, and I feel because of my experience that I can help other people, which is very uplifting for me.

Dr. Burzynski is a wonderful man. So is Dr. Orlam, who works with him. After having had recurrence after recurrence, I feel with Dr. Burzynski that I finally have gotten control over my cancer. My tumor markers are great so far, and I am grateful each day that I am alive.

—Lolli D'Orisio, breast cancer survivor

Chapter 8

DR. NICHOLAS GONZALEZ

After all, and for the overwhelming majority of the cases, there is no proof whatsoever that chemotherapy prolongs survival expectations. And this is the great lie about this therapy, that there is a correlation between the reduction of cancer and the extension of the life of the patient.

—Philip Day, *Cancer: Why We're Still Dying to Know the Truth*

What if it was much simpler than we ever thought?

What if it was a change in the way we were eating? What if it was about detoxification and enzyme replacement? What if it wasn't about harsh drugs? What if you could live with your tumor and not have it bother you? What if you could live your life as a normal, healthy person after being diagnosed with stage IV cancer?

The patients of Dr. Nicholas Gonzalez are living testimony to exactly that. Many are well and happy and healthy—and living long lives.

Nicholas Gonzalez is a renegade. It takes great strength of character and a fierce personal belief that you have a better way to be able to stand up to big business, the media, and your peers. Dr. Gonzalez has done just that.

He graduated Phi Beta Kappa and magna cum laude from Brown University and completed the premed curriculum at Columbia University. He received his M.D. from Cornell Medical College, where he was named a Teagle Scholar, and he has been awarded numerous honors for performance in internal medicine and research in cancer immunology. But his honors don't stop there. He also received the Ernst L. Wynder Award from the Center for Mind-Body Medicine in 2000 (Dr. Wynder was the first scientist to confirm the link between cigarette smoking and cancer).

Dr. Gonzalez's personal journey in looking at cancer from another viewpoint began as a second-year medical student when he met Dr. William Donald Kelley. Kelley was an eccentric dentist who during the 1960s and 1970s had developed a very intensive program for treating advanced cancer with great success utilizing pancreatic enzymes and nutritional approaches.

When Dr. Gonzalez met Dr. Kelley, his research mentor had been Dr. Robert Good, who was then president at Sloan-Kettering and who encouraged Dr. Gonzalez to look into Dr. Kelley's patient charts. His investigation of Dr. Kelley's work took five years of intense research into thousands of records, not only Kelley's successes but also his failures. And what he found was patient after patient with appropriately diagnosed cancer who after five, ten, or even fifteen years still appeared to be in good health. After speaking with many of these patients himself, he felt that something very profound was happening.

Dr. Gonzalez's treatment protocol is controversial. Anyone who goes against "standard of care" is controversial. But read his patient testimonials and you will probably agree: his results are impressive.

The clear bias against acceptance for natural remedies to treat cancer boggles the mind. There is a double standard that reigns supreme in medicine. Chemotherapy drugs such as Gemzar make headlines as the new wonder drugs, while other voices go unheard. As I spoke with each of Dr. Gonzalez's patients, it seemed to me that their stories should be headline-getting, earth-shattering news.

Research should be unbiased, but in the medical world there is a bias against anything developed outside academic centers, particularly anything natural. As a result, we patients are the losers.

Penicillin comes from mold; digitalis comes from foxglove; Adriamycin, a major chemotherapy drug, comes from a bacterium—and these drugs have great acceptance today. But the present perception is that if the idea or the medicine wasn't developed within the academic club, it can't possibly be of benefit.

Considering the billions of dollars and thousands of highly trained researchers in the cancer wars, there should be a lot more success to show for it. Yet even with this poor track record, traditional medicine's gatekeepers are arrogant toward natural therapies.

You never know when a new idea offers promise.

SS: Thank you for your time, Dr. Gonzalez. In what I've read about you, it seems that what started as a simple student project of Dr. Kelley's work developed into your life's work. How did that happen?

NG: Well, I completed this investigation of Dr. Kelley when I was an immunology fellow under Dr. Good, and when I put the findings together in a monograph in 1986, no one would publish it. They thought it was absolutely impossible that a crazy nutritional program could be useful against cancer. But I was so impressed with what I learned that I turned down a job at Sloan-Kettering and opened up a practice to start using the therapy. I always had the intention of getting research money— thinking, hoping that the strength of the results would convince my conventional colleagues that we at least had to start looking into this.

SS: This program mainly involves pancreatic enzymes, right?

NG: Yes, but Kelley's program had three basic components: first an individualized diet, different from other alternative approaches in that there isn't one diet. There are ten basic diets ranging from pure vegetarian nuts and seeds to an Atkins-type red-meat diet, and about ninety variations of the ten basic diets. For each patient he would individualize the diet. But the main anticancer elements were the large doses of pancreatic enzymes. We know they serve a digestive function; that's how we break down our food. But 107 years ago Dr. Beard, the Scottish embryologist, said that pancreatic enzymes are also our body's main defense against cancer. He put his thesis and supporting evidence in a book in 1911 that should have changed the course of medicine, but it was so far ahead of its time that people thought it was insane. He died in obscurity, angry and bitter. Then Dr. Kelley resurrected the enzyme therapy.

SS: So it's an enzyme therapy, large doses, not a vitamin program. But as I understand it you do also use vitamins and minerals, right?

NG: Yes, the first component is diet, the second includes supplements with large doses of enzymes, and the third component is detoxification routines like the infamous coffee enemas, juice fasts, liver flushes, and other things. It's a three-pronged approach, but essentially it's about pancreatic enzymes.

SS: You must take a beating. Coffee enemas, enzymes?

NG: Yes, about two cents' worth of coffee a day. When I met Kelley in 1981 I went on the program preventatively. I was burned out from being a medical school student living on pizza and junk food. It really changed my health. I had thought I was in good health, but as I always tell my patients, never trust a doctor who doesn't live by his own rules. I've been doing coffee enemas now for twenty-eight years. The whole program is inexpensive, and when you are talking about cancer, compared to chemo it's nothing. The first year on our program is the most expensive, as there are some initial costs: you buy a juicer, a water filter, and all the supplements. Then there are the enzymes. The whole thing might run you $12,000, including office visits and initial evaluation, which takes four to five hours. It gets less expensive after that. Chemotherapy, on the other hand, can run $50,000 to $70,000 easily, and radiation $25,000 easily.

You can't patent enzymes, so there's no incentive for any drug company to get interested in what we do, even though I've been told drug companies know about my work but hope I get hit by a bus.

SS: It must be because it seems what you are doing works. You are affecting their bottom line.

NG: Last year just the chemotherapy alone, without considering radiation, brought in $100 billion.

SS: Add to that doctors' fees and hospitalization, lost work, and it's actually up to $200 billion.

A cancer diagnosis is frightening—you see your own mortality and it takes courage to go against the common course of chemo and radiation and say, "No, I think I'll do this instead." Walk me through it: If I came to you with stage IV pancreatic cancer, could you help me?

> **NG:** *A stage IV patient who has metastases, has had no chemo and radiation, and has been diagnosed within two months of seeing us has over a 50 percent chance of doing real well. As soon as patients have chemo and radiation their chances of success, although not completely eliminated, are lessened.*

On our website we have half a dozen pancreatic patient case reports, some of whom have been alive in excess of fifteen years now. These patients have been appropriately biopsied and had extensive disease. One of them actually had chemo for liver metastases and he's alive eight years now and doing so well with us. So more than 50 percent of our patients with stage IV pancreatic cancer do very well long-term, and by real well I mean seven or eight years down the line.

SS: Well, that's certainly better than the present survival rate of pancreatic cancer in traditional cancer care. My sense is that most people don't survive longer than four months and they go through a living hell before they die. What is the first thing you would have this patient do?

NG: Before patients even come in we get all their medical records and assess whether we think we can help or not. We turn away patients we don't think we can help because there's no point, there's no benefit to them.

SS: And what type of patient would that be?

NG: For instance, we had a patient today, stage IV pancreatic, had about three months of chemo which didn't work. The person couldn't eat, his belly was swollen from fluid, tumors are all throughout the liver—I mean, the cancer was everywhere. The main problem is that this patient can't eat. If a patient can't eat, there is nothing we can do. Our program is all nutritional. If a patient can't eat, they cannot do our therapy. So that's a limiting factor. If we had drug company support, we could actually develop injectable forms of enzymes, which have been available in the past but currently are not available in the United States by FDA edict, which is too bad because if we could use injectable enzymes we would implement them as a kind of natural chemo.

SS: Do you know how awful that sounds to me, a layperson, that lives could be saved but are stymied by our government?

NG: I have to let that go. Otherwise it would just be too frustrating. Yes, it would be nice to have the treatment available for everyone, but we are not allowed right now. But we are saving so many. So we give our enzymes orally. Frankly, it's so simple it's unbelievable. And that is what makes this treatment so nice. The patient takes the enzymes at home.

SS: What happens on the first day?

NG: It's very simple—the first evaluation is in two sessions. Most of my patients are not from New York. They're from all over the world, from Singapore to Israel. They have to spend two days in New York and we spend about four hours with them total, two hours the first day, where we do a history and a physical like any other doctor's visit. Before they come in we have to have all the records here, so I will have already reviewed them, and we also use a controversial hair test, which gives us a lot of nutritional information. Based on the results of the records, my experience, the hair test, the blood work that has been done, we design a diet and the specific supplement protocol. Each protocol is individualized.

That evening after I've seen the patient, I design the program on my computer. The next day we spend another two hours going over everything. There is a diet to follow, a supplement protocol, and what dose of enzymes they require—all of which has been individualized.

The third part is the detox: how they do the coffee enemas, how they do the liver flushes. And we teach them how to eat organically, what juicer to use, and what water filter to buy.

SS: So the second session is like a training session, and you spend about four to five hours with each patient over the two days.

NG: Right. Then they go home and start the program. They order the supplements, follow the diet, eat organically, drink filtered water, use their juicer, and start on coffee enemas.

SS: And what is the purpose of doing this?

NG: It's to flush the liver. One of the keys to success with any program is a healthy liver. We have a five-day liver flush that really cleans out the liver. It's a wonderful procedure. Once they have done the liver flush they dive into the supplements.

SS: Is the liver flush the enema?

NG: No. The liver flush takes five days. During the first four days they take something called Phosfood, a Standard Process product that dissolves gallstones and emulsifies bile. They take it in apple juice for four days, and on the fifth day there are a series of things to do: two doses of Epsom salts, which relaxes all the bile duct tubes and ducts of the liver, then they have a fruit dinner with lots of heavy cream, and before they go to bed they drink half a cup of olive oil on an empty stomach, which stimulates the gallbladder ducts.

The gallbladder contracts vigorously and all this junk in the liver and gallbladder gets squeezed right into the intestinal tract and they just poop all the waste from the liver right into the toilet. It's a way of cleaning out the liver done orally. That's in addition to the coffee enemas.

SS: When they take this flush, which stirs everything up, does it make them feel sick?

NG: Usually not. After they take half a cup of olive oil, well, no one, I mean no one, likes it. I've been doing it for twenty-seven years and it's not fun to drink that much olive oil. It's possible that you might feel a little queasy, but nothing serious. The first time I did it I passed what looked like gallstones.

SS: Is coffee good for you? I mean, if coffee enemas are such an important part of your regimen, could we drink a lot of coffee and get the same result?

NG: No. It's interesting—when you drink coffee, it actually turns on the sympathetic nervous system. When the sympathetic nervous system turns on, it shuts the liver down. When you take coffee rectally as an enema it stimulates certain nerves that are only in the lower bowel that turn on the parasympathetic system, which through a reflex causes the liver to release all its toxins. When you drink it, it shuts the liver down temporarily, but when you take it as an enema it turns on the liver and increases its efficiency. When the liver works better, everything works better. So drinking it and taking it rectally work completely differently physiologically. We never allow our patients to drink coffee ever.

SS: From what I hear from my readers, everyone has gut problems. Sounds like everyone should be on this diet.

NG: *Dr. Kelley said cancer and all diseases begin in the gut—poor nutrition, poor absorption, poor digestion—and I believe he's right.*

One of the things we try to concentrate on is getting all the digestive organs to work properly, including the liver and intestines. We have an intestinal cleanse that all our patients do, and periodically we repeat these things. Unquestionably, the key to success with any disease and with any therapy is to keep the gut working. If it isn't, then you can't absorb anything and nothing is going to work, no matter how good your nutrition is. If your digestive system is compromised, nothing is going to happen.

SS: So if your gut isn't working properly, you are not going to succeed. You are not going to get well.

NG: We have to get everything working properly: the accessory organs of digestion, the liver, the gallbladder, pancreas, the stomach, and the small and large intestines.

SS: But everyone thinks regarding cancer that there is only one protocol, "standard of care": surgery, radiation, chemotherapy, and the aftercare drugs. What made you walk away from that?

NG: A lot of people ask me that, especially my colleagues from twenty years ago. I went to Cornell because they are associated with Sloan-Kettering and I wanted to spend the rest of my life in basic science research in some lab at Sloan. But then I met Kelley. And you will hear everything good, bad, and indifferent about him, and it's all true, because he is like a lot of geniuses—extraordinarily eccentric and kind of half-crazed. And when I started going through his records, whatever my preconceived notions may have been and whatever my career path was to be, I knew that the guy was reversing cancer.

There was no question about it, and he was hated for it.

SS: I am familiar with the story of Steve McQueen's cancer, and I do remember in the press Kelley was blamed for killing him.

NG: Right, Kelley was involved in a peripheral way in 1980. But McQueen had failed radiation and immunotherapy, and he was smoking and wasn't really following the program. But Kelley was blamed.

Despite the fact that Kelley was considered a lunatic, I kept seeing patient after patient with advanced cancer who got well. For me there was no choice; as a scientist you can't walk away from that. Frankly, it would have been a lot easier if I had. My career would be much nicer and calmer. But if you are an honest scientist, it doesn't matter if it's moondust—if it's working, you have got to follow through. Kelley was difficult to be around—I would never choose him as a friend—but he was curing cancer, so I didn't care if he had six horns on his head. He was getting cancer patients well.

I made the commitment to go into cancer research because I met somebody who had the extraordinary capability of reversing cancers with a nontoxic approach. I would have to be a dishonest idiot not to follow up. I did what I thought was the appropriate thing.

SS: Back up one minute. You said he was curing cancer. You used the word *cure!*

NG: I would have to say he was, and I am very cautious about using that word for all the obvious reasons; medical, legal, and of course I don't feel like getting attacked. I am saying he was curing cancer. We followed one patient who was diagnosed in 1982 with pancreatic cancer with metastasis in the liver. The liver lesion was biopsied and confirmed at the Mayo Clinic that it was, indeed, metastatic pancreatic cancer. The worst kind. They gave her two months and maybe if God smiled on her she might live a year. They didn't even want to do chemo. I have the doctor's notes from Mayo and to his credit he did not push chemo on her, because he told her honestly it would do nothing for her, and that's rare. So she went home, learned about Kelley, went on the program, and soon she was back helping run the family gas station, working eighteen hours a day, with metastatic pancreatic cancer.

In the meantime we were continuing our research on Kelley's program. Dr. Good, president of Sloan-Kettering, who is one of the world's experts in cancer, said he'd never seen a patient like that. At that point she had been alive four years. About six weeks ago—I hadn't spoken to her since the midnineties, when she referred a patient to me—she called my office to tell me how well she was doing. It has been twenty-seven years since her diagnosis.

That's a cure.

SS: Well, no matter what, no matter how they want to criticize alternative medicine, no one could say that was not a cure.

NG: When I heard from her, I just felt so good. I mean, here's a woman who, tragically, had a terrible diagnosis. But she had a very honest oncologist who did not push chemo down her throat, which gave her the freedom to start investigating alternatives because she had no option. She hadn't been interested in alternatives until the authority at the Mayo Clinic told her there was nothing he could do, and she fortunately found a copy of Kelley's book at a health food store, and that's how it happened.

If she had been a chemo patient with this kind of success, the orthodox oncologists would have paraded her around all the talk shows. Kelley was a dentist; he wasn't even a physician. He had no legal right to treat cancer. To be treated by a dentist with no academic standing, no research grants, no big buildings, no academic staff, and reverse a disease that the Mayo Clinic said they couldn't touch—I mean, that's an astonishing story that no one has heard, as it hasn't been told.

SS: Everyone points to Lance Armstrong and his remarkable success with testicular cancer and chemotherapy. He is literally the poster boy for the success of chemo. The way I found out about you was reading an article you wrote that chemo really only works for three kinds of cancer: childhood leukemia, some lymphomas, and testicular cancer.

NG: The way Lance Armstrong has been promoted by the chemo industry is really unfortunate, and I'm really saddened that a man of that character would allow himself to be promoted that way. Testicular cancer is a rare cancer, not that many cases each year. There are 210,000 cases of breast cancer diagnosed yearly, and only 10,000 to 15,000 cases of testicular. It's just not that common, and you are correct that it is one of the few cancers that responds to chemo. Hodgkin's is the other aside from the three you mentioned. The fact of the matter is that for all the major cancer killers—metastatic breast, lung, prostate, and pancreatic—chemotherapy does absolutely nothing . . . zero. There's no evidence that those chemo drugs in metastatic disease prolong survival significantly. If they do, it's a couple of months. So to generalize his experience to chemotherapy success in general is a disservice. It's not scientifically accurate nor honest. It truly gives false hope.

There's a German mathematician by the name of Abel who in 1992 published a monograph on the effects of chemotherapy. He was hired by the German government (they chose a mathematician with a Ph.D. in math rather than oncology because they wanted someone who wasn't tied into chemo) to review the world's literature on chemotherapy used against solid tumors like metastatic breast, colon, lung, and pancreas, and he found there was absolutely no benefit to any of it except for these few rare cancers we've mentioned. He published his monograph in German and in English but the American oncology community got it suppressed in the United States. There is an updated version from 2001 which only confirmed what he'd said earlier: that for most cancers chemo does nothing. That version was never translated because of the political pressure against it. I spoke with him and he said he was just tired of being attacked as an independent scientist reviewing scientific literature. You would think everyone would be happy to review that effort, but it's so contradictory to what the oncologists wanted to believe that he was continually harassed about it.

SS: Without chemo no one knows what to do about this epidemic. They've bet the farm on it. Medical schools have bet the farm on it and the makers of the poison own the lottery.

NG: It's hard for me to believe that an oncologist who has gone through four years of college, four years of medical school, three years of residency, and then three years of oncology postresidency training can't connect the dots. You have to be an idiot not to be aware that for most of the cancers chemo isn't doing anything. It's in all the journals. It's not like it's a secret.

I suppose a lot of them know it and will admit it publicly in articles, but they all like to point the finger at doctors like me and others practicing alternatives and say we're stealing patients who could be cured from the orthodox people, and that we're luring them in for financial reasons. The fact of the matter is that 95 percent of the patients who call my office have been brutalized by the orthodox system. They have had regimens that never offered any chance of working: chemo, radiation, all kinds of grotesque surgical procedures. A lot of these people are actually very debilitated by the time they even call my office, and sometimes my staff just sits there dumbfounded by their stories, story after story, over and over again. Every day.

Spend one day in my office listening to the dozens of people who call in with these horror stories about the conventional therapies that were pushed on them with false hope, and then you will see why we get upset when we are criticized as alternative guys offering false hope. These people come to me half-dead because they were promised that these treatments could work, and we see this in particular with patients diagnosed with pancreatic cancer because we are known for treating pancreatic cancer. These people were given regimens that never could have worked, and so often they're dying and we cannot help them because it is too late. They lost their window of opportunity.

SS: Clearly these oncologists really must know in their hearts that what they are offering is not going to work. I mean, look around. The success rate is dismal. So, what's all the hoopla about the new wonder cancer drug Gemzar?

NG: They have compared Gemzar to the previous "best" chemo in pancreatic cancer, and median survival improved from 4.2 months to only 5.7 months—about one extra month of life for this expensive drug. Not a single patient out of 126 in the study lived longer than 19 months. But Gemzar has been considered such an advance that the FDA approved it, and now it's a billion-dollar industry. Gemzar, it's used all over the world. One month improvement in survival and not one patient in the clinical study lived longer than 19 months, and that has been considered a major advance. How can you tell a patient that this is really going well when they know the data doesn't support that?

SS: I have buried two people in the last week with pancreatic cancer. I begged, begged one of them to try another way, your way, but they were both sold this bill of goods. One died in four months, the other in a year. Why do patients go for it? I watched my friends degrade before my eyes.

NG: You can't save them. You just have to love them and let them do what they want to do. A lot of oncologists use the word *response*. They say, "You've got a good chance your tumor will respond," but patients interpret that to mean cure.

SS: What does *respond* actually mean?

NG: It means that you have tumor regression that lasts four weeks. The official definition of partial response at the National Cancer Institute for decades was a 50 percent decrease in tumor size that lasts four weeks. Hallelujah! Four weeks, and if you die in the fifth week you are still considered a "responder." Chemotherapy can shrink tumors; what it generally doesn't do is prolong life for most cancers other than the few we discussed, where you can get long-term survival, like Lance Armstrong.

SS: Why is there so much cancer?

NG: Clearly, it's usually wrong diet. People don't eat the right foods. Then there is the increasing chemical contamination in our environment, plus the electromagnetic contamination and radioactive contamination. It's everywhere.

SS: You mean like cell phones?

NG: Yeah, cell phones. There are thousands of towers giving off electromagnetic fields. Twenty years ago they didn't even exist. Computers give off electromagnetic radiation. I work with a computer, but we have safe screens. There is this extraordinary exposure to carcinogenic chemicals that only increases every year. There are thirty thousand synthetic chemicals in the environment and nobody knows what they do or what they do in combination. The food supply for most people, unless you eat organically, is only decreasing in its nutritional content. It's loaded with chemicals, and the American diet consists of a lot of refined, processed, chemicalized food that couldn't support a paramecium, let alone a human.

So we are getting more and more exposed to more and more chemicals and more and more electromagnetic fields, the effect of which no one really knows. Just when we need our bodies to be stronger to deal with all the environmental changes and threats, most people's bodies are taking in junk that they can't process. It's disastrous. Wrong diet, not enough nutrients in the food we eat, coupled with a lot of environmental exposures, and you get the present cancer epidemic.

SS: And I fear it's only going to get worse. Tell my readers what diet soda will do to them.

NG: I could really get worked up on this one. But I'll calm down. I'm not a fan of synthetic sweeteners. Richard Wurtman at MIT, a physician-researcher, has done extensive research into aspartame and says it is neurologically toxic and it increases your appetite. So you end up gaining weight when you are eating or drinking these diet sodas. A single can of nondiet soda has ten teaspoons of sugar. The average American eats 160 pounds of sugar yearly. There are no vitamins or minerals in these foods, and the extraordinary intake of white sugar in the Western world, which correlates with the accelerating rates of diabetes, is now a clear indicator that we are killing ourselves.

SS: I read recently that high school kids are getting 30 percent of their calories from soda pop.

NG: It's tragic. Their main vegetable is potatoes, but not baked potatoes—they mean french fries or potato chips. Soda pop and french fries!

Worldwide cancer is exploding. In the next ten, fifteen years it is predicted it's going to become an epidemic nightmare. Developing countries don't have the funds to deal with this avalanche of cancer. Ever since these developing countries adopted a Western diet and habits, their health has deteriorated.

SS: In this country there are a lot of people who consider ketchup a vegetable.

NG: Yeah, I love that . . . in what universe is ketchup a vegetable? So now you wonder why childhood obesity is becoming an epidemic? How can their brains function? If you are not providing your brain with the absolute ideal nutrients, it's not going to work right. We treat our cars better than we treat our bodies. No one would think about putting the wrong fuel into their expensive car, but they will go out and put the biggest pile of junk into their mouths.

SS: I think we are just naive about nutrition. But you are all about nutrition. So when a patient comes to you, are they already health nuts like me or are they just desperate?

NG: We want patients here because they want to be here and believe in what we are doing. If they don't believe it, they are not going to follow it, and it's a waste of time for both of us. Desperation can breed faith, that's true. They get desperate and look for alternatives because all the conventional therapy they believed in failed. Some of my best patients are the ones who did conventional therapy and failed, and they end up in my office. A lot of my patients have had a long-standing interest in nutrition and they ended up with cancer, so they were halfway there, and we just try to take them the rest of the way.

SS: Explain the autonomic nervous system and why we should care about it.

NG: It's really one of the basics of how we use diet and supplements. The autonomic nervous system is basically the collection of nerves that go out to all the various organs and glands and control their function. For example, the autonomic system ultimately controls all the endocrine organs that secrete hormones, like the thyroid, the adrenals, the ovaries and testicles. It controls cardiovascular function: heart rate, blood pressure, and pulse. All digestion is controlled by the autonomic nervous system: secretion and release of enzymes, bile, the function of the liver, the peristalsis in the intestinal tract [the function of moving food by the digestion and elimination process].

The autonomic nervous system is divided into two branches, the sympathetic and the parasympathetic.

SS: How do these two branches work?

NG: They work in opposite ways. The job of the sympathetic nervous system is to help your body deal with stress. It diverts the blood to the brain and the muscles, so in a time of stress you can think quickly and your muscles can react quickly as well, and it shuts down the entire digestive system.

SS: So when you are under stress your digestive system is kaput?

NG: Yes, sympathetic nerves divert energy away from the gut to the brain and muscles to help you deal with a stressful situation. The parasympathetic is the opposite. The parasympathetic system repairs and rebuilds, and it turns on at night when we're asleep. It's responsible for digestion and increases the efficiency of digestion and secretion of hydrochloric acid, enzymes from the pancreas, the bile salts from the liver. It increases the absorption of nutrients, stimulates the repair of damaged tissues, and basically is a reparative system.

SS: So these two systems work in opposition to help you get through the day?

NG: Yes. Every minor or major stress you have signals the sympathetic system to divert energy, whether it's a job interview or a project you have to finish. And then the parasympathetic allows the body to repair from the day's damage.

SS: Which all brings up a question: What does this have to do with cancer?

NG: [Laughs] Dr. Kelley believed certain people have a strong sympathetic system and a weak parasympathetic, and these people are prone to solid tumors of the breast, lungs, stomach, pancreas, colon, liver, prostate, uterus, and ovaries. People with strong parasympathetic systems tend to get immunological cancers like leukemia, lymphoma, myeloma, sarcomas.

SS: Are any people balanced with both systems?

NG: Yes, they are the lucky ones and they usually don't get cancer. They have to work really hard to get cancer. And diet is how you bring the autonomic system that is out of balance into balance.

SS: You mean we can reprogram our tendency to cancer with diet?

NG: Yes, that's the good news. For example with a sympathetic system that's too strong we put them on a vegetarian diet, because there are certain minerals and vitamins in vegetarian food that will turn down the sympathetic tone and turn up the parasympathetic. Parasympathetics are the classic meat eaters, and these are the people who would actually do well on an Atkins-type diet. We call them our Eskimos because that group traditionally ate nothing but meat and fat. Meat turns on the sympathetic system and turns off an overly active parasympathetic system and brings the nervous system in balance.

SS: What do you give the balanced people who do get cancer?

NG: They need to eat fruit, vegetables, plant foods as well as animal foods. The one commonality for all three types of systems is enzymes. There are benefits to having a strong sympathetic or parasympathetic system; it's when it gets out of control that it's a problem. Sympathetic dominants are going to be very smart, organized, good leaders, good engineers. Parasympathetics don't tend to be as disciplined in school or organized, but they can be very creative.

SS: How do you determine what a person's type is? By the kind of cancer that they have?

NG: After twenty years of experience in the clinic, you get to know right away. If they have colon cancer, you know they are a sympathetic dominant, but there are also certain characteristics in the blood work, the way they look, their personalities—and the hair test tells a lot. It gives us the profile on the autonomic nervous system which is critical to how we design the diets and the supplement protocols.

Sympathetics need a lot of magnesium and potassium and do terribly with large doses of calcium, whereas parasympathetics need huge amounts of calcium and do terribly on magnesium, which makes them very depressed.

SS: Interesting, because I had breast cancer and I do terribly on calcium and feel great on lots of magnesium.

NG: There you go. And most women are overloading on calcium— 1,500 milligrams daily is a sure way to make your breast cancer come back if you are a sympathetic type. It will make you sick and is actually a kind of poison for this type, but the parasympathetic is exactly the opposite. Give her some steak and bacon and some calcium and she is happy as a clam and starts doing better.

SS: More and more patients are developing multiple myeloma. Do you think there's a connection to weed killers and toxins in and around the house?

NG: I think even orthodox physicians are beginning to suspect that myeloma, like lymphomas, might be tied to environmental exposures. I think unquestionably it is. We've seen a real increase in people coming to us with myeloma, and with some people it's heavy metals, and with others it's radiation exposure in the environment and low-dose chronic radiation exposure, like radon. To me there's no question there are increasing instances of myeloma and an increase in brain tumors.

SS: In my last book, *Breakthrough*, Dr. Blaylock made a correlation between diet soda and brain tumors.

NG: Yes, and cell phones. I had a patient, thirty-three years old, a lobbyist in Washington, had three kids, and had glioblastoma, which is the worst kind of brain cancer. He lived on his cell phone eight hours a day. I told him he had to give it up. He said he couldn't do that, and ultimately didn't do my program. Three months later he was dead, having done chemo and radiation. I can't prove it was his cell phone, but I'd be willing to bet that was the root of the problem. How can you have that electromagnetic force field two inches from the brain, which is the most delicate organ in the body, and not expect to have a downside to it?

SS: And then birth control pills that give women only four periods a year . . . that doesn't make sense to me at all.

NG: Yes, trying to eliminate periods—why not try to get rid of your

heartbeat at the same time? It's just ridiculous. This is normal physiological function. There's a lot of debate about birth control pills; some of the
experts I've talked with think they are a problem.

SS: And who is going to do the studies? The makers of birth control
pills?

NG: When I was in medical school—I graduated in 1983—we were
taught that breast cancer affected one in twelve women. Then it was one
in eight. They are just getting ready to readjust again . . . there's got to be
a reason. They keep denying that it's birth control pills.

SS: I want to ask you a question that will make you nervous. What is
your cure rate?

NG: Unquestionably, Kelley was curing patients. I would never say
that about myself, for a couple of reasons. First, I'm not trying to be cagey
and avoid making a provocative statement, but Kelley taught me to look
at cancer as a kind of chronic disease that can be managed indefinitely.
He was one of the first people to actually use the analogy that cancer
should be approached like diabetes. Diabetics can live a hundred years if
they follow the right diet, take insulin if they need to, but they can lead a
normal life.

SS: That's an interesting analogy.

NG: I have patients who have been with me now for ten, twenty years
and some of them still have tumors. Very often tumors don't go away.
One patient of mine with lung cancer was eighteen years out and he still
had tumors in his lung. The tumors could be dead or scarred over, but
he's not going to let them be biopsied at this point—he's just living at
peace with his cancer. Is he cured? I don't know that he's cured; he may
still have cancer left. It does look good. But when we look at his X-ray
he's got a tennis ball sitting in his lung. His body has controlled it nicely.
So, like a diabetic, he's living in peace with his disease. If diabetics go off
their diets and stop taking insulin, they can be dead in a week.

SS: So cancer patients have to take their enzymes and follow your
protocol and then they can live with and manage their cancer throughout
their lives. In essence, it's controlled and they have quality of life.

NG: Exactly. There are patients we have where the tumors are completely gone. So by orthodox standards they would be considered cured.
But I hesitate to congratulate myself that we are curing people. We do
have people who have been with us over ten years with a terrible stage
IV disease, all appropriately diagnosed and proven with biopsy, who have
no evidence of cancer by scans. There might be a microscopic nest left
that you can't see on the CT scan, but they are leading normal lives, and

whether we got rid of every cancer cell is not relevant. They are leading normal lives after having been given six months to a year to live.

SS: That's all anybody really wants. Having had cancer, I know it doesn't hurt until it has taken over, so if you just have your quality of life, that's enough for me. What do you think of the present chemo drugs Adriamycin and Taxol? My oncologist says they've been proven ineffective.

NG: These are not miraculous drugs. With metastatic disease you might expect tumor shrinkage, but it doesn't last. We are constantly dealing with women who come to us all messed up from these drugs. We have about three hundred women with breast cancer in our practice. One woman in particular I am thinking of took Adriamycin and got so sick on it that she stopped the treatment. She came to us when it had metastasized to the liver and brain. Today she's alive and well.

SS: Do you call this cured or controlled?

NG: I think if she got real careless she would be in trouble again, so let's call it controlled. I have some patients I haven't seen for years who send me Christmas cards, so I know they are doing fine. I know they continue with their coffee enemas and eat organically and are doing the right things. But with cancer, no matter whose therapy you follow, even if you've had success, there is always a risk that if you get careless with your life it's going to come back.

SS: So you have to be realistic, and you have to live a cautious life.

NG: There's no question. I know you've interviewed Dr. Burzynski, and he is unquestionably turning cancer around. He works completely differently than me, but I know him very well and I have nothing but enormous respect for him. He's one of the great scientists of our time.

SS: I am sure he will appreciate your saying this about him. It's two different approaches—he's identified a missing peptide and is putting it back, and you are building up with enzymes and nutrition. In the end, the patients I've interviewed from both of you are well. That speaks volumes to me.

NG: One day I'd like to sit down with him and compare how enzymes work versus antineoplastons. I know he is unquestionably getting responses. A very smart guy.

SS: Talk to us about fatty liver disease. It seems our livers are groaning from all the toxicity from our environment.

NG: Right. The sugar we're taking in is creating fatty infiltration of the liver. We take in so much extra sugar that the liver in its wisdom doesn't know what to do with it. So it converts it into triglycerides, a form of storage fat. So then, ironically, eating sugar will raise your blood fat and the liver has no choice but to store it. People walk around with fatty livers now because of their sugar ingestion.

SS: And these are people who don't drink alcohol?

NG: Right. I've had many people who have fatty infiltration of the liver and the only correlation we could make was the prior ingestion of the typical American intake of sugar. The liver is the main detoxification area of the body. That's where the environmental chemicals are neutralized and processed. The intake of toxic chemicals in the typical American diet coupled with the polluted air we breathe is all toxic and damaging to humans. Most people don't drink filtered water and you can't filter the air we breathe, and then there is the junk food that is loaded with chemicals and it's going to stress the liver. Add to that more sugar, more refined products, all of which go to the liver, and you see why we have problems.

SS: What kind of water and what kind of filter should we be using?

NG: There are many debates on which water filtration system to use. I'm kind of traditional: I use reverse osmosis. It isn't a perfect system; it removes heavy metals, but it also removes all minerals. In this day and age, that's the way it is. You just have to take supplements to make up for it.

SS: There's always debate on how much water to drink. Six glasses a day? Eight?

NG: Water flushes out toxins and I drink eight glasses a day. It's very important.

SS: What about alkaline water?

NG: It's great for the sympathetic dominant, but for parasympathetics it's too alkaline. They need to be more acid, that's why they do well on red meat. Red meat is very acid. With every patient I want the acid base to be in balance. Sympathetic dominants tend to run on an acid metabolism—they produce lots of acid, metabolic waste. People who get breast, colon, and liver cancer are always too acid. We get them alkaline, so for these types alkaline water is good.

But if you put parasympathetic dominants—they're already too alkaline—on alkaline water, they're going to end up so depressed they won't be able to get out of bed in the morning, and their leukemia is going to get worse.

SS: Is cancer acid?

NG: Parasympathetic tumors exist only in an alkaline environment. These are the leukemias, lymphomas, and myelomas. We believe myeloma and sarcomas are occurring in people who are too alkaline, and that's why getting everyone alkaline is not a good thing. I've had some patients decide, because they have cancer, that they want to become vegetarians, but if they are parasympathetic, it is the wrong fuel for the body.

SS: Interesting. Like putting regular gasoline into a diesel car.

NG: This was part of Kelley's genius—he recognized that being too alkaline creates a whole other set of problems, like catastrophic depression, leukemias, and myelomas.

SS: It's difficult in today's world to get perfect balance. It's a lot of work. It's worth it, but it's a lot of work.

NG: The human body is the most exquisite engine ever designed, and you have to put the very best fuel in it for it to run properly. Yet most people don't tend to think of it that way. As you said, people feed their dogs better than they feed themselves. Everything in our bodies comes from one place: our diets. From our bones to our brain cells, we are made up of nutrients that come out of our diet. And when you consider the exquisiteness of our brains, I want to feed it the best of everything I can for my benefit. Nutrition is key. It's the foundation. It's not the end, it's the beginning. It's the ultimate foundation for good health. If you don't have that, nothing else is going to work too well.

SS: What is your feeling about biopsies? They make me nervous, and I had one that I describe in the beginning of this book, when I was under much duress. I have since read that if it is cancer, a biopsy could spread it further. Is that correct?

NG: Traditionally orthodox surgeons and conventional oncologists would laugh at that and say you are worrying about silly things, but there was a study about ten years ago with biopsies of the liver confirming that when you biopsy a liver tumor to find out what it is, you actually increase the rate of spread, and it has a negative effect on survival.

In America every urologist is biopsying prostates every day of the year. That will increase the rate of spread and now they can confirm this to some extent from a study I recently read. The same seems true with breast cancer.

Biopsies are so cavalierly done, but we now know you can create a worse problem. The legal system has set it up this way. You have to have a biopsy before you can be treated.

SS: What do other doctors think of you?

NG: I had a referral today. I have this pancreatic cancer patient and his son is a very well-established conventional physician. He wrote me the most gracious letter about his dad. This guy had read my website and he really felt the cases were impressive, but he wondered why I am so criticized. I always say critics need to get a life, stop worrying so much about me.

I love coming to work. It's not easy. I treat mostly advanced patients and not all of them make it, but most of them do. They're very sick and I spend two hours each night returning phone calls. I have patients all over the world and they are all desperate to keep in touch with me by phone. It's an enormous amount of work, and there are other ways of making a living.

SS: Do you do it for the money?

NG: [Laughter] If I wanted to make money, I'd become a cardiovascular surgeon making $60,000 an operation. They do two a day. That's how you make money in medicine, not doing what I'm doing. I do this because the patients get well. Same reason I followed up with Kelley twenty-five years go. I don't care what critics say.

SS: Do you think your kind of medicine will ever see the light of day?

NG: I think it's already seen the light of day. That's part of why I am criticized—what we are doing is a threat. This book is coming out; we have one that is coming out about the theory of our protocol.

SS: Well, I guess they're not going to put you on TV unless you are being attacked for going against the grain. The pharmaceutical companies fund everything: every TV show runs their ads, all the airwaves, they even fund Hollywood. That's what I mean about seeing the light of day.

NG: One of the big problems is that our medical and political leaders could care less. They talk about global warming, but they never get into nutrition or alternative medicine. The drug companies control medicine, and they are very powerful. There are a thousand full-time, paid drug industry lobbyists in Washington, D.C.; that's not counting state capitals. That's two for every senator and congressman. A thousand full-time drug lobbyists and they are all getting six-figure salaries.

But I think truth is very powerful. And I also believe that truth always comes to the top.

SS: How much of surviving cancer is faith and how much of it is nutrition?

NG: I asked Kelley one day after I'd seen these miracle cases, "What percentage of cancer is physical, what percentage is nutritional, and what percentage is psychological-spiritual?" He said, "That's simple. It's 100 percent physical and 100 percent nutritional." He waited about two seconds, and then he said, "It's 100 percent psychological." And then he waited two more seconds and said, "It's 100 percent spiritual in every single patient."

Nutrition is just the foundation; the psychological and the spiritual are what patients have to deal with. It's about faith and having to confront what life is really all about. He said nutrition is just the building block. He was very humble regarding his work.

Most of our patients come into our office so sick that just to get them to make carrot juice is a major effort, but interestingly enough, as their nutritional foundation improves, they feel stronger and the brain starts working better because it is getting the nutrients it needs. They then start thinking about the psychological issues in their lives and it helps them get better. They start becoming more spiritual and may express themselves in different ways with different people. It's quite wonderful to see. Good nutrition is not going to help your kid get off drugs or make your marriage better, but spiritual issues for human beings are critical for finding who we are.

SS: How do you feel about what you have chosen to do?

NG: I don't look back. Sometimes I think maybe I should have taken a different path with the research or something like that. I know what I'm doing works. I'm not crediting myself as someone who found the answer to cancer. Dr. Beard is the one who first said pancreatic enzymes have the anticancer effect. I'm just following his work. He was right, and if I have any intelligence at all, it is to realize that Beard was correct, and that is what I am trying to bring to the world. Kelley was as eccentric as they come, but as crazy as he was, he was right too. Enzymes do work, and the world needs to know this and have the option to use the treatment. I have done what I have done because of the truth of it, and the truth has proven to be only truer as I've gotten further into the journey.

SS: They say the most important thing we can do with our lives is to do what we love. It seems like you love your work.

NG: Absolutely. I do. Fundamentally, in my heart, I am a scientist. I want to find the truth. I'm not interested in promoting drugs or being a famous surgeon; I wanted to find the truth and where it would lead. That is why I was willing to look into Kelley, even though it was an odd truth and not what I had been trained to think about. But this quest and the results have been my greatest joy. We have found the fundamental way in which nature works with cancer, and it's extraordinary. It is the greatest reward I could ever ask for.

SS: I am deeply moved by you. Thank you, and God bless.

DR. GONZALEZ'S PATIENTS IN THEIR OWN WORDS

Twenty-six years ago I was diagnosed with stage IV pancreatic cancer and at that time they told me chemotherapy and radiation would do me no good. This was probably the best news in retrospect, but at that time it was devastating because they told me there was nothing they could do and I should prepare myself to go home and die.

Well, that pissed me off. I mean, I was forty-six years old at the time. I wanted to live. I was married and I had six kids. I am from the old school where only the good die young and I wanted to stick around a long time.

I was told I could try going to the Mayo Clinic. But when I went there, they said the same things the first hospital did and essentially told me to go home and get my things in order and enjoy what good days I had left.

Now I know I can talk smart, but really, I didn't know what my options were. My doctor told me I was going to starve to death, the shriveled-up shrimp that he was. I looked at him and said, "You are going to tell me that I weigh two hundred pounds and I am going to starve to death?" He said, "Yep." Well, guess what? It didn't happen. I didn't have anything better to do, so I roamed around the stores looking for answers and I found a book at Steins' Natural Foods in Appleton. The name of the book was The Answer to Cancer *by Dr. Kelley. I splurged and bought the three-dollar book. In it was the name of the Dr. Kelley program and at that time it was headquartered in Grapevine, Texas.*

So I called to make an appointment and they told me where to go in Wisconsin, to get this treatment from James Kolner. The next week I was in his office and he looked at me and said, "You're not going to die." I then said, "Well, Mayo just told me I was." And he said, "Do what I tell you and you will have good years ahead of you." He gave me a book about an inch thick; they wanted to know how much I ate, how often, how it was fixed; if I had ridges in my fingernails; if I had calluses on the bottom of my feet. All my answers pertained to something.

After I got the blood work done, he sent it into the Kelley program, and then my regimen started: how to fix food, how often you are supposed to eat what, and then there was a list of pills I had to order and take. When I counted them up there were 357 pills a day. Ninety of them were pancreatic enzymes, and they were to do the work of the pancreas so the pancreas could rest and heal itself. The rest were vitamins. I took 10,000 units of vitamin C daily. There were several things I was told I could not eat: no red meat, no white flour, no dairy products, no citrus, and no sugar. I ate and did everything they told me to do, including coffee enemas. But nobody told me how strong to make the coffee. Dummy me made it like I like to drink it. Three days later I was still high. Now I know that you have to make weak coffee, honey.

I realized the hard way that you have to take the treatment seriously. I started in August (that was when Mayo told me I had six months to live) and at Christmas I had company and ate like a pig. And I ended up throwing up all of it. It was then I realized I had to take the vitamins and all of it seriously. You see, I hadn't started taking any of the vitamins yet, because they had given me a list of what the side effects were going to be and I didn't want to feel badly at Christmastime. Funny, by not doing it, I felt real bad.

It was then that I made up my mind that I was going to pull myself up by my bootstraps and keep going with this thing. I didn't like the idea of coffee enemas or 300 supplements a day, but then I realized I didn't like the options. . . . I stayed on these pills for five years.

For fifty-four years and eight months we worked our gas station. I lived on candy bars and sandwiches and soda and ice cream and tomato juice, you name it. So I've had more than my share of garbage.

But I changed my ways. You can do anything you want, especially when you look at your options. Dead was my option. That's pretty motivating. So when they told me I had to eat raw liver, I've got to say the idea turned my stomach . . . but then I had an idea. I put that liver into the freezer on a cookie sheet. And just before it was frozen solid I cut it into quarter inch squares like ice cubes. Then I put it back into the freezer and I let it freeze. When I'm supposed to have my handful of raw liver, I pop the liver into my mouth and down it with a glass of water. Because you see, you can do anything you have to do.

Several years later Dr. Gonzalez wrote me a letter saying he wanted to put my story in a book. But I don't do anything anymore. I feel I'm better, so no coffee enemas, no vitamins, nothing. Whatever happened in the five years has kept me healthy because I'm still fat and sassy. And I never went back to the original doctor because he has been dead a long time now. I had told him, that gray-haired little B., "I'll be alive when you're dead and gone." He's been dead close to ten years now.

—Arlene Van Stratten, patient utilizing Dr. Kelley's protocol, stage IV
pancreatic cancer, cancer free for twenty-six years

I'm a nurse. And I was very lucky that when I was diagnosed with stage IV ovarian cancer I had a friend who had done a lot of research, because her father had had pancreatic cancer and she found Dr. Nick Gonzalez. She said to me, "You know, there's another option."

I had been in the hospital for five days and had a total hysterectomy, removal of tubes, everything. I figured it was worth a try, so I called Dr. Gonzalez and thought if worse came to worst I could always go back to the chemo route.

I have to say I was shocked to hear how in-depth the program was; there was so much involved in it and a lot of work. It would have been so much easier to just lie down and stick a needle in my arm, but something inside me told me that I had to try this. First I had to shop and buy all this organic food, and then there were all the pills. It's a lot of work.

Dr. Gonzalez gave me a diet plan based on my hair sample. My diet was prescribed as moderate vegetarian, and it listed all the fruits and vegetables I was supposed to eat. Then I ordered my pills, at least 150 pills a day, including pancreatic enzymes and vitamins C, A, D, B complex, calcium, liver supplementation, hypothalamus, and supplements for other organs that were weak.

When you have cancer your organs become weakened in so many areas— it's not just localized. Plus, I took certain other chemicals—sodium, potassium. And other elements—magnesium, selenium, zinc. You know, all my deficiencies.

I'm Italian, so my diet had never been bad. I never ate fast food. I ate a lot of fruits and vegetables—I wasn't a White Castle kind of person—but I did smoke and I did drink excessively, so I had a lot of bad habits to turn around. And the food I had been eating, though not highly toxic, was not organic.

Then there was my work, a lot of stress. So I decided to do consulting work and leave the high stress of the hospital and the nursing homes.

The detoxing procedures were horrible. I did not enjoy doing them at all . . . I had to hold my nose when I had to drink the olive oil. But it was all for a good reason; I was getting stronger and healthier and every time I went to see Dr. Gonzalez, which was every three months, the cancer rate was coming down. After a couple of months went by I saw my sister one day and she said, "Wow, your skin is so clear." It was because all the toxins were just oozing out of me, and she was so impressed.

The people in my life were impressed that I was alive having had such a horrible diagnosis, because stage IV ovarian cancer is usually a death sentence.

I am deeply grateful that I am alive today and feeling better than ever at

*my age. People are totally amazed when they see me and how well I look. It
has been hard work, but life is about the choices we make.*

*When I went back to my gynecologist's office she could not believe it. She
assumed I had gone on the chemo regimen. When I told her I didn't do it, she
just shook her head in disbelief—in fact, such total disbelief that I couldn't go
back to her, because she was so unsupportive even in the face of my success.
Same with the surgeon.*

*My liver had been in such bad shape, and I had evidence of metastasis, so
my success is quite a miracle. And yes, I do the coffee enemas twice a day
still. And I will do them for life.*

*It's been seventeen years. Why mess with success? I am not going to take a
chance and not continue with the program. I can never say I am cured, but
at present I have no evidence of disease.*

*I have energy all the time. I go to tai chi, I go to yoga, I go to Curves. I am
always exercising. I love to dance. I think if people saw me they would say I
am a happy, joyful person. And I am. I feel upbeat, very positive, and I
always see the glass as half-full.*

*Dr. Gonzalez is very, very smart. He did a lot of research on this when he
discovered Dr. Kelley's program. He's the bravest man I have ever met. You
know he really cares, but he doesn't get emotional. You can call him about
anything and he is there for you. I see him as a knight in shining armor, even
though he'd kill me if he knew I said that. But he really is, and I'm so sorry
that other people can't get to know about his program and understand that
they have a choice.*

*If there is such a war on cancer, how many years do we have to play this
war before we get somewhere? I resent when people ask me to give money for
cancer, because it's going out the window. It's all going to the drug companies
and they are making huge profits but no one is getting well. In fact, it's getting
worse.*

*In November I will be seventy years old and I just thank God every day
for Dr. Gonzalez for taking on the cause. I was very lucky to meet him at that
time. I believe it was all meant to be.*

—Raphaela Savino, stage IV ovarian cancer, seventy years old,
cancer free for sixteen years

*In 1988, I had severe back pain, and when they did a CAT scan they
discovered that I had several tumors, and immediately wanted to take them
out. It was very serious. I had a double surgery; a total hysterectomy as well*

as removing the cancers that were attached to the transverse colon. Both the gynecologist and the surgeon assured me that I then needed to take chemotherapy, six months of it. So I braced myself and went ahead and endured strong chemo of seven different drugs. I was nauseated and sick as can be and in bed most of the time. Then in July '91 I finished chemo and did a follow-up CAT scan and there was a recurrence in my lungs, which was a death sentence.

Fortunately, at the time I was attending a meeting at a health-related business and a doctor who was a nutritionist told me I needed to get on Dr. Nick Gonzalez's program. I let it pass because he told me it involved taking a whole lot of pills. Strangely, a month later I ran into this same doctor in Texas at another meeting and he asked me if I had thought about going to Gonzalez, and I said, "I can't afford to go to New York." And he said, "Joy Lee, you can't afford not to go to New York—your life depends on it." He knew this because his wife was a patient also. I truly believe the good Lord led him to me to make me aware.

At that time, the oncologist told me I was going to need to do another eight months of chemo to deal with the recurrence, plus they wanted to surgically remove part or all of that lung. It was the first time I asked the Lord to take me home, it was so bad. I don't believe my body would have stood up to all that treatment.

So we went to see Dr. Gonzalez. I took all my records and we sat in his office, and later that evening, my husband, Gary, said to me, "I wish we had known about this three years ago."

The initial visit was two days: a two-hour session the first day and one hour the next. He had to meet with me to discuss the history. Then he formulated my program. All of his programs are individualized for just that patient because each person and each cancer is different. On the second day he told me what my personalized program entailed, what needed to be done, and how to do everything.

The one thing everyone questions are the coffee enemas every day. Well, I had never heard of it before, but I decided to do whatever needed to be done on this program because I wanted to stay alive. And if this is what it took, this is what I was willing to do. I was very positive about it, and I certainly didn't want to go back to the other way ever again.

I was surprised by the diet. I mean, I had been brought up to eat healthy meals, but I was not eating organic. Then there were about 130 pills I needed to take daily, which included pancreatic enzymes. He put me on a lot of vitamins, minerals, and enzymes. I'm still on them. And then there's the monthly detox, which is not my favorite thing, you know—drinking the olive oil and the liver flush, which you prepare by taking phosphoric acid in apple juice and this stimulates different parts of the body to do different things. It's very nauseating, but this helps to flush all the toxins from the liver.

Sometimes I am slightly nauseated through the night, but it doesn't even compare with chemotherapy. It doesn't make sense to poison the cancer with chemotherapy. They gave me Adriamycin and leucovorin, which affects the heart and lungs, and now twenty years later I still have residual effects from these terrible drugs.

I guess when I was diagnosed, I was just afraid, and I let them do things to me that I would never let happen today.

As for Dr. Gonzalez, I would recommend him to anybody. Sometimes I try to talk to people, but they won't listen. I've had people say to me who were very, very close to the end of their lives, "I wish I had gone to your man."

It's been seventeen years that I've been on this program and I'm feeling pretty good. I'm one of the rare patients who have had chemotherapy, and he was able to save me in spite of the fact that my liver and my immune system had been compromised. I will be on this program for the rest of my life and I am fine with that. My goal is to stay alive and be with my children. I have a very supportive family. They believe in this with me.

We have insurance, but they won't cover anything alternative, because they say this is all experimental. Experimental! Yet I've been alive with what was horrible cancer for seventeen years. The insurance would have paid for the medicines to kill me. It all just doesn't make sense. But you do what you have to do. We don't take vacations. We don't have a whole lot, but we manage to buy the supplements and we absolutely feel this is money well spent. I am sixty-six years old. I'm proud to be this age; because there was a time I never thought I'd be here.

—Joy Lee McCoy, stage IV diffuse mixed lymphoma, sixty-six years old,
cancer free for seventeen years

Ten years ago, I was diagnosed with stage IV lymphoma. It was totally unexpected because I had been misdiagnosed for two years before that; in fact, I had been told that it was just a fatty tumor. No one even told me to take care of it until I went to a gyn who said, "You might want to get rid of that, it could get ugly." So when it was diagnosed as lymphoma I was totally shocked. My nature is to be courageous about my health, but going to Dr.

Gonzalez took a leap of faith. But thankfully, my husband encouraged me. He had been working with a man who was very into alternatives, and he kept pushing my husband to get me into the land of alternatives.

I waited about a year and a half before I went to Gonzalez, and even then it was still a leap of faith. In the beginning it was so much to think of . . . meaning all I had to do to embrace this program; the amount of pills, trying to figure out how I would take it during the day, the enemas, the gallbladder flushes, the whole program. It was truly overwhelming, but I was determined to give it a shot.

He gave me a diet in the beginning that was acid-based because I was very alkaline. His theory is this kind of blood cancer does better in an acidic body than an alkaline. So it was a lot of meat and very little greens. Now I'm on a moderate diet where I can eat just about anything—organic, of course—so that's a joy. I had always tried to be healthy, eat whole grains, whole wheat, and exercise, but I know there were times I was exposed to chemicals in the garden or in the air.

So I took his program seriously, I took the vitamins: the As, the Bs, the Cs, all the pancreatic enzymes. I would break it down to a system: breakfast, lunch, and dinner. Now I just do it automatically; I can go out with friends and they don't even know I am taking them. I feel had I gone the other route of chemotherapy, I probably wouldn't be here today. I think about that often and it's only by the grace of God that I have lived, and I am thankful every day.

Dr. Gonzalez is a great man. We all have our heroes, and on earth he is one of my heroes. He's just a very loving, caring man for his patients. He calls me back when I have a test as soon as he gets the results. Sometimes I've waited for doctors for over a week to get results; but when he gets them, he responds right away. He just shows how much he really cares for each one of his patients. I feel it, and this makes such a difference when you are dealing with a doctor. It makes you feel kind of special.

Dr. Gonzalez says we all have cancer cells in our bodies. It's just that some people have a stronger immune system, and I know I had been going through a lot of stress. So it all adds up. You just don't know the toll it's taking on your body until your body starts to shut down in one form or another.

Whenever I get a little down Dr. Gonzalez will give me a gentle push, remind me how well the program is working, and usually that's the jolt I need. I'm so thankful for him because I can't imagine where I would be if he didn't give me that push. I am so grateful to him.

—Esther Devito, stage IV lymphoma, cancer free for ten years

I'm a voice teacher and that is my life's work. I have degrees in medical areas; I even spent seven years in college and was an officer in the army. Yet it seems my biggest accomplishment is surviving cancer.

When my third cancer was diagnosed, I said to myself, "I will not go through chemotherapy again." I had been so sick I could not sit up. Then I remembered this article about a Dr. Gonzalez. So I got in touch with them and they said, "You know, Dr. Gonzalez only takes a small percentage of patients who call him." They asked if I had any other health issues at that time, and I said, "No, I am absolutely healthy. The only thing I have is cancer." She went on with her questions and then I stopped her and said, "Let me tell you something—if you tell me I have to stand on my head, I will do it."

Later that day, Dr. Gonzalez called me and took me on as a patient, which to me has been phenomenal.

When I was diagnosed with my second cancer, my doctor at that time told me that only 20 percent of people with rectal cancer survive, and I was so astounded that he would say that. I said, "Where did you go to medical school?" I mean, he was very nice, but I thought that was a terrible attitude.

When I met Dr. Gonzalez, he walked in and said, "Let's see what we can do to get you better." I tell you, it was love at first sight. He's adorable—he looks thirty but he's got to be at least sixty, he's charming, and he has a lovely sense of humor. I am a good patient and I was willing to do anything. I knew my options were running out. This was my third serious cancer. My mother had a double mastectomy, my grandmother had uterine cancer, my father had colon cancer—I think it's in our genes.

I've thought a lot about my cancer and how I got it. I was under a lot of stress all the time. But I thought I was handling it. I was so busy all the time, but I enjoyed all my careers. I had a wonderful service career.

For my second cancer (not with Dr. Gonzalez), I had chemotherapy, which was dreadful. I also had radiation on my right breast and there were all kinds of burns with radiation. The doctor who treated me at that time was my ranking officer in the army, so he knew me very well. One day he said to me, "Hester, I feel calcium deposits; that usually means trouble." Now, I'm a 38DD, and I didn't think I'd miss a breast, so they removed that one. Three years later, they diagnosed rectal cancer. It was then they decided I had a little cancer machine in me, so they hit me with radiation again and then aggressive chemo.

I was told this would be nothing and that I could go back to work. Well, I couldn't even stand up, let alone go back to work. I was so nauseated, and that went on for months. Then after months of chemo, the cancer came back again, this time in the lungs. Spread all over my lungs like little pellets, and that's the point when I went to Dr. Gonzalez.

I followed his regimen perfectly. I knew this was my one chance, and I believed in him. I do it all—the 150 pills a day, the olive oil, the coffee enemas, the organic food—and I'm strict about that.

Dr. Gonzalez's treatment program literally saved my life. If you have a negative attitude, it's not going to work. You have to do his regimen and believe it will work.

I was ready emotionally and philosophically to receive this treatment. I'd been through the other orthodox treatment and it almost killed me, plus it didn't work. It's a mental acceptance of what you are doing, and you have to have faith. Oh, Lord, at eighty-two you better believe in something!

—Hester Young, eighty-two years old, breast, rectal, and lung cancer free for twelve years

I am fifty-three years old and I should have been dead. In January of '01, a little over eight years ago, I was diagnosed with stage IV metastasized liver cancer at age forty-five. Pretty devastating. I took a few rounds of chemotherapy and the tumor had shrunk, but my doctor wasn't very encouraging. He said he thought the cancer would come back and probably very quickly, and that we could try another kind of chemo. But he felt I would either die of the cancer or die of the chemo. He really didn't have any hope for me.

So I thought, Well, it's silly to wait around. And I had been researching other options. But it was my mother who came up with Dr. Gonzalez's name. We went to New York, and after talking to him for a short time I decided to give him a try.

Chemo isn't fun stuff. I didn't have as bad a reaction as some people report; I was mainly tired, cramping, that type of thing. And my hair fell out, but I dealt with it because I felt at that time it was my only option.

Dr. Gonzalez's program was about carrot juicing, taking a couple of hundred pills a day, skin brushing, saltwater baths, coffee enemas, a variety of different detoxing therapies, and of course eating well. When I first started on this program I can't say it made a lot of sense to me, but over the years I now feel it makes total sense.

Strangely, when I go back to my original oncologist and tell him I've been well all these years and that I am on Gonzalez's program, he tells me I am insane. I think it's fear and embarrassment that maybe he spent so much time learning his craft and maybe it wasn't the answer.

My regimen now is quite easy. I take about 130 pills a day; instead of coffee enemas twice a day, I typically do it once a day now; I still follow the same diet; and that's about it. My health has improved. This all happened because I had such bad acid reflux that they were going to do a procedure to try and fix it laparoscopically, and that is when they came across all this cancer in my liver. I guess if they hadn't done that I'd be dead.

But my overall health has improved since I have been on this diet. After three months on his regimen, my tumor had shrunk quite a bit, and at six months it was totally gone. Gone! And it's been gone ever since. I'm still thin, I still have a little acne, but you know what? The coffee enemas really make you feel very good.

I'm able to do whatever I want. I have a lot of energy. And I did retire, so I don't have that stress anymore. I enjoy each day—I have two teenage daughters, and they keep me very busy.

Dr. Gonzalez is a wonderful guy, and I can't recommend him any more highly. He is very accessible, and whenever you need him, he'll call you right back. I think it's a shame the medical community won't take him more seriously.

I'm well, that's all I know. I have my life and my daughters, and I take my diet seriously because it is what saved my life. Sometimes I think of what could have happened, and I feel great that this is the regimen I have chosen. It's been eight years. Liver cancer is usually always deadly. I feel pretty lucky.

—David Yoffee, stage IV liver cancer, eight-year survivor

So many women die of aggressive breast cancer, but I refused conventional therapy. I had a needle biopsy which confirmed the microcalcifications that were spread throughout my breast. It was DCIS [ductal carcinoma in situ]. They recommended a radical mastectomy with follow-up radiation, and the first thing I did was go home and pray.

Then my daughter heard about another woman who was on Dr. Gonzalez's program and my daughter insisted that I call her. As I listened to her story I thought, That's what I want. It made absolute sense to me that the body would cure itself if it was given the right support. I lived in Ohio at the time. It was exactly one month from the time I had my diagnosis until I was accepted by Dr. Gonzalez, but he said not to worry, this cancer is slow growing and I had time.

I knew all about the program going in—the coffee enemas, the diet, the enzymes—and I was ready and willing to do anything to save my life. I did the program religiously and did not deviate for any reason. It took over my life for quite a while, but I needed to do it and do it right.

After two months I sent in a hair sample and my cancer rate had come down three points. That was huge. It's like losing weight; if you lose fifty pounds, you know it's working. The longer I continued on the program the better I felt. It wasn't instantaneous. I could feel the movement of it, the war that was going on in my body, and it took every bit of my energy.

I stayed on the program intensely for six or seven years without any kind of deviation. I still do the program; I just don't take as many enemas as I did. I feel great when I do the enemas, and I still do the carrot juicing once a day, whereas I had been doing it four times a day, and I continue to eat 90 percent organic. I found that after I had detoxified if I put anything in my body that had chemicals in it, I would have a headache within a few minutes.

I will do this for the rest of my life. I don't know if you have seen any of Dr. Gonzalez's patients, but the program itself has turned back my age at least ten years. I'm sixty-three but people think I'm fifty. It's absolutely antiaging. I just led a group on a cruise and I was aware how grateful I was to have my good health and energy.

Dr. Gonzalez saved my life. God used him to save my life. I'll be indebted to him forever. I love the man. He's just incredible.

—Wanda Flick, metastatic breast cancer, cancer free for sixteen years

Pancreatic cancer is usually a death sentence, but today, nine years after my original diagnosis, I would say I am cured. The reason I say this is because of a surgery I had in '95. I had a hernia in the abdominal area, and I had this surgery done by the same surgeon who had done my original cancer surgery. He looked at my pancreas and was amazed to see that it was clear. I know Dr. Gonzalez doesn't use the word cured, *but I do.*

Originally, the local oncologist in Kalamazoo told me there was nothing they could do. He said, "We can give you chemo but it doesn't really help." Then he suggested I go to the Mayo Clinic and see if there was anything new. We did and talked to the head of oncology there, who said there weren't any new alternative methods, so I went home thinking there was nothing available.

But my wife and I started searching, and one day we heard this guy talking on the radio about pancreatic cancer and it was Dr. Gonzalez on an NPR program called Sunday Rounds. *I listened for a while and then a lightbulb went off, and I said "There's my guy." My father was living in New York, so I went and stayed with him. I knew I didn't have a whole lot of options at this point, and what Dr. Gonzalez said made sense, so I went with it. I thought his theory of cancer—that it was a failure of the immune system to react properly—made sense.*

As Dr. Gonzalez laid out the program, I thought, If this is what it takes, this is what I am going to do. I dove right in. My wife was behind me, and we did everything the way he told us to do. We called him back a lot to be sure we were doing it right. He's so dedicated to this.

My diet wasn't horrible before I was diagnosed, but I did drink too much pop, too many sweets, so we cut all of that out, and of course we cut out anything white.

You know, when you have cancer you try to figure out where you got it. I was exposed in my work to asbestos and some of the electrical transformers on poles that contain some really bad stuff—that's the only thing I can think of.

Eating this way now is great. I always feel good and I will eat healthy like this for life.

When people come to me for advice I say, "Look to Dr. Gonzalez first." I watched my mother go through traditional cancer treatment and die. That was my biggest fear when I had cancer. I thought, I hope I don't have to go through what she went through. I was even kind of relieved when they said, "There is nothing we can do."

I feel lucky to have found Dr. Gonzalez's program. I was with my gastroenterologist recently and he said, "Well, it's either a miracle or it's Dr. Gonzalez." I think it's Dr. Gonzalez because I started getting better from day one. It was pretty amazing. I live a happy life; I have a great wife and a lot of interests. I play in a couple of bands in the area. I have a sailboat and we sail out on Lake Michigan . . . so life is good.

—David Johnson, pancreatic cancer, cancer free for nine years

I was diagnosed with invasive breast cancer seventeen years ago, and the MRI clearly showed two lesions on the bone, one on each leg bone. To get a reliable biopsy would have meant taking a chunk out of the bone and putting in hardware to make the bones strong enough. It was a big deal and I didn't want to do that.

I did agree to a lumpectomy, and then I talked to the orthopedic doctor about the leg, and he pushed to do the biopsy. I asked him, "What are those things on my leg bone?" and he said, "Tumors." And he also said he expected it to be cancer. And then he asked me how I wanted to proceed. I told him that tomorrow I had an appointment with a physician who treats cancer metabolically. The doctor smiled and said, "Wonderful." He gave me my X-rays and wished me luck. I think he was grateful to have me go elsewhere so he didn't have to watch me die. I think he genuinely thought it was my best shot.

When I got the news that the mammogram was not good, first thing I did was pull out Max Gerson's book, and simultaneously my mom ran into a patient of Dr. Gonzalez's, so it was serendipitous, meant to be. We went to see him, which was a very good decision for me.

I was familiar with his protocol, but when I got home that first night I just kind of sat there at the table, overwhelmed. I had been on Premarin for quite some time, and of course I had to stop that, and as a result I crashed emotionally. I didn't have any hormones to make me feel good.

A few years into the Gonzalez program a chiropractor did an adjustment on me and cracked some ribs. Just like that, Dr. Gonzalez said, "I didn't realize it was that bad," so he put me on bioidentical hormones, which I have been taking ever since.

I'm not going to say I became twenty years old again, but I began to feel as though I was back in my own body again. I didn't feel this self-hatred that I was all swollen and ugly. It's hard to describe.

I believe I got cancer from this cruddy environment we all live in. But being on the Gonzalez program has been the greatest thing in my life. I have energy; I can run down to the end of the walk. I feel I'm part of life, rather than watching it; so many are just watching life. I paint for enjoyment. I haven't settled into what I'm going to do in retirement because unfortunately my partner came down with cancer just around the time I retired. He did not survive; he did what he could with the Gonzalez program, but it didn't save him. That's the sad fact of cancer. It kills, and some people die. That took a couple of years of our life. But I always believed this program was going to work for me. Maybe my partner didn't really believe it. Belief is very important in healing.

I don't feel that I am cured. We are managing my cancer. My numbers seem to go up when I get stressed, so I know that it is still in me. But with the diet and the enemas and the enzymes and the belief that I am well, I am managing it, and I don't think it is ever going to give me any more problems. After all, it's been seventeen years.

—Carol Wycoff-Fields, invasive breast cancer,
cancer free for seventeen years

Chapter 9

DR. JAMES FORSYTHE

Cancer patients suffer twice: first with fear and suffering caused by their disease, and second from the ravages of a malignant system that forces toxic drugs of dubious value on frightened and gullible people.

—Majid Ali, M.D.

Dr. James Forsythe is a Renaissance man in the area of cancer treatment. He is a board-certified oncologist and also a board-certified homeopath, which makes for an interesting mix of Western and alternative medicines. The combination of the two allows Dr. Forsythe to be extremely creative in his approach to cancer. He is an integrative oncologist providing, in his words, "the best of what both worlds have to offer."

Today, Dr. Forsythe enjoys a successful career as a medical oncologist who utilizes alternative treatments, and patients flock to him from all over the world for his cutting-edge treatments.

SS: So nice to meet you, Dr. Forsythe. Tell me how you got started in medicine.

JF: I did my undergraduate studies at the University of California, Berkeley, and graduated in 1960. There's a movie called *Berkeley in the Sixties* which said that this was the last normal graduating class from Berkeley, so we were before all the freedom movements, the antiwar movements, the women's movement, and all the angst that came about at that time. When I was there it was more like an Ivy League school. I then was accepted into medical school across the bay, at the University of California, San Francisco [UCSF].

After graduation in 1964, the war was heating up in Vietnam, so I decided to go into a pathology residency at Tripler Army Hospital in Honolulu, Hawaii. I felt that it would be a good background for just about any specialty. I became an army pathologist and eventually did end up in Vietnam for a year in 1969. I was head of several laboratories, head of malaria control, tropical medicine, blood banking, and forensic pathology. I had quite an experience in Vietnam. I came close to death a couple of times, went down on a Chinook helicopter when we were treating refugees on an island, and somewhere in all those close calls I decided I didn't want to spend my life as a pathologist. I'm a people person, so I went into internal medicine residency in San Francisco.

From there I decided I wanted to go into the new field of medical oncology. There were only a few drugs, as you know, at that time for treating cancers, so I entered a fellowship at UCSF and became certified in medical oncology. I practiced in San Francisco for a couple of years and saw the first cases of AIDS and didn't really know what was going on. We were all befuddled. We thought they were being poisoned, maybe heavy metals in the water system or something; we couldn't figure it out. If you read the book *And the Band Played On*, you know how difficult it was in those days to diagnose that disease.

SS: Well, actually about thirteen of my books ago, I wrote *Wednesday's Children*, where I interviewed Randy Shilts, who wrote that book, about AIDS and what was going on at that time.

So then what happened? Where did you go?

JF: I moved to Reno, where they had no oncologists. So I set up cancer wards at the three existing local hospitals and was medical director of the VA hospital medical oncology program. I also taught at the University of Nevada, Reno, as an associate professor of medicine. After treating thousands of patients and having a very large practice (being the only one in town), I became concerned and depressed by my patients' long-term results. After five, seven, or ten years, counting the number of surviving patients was hard to do. I mean, I thought I was doing everything right. Yet I knew I was creating toxicity, and often without benefits.

SS: It says a lot about you that you felt disappointed in the treatment you had learned. Tell me about your work today.

JF: Well, I got interested in homeopathics because in Nevada they had homeopathic and naturopathic boards, and I started to see that cancer patients from the alternative therapies were getting impressive results. And these doctors did not follow the usual paradigm that I was used to: surgery, radiation, and chemotherapy. These cancer patients were getting alternative treatments and doing better than many of my patients. That's when I decided I had to study this more, and started going to conferences. Eventually, I purchased an alternative/homeopathic clinic, took my state boards, and became a certified homeopathic doctor.

I felt by taking my boards I would be protected and would also be able to push the envelope into the area of integrative oncology and do other things mainstream oncologists couldn't do, which is to give dietary supplements and vitamins intravenously. I also wanted to do outcome-based studies on alternative treatments, which were precious and few at the time. In the nineties there were almost no studies on alternative treatments for cancer.

SS: So now you are an integrative doctor?

JF: I'm what's called an integrative medical oncologist. I trained at UCSF, University of California at San Francisco, and they now have a department of integrative oncology, so I don't think I am that far out from mainstream medicine, professionally speaking.

SS: What I am getting from interviewing all of you wonderful doctors is that we can protect ourselves from getting cancer. And walking the fence between conventional and alternative seems to give the doctor more options. Is that correct?

JF: Absolutely. It is a tightrope and sometimes a minefield. I am dually boarded. I have my medical license and homeopathic license in the state of Nevada. I have to follow the medical board's regulations, as well as those of the board of homeopathic medicine. Some treatments which are legal under homeopathic regulations are not under the provisions of Chapter 630 of the Nevada Revised Statutes, which regulates the practice of medicine in Nevada. So I have to be very careful. I have found a compromise so that I can accomplish my clinical medical investigations and keep all transparent.

Physicians in the community know what I do, and some respect it; others do not. I get patients from all over the world, from as far away as Perth, Australia, who are searching for more integrative cancer treatments.

SS: I think people are fed up. I think we are all watching these horrible deaths by chemotherapy and are realizing that the war on cancer is a dismal failure. The *New York Times* recently said as much.

JF: You are right. In the 2004 *Journal of Oncology* a large retrospective study showed that any patient entering into a five-year chemotherapy program in the United States has a 2.1 percent chance of surviving after that five-year period. In Australia results are similar. So if you were to enter chemo today, in 2014 only two out of one hundred patients would be alive. That's nothing to brag about.

SS: Is this what happened to you? Is it what made you change the way you approach cancer?

JF: You know, Suzanne, it's much easier to be a conventional oncologist, because you just tell the patient to be in the infusion center on Monday and the protocol is recommended. We give them their dose schedule and we don't deviate. As an oncologist doing it this way, you'll never get in trouble even if the patient dies from your treatment. But if you go outside the box at all and add vitamins or anything alternative, that's when the criticism comes down on you. It's just much easier for oncologists to follow the straight party line.

SS: But if the outcomes are so dismal, it's hard to believe that so many doctors are still walking that party line. I guess the pressure is so intense and medical school is so arduous and difficult, it's hard to return to school to learn something new. I am not impressed with that aspect of traditional medicine. I understand we're all human, but my great respect is for doctors like you who have stood back and courageously said, "Hey, it's not working."

What kind of successes have you had?

JF: I've done studies on a number of natural supplements, including a substance called pawpaw from Nature's Sunshine. It's from the pawpaw tree in the southeastern United States and it affects the energetics of the cancer cell. It is now used internationally and even in animal cancers.

After that I became intrigued with Poly-MVA, which is a complex of palladium and lipoic acid. It's a tightly bound complex of both of these substances, plus it's got a number of vitamins. It comes as a liquid. I kept meeting people at alternative conferences who have been on this treatment and said, "You've got to study this—my cancer's been in remission for over five years."

But individual case studies hold no credence. No conventional medical oncologist would take an individual case seriously. So we got 225 patients to participate, all with stage IV cancers, and Dr. Albert Sanchez out of San Diego supplied the Poly-MVA free to my patients. At five years out, our response rate is much better than conventional chemotherapy, which is at 2 percent. We are getting 35 percent to 40 percent survivorship, and these are all stage IV cancers. This excellent response rate does not carry with it any adverse side effects on any organ system in the body, even five years later.

After that study was completed I was introduced to a new homeopathic remedy called Salicinium. This product was discovered by a retired chemistry professor at the University of Nevada, Reno, and marketed by Perfect Balance. Actually the name is glyco-benzaldehyde, sometimes known as "Chinese aspirin." It has some actions similar to laetrile but doesn't have the toxicity of laetrile. It's very nontoxic. I've been doing studies on this now for over four years. We have 350 patients, all with stage IV cancers, and our responders are especially high in breast and prostate cancers, having over an 85 percent response in prostate cancer, stage IV, at four years out.

SS: How are you combining conventional and alternative therapies at this time?

JF: We give our natural product Salicinium in a loading dose in the Forsythe Immune Therapy, an intravenous cocktail where we give a number of immunoboosting substances; and then we send them home on oral Salicinium, which includes six capsules a day until their tumor is in remission. We've seen no toxicity with any of these alternative therapies. Sometimes I use very low-dose chemotherapy with the treatment or use insulin-potentiated therapy. The insulin is given along with low-dose chemo—by low-dose I mean 10 to 20 percent of the usual dose—so it's very nontoxic.

SS: Why do you do this?

JF: Because cancer cells are so rich in insulin receptors on their surface. It's kind of like a smart bomb. When you give this mixture intravenously along with the low-dose chemo, the cancer cell thinks that a simple sugar is available, so the cell becomes very receptive, opens its pores, and is more accessible to the low-dose chemo.

SS: So it tricks the cancer?

JF: Yes. Cancer cells only thrive on simple sugars. They cannot metabolize complex carbohydrates, fats, or proteins.

SS: So you put your cancer patients on a sugar-free diet?

JF: Yes, of course, a very strict low to no-simple-sugar diet. It's very difficult because that means no fruit also. We stress alkalinization, which is a big factor: alkaline water and the green powders that contain wheatgrass, ryegrass, barley grass, and algae. These substances alkalinize the body. Cancer cells thrive in an acid environment, and they don't do well when the body is more alkaline.

We also talk about various oxidative therapies which can be helpful, such as ozone, hydrogen peroxide, or hyperbaric chambers, and then we talk about the fact that the cancer cell is a low-energy system. As I describe it to my patients, it's like outside patio lights, which are low-voltage, and if you were to turn up the voltage on those transformers you'd burn out the system. Cancer cells produce 5 percent of the energy of a normal cell. Poly-MVA works on the energetics, the pawpaw works on the energetics, the Salicinium blocks the sugar metabolism called anaerobic glycolysis.

SS: Do you approach each patient exactly the same or is this individualized? Do you take their genetics into account? Is it all about the differences in the severity of each individual's cancer, or is it the age of the patient?

JF: I take all those things into account, and I always give them options. Because I am a conventional board-certified oncologist, I offer conventional protocol chemo first. Basically, I do that because it is a legality. I am required by law to offer "standard of care." I once had an FDA agent tell me that I was depriving patients of the benefit of conventional chemo, and I kind of had to laugh under my breath at that. That's how they think. I offer the low-dose chemo with the Salicinium. The third option would be to do the two different agents which vector in differently; this is Salicinium and Poly-MVA.

The Poly-MVA is given orally and the Salicinium is given in a three-week loading dose, where they get two hours of IV a day for three weeks. Then they go to the oral.

SS: So essentially, a patient comes in and you are required by law to first offer "standard of care."

JF: I have to do that, right.

SS: But if I were coming to you, let's say, with stage IV pancreatic cancer and I tell you I don't want chemotherapy, would you take me as a patient?

JF: Absolutely, but I would certainly chart that the patient refuses conventional chemo. That way I am covered.

SS: Would you be happy to treat me that way?

JF: Absolutely. In fact, very few patients I see come in for conventional therapy. They know what I do and they are not in my office for conventional. Less than 5 percent are requesting conventional therapy only.

SS: Your greatest successes have been with what types of cancer?

JF: In the Salicinium study, breast, prostate, and lung cancers were all high responders. We've treated 350 cases with leukemia, bladder, brain, breast, colorectal, esophagus, gastric, gallbladder, head and neck, mesothelioma, melanoma, gliomas, all the Hodgkin's and non-Hodgkin's lymphomas, ovarian, uterus, pancreas, prostate, renal cell, sarcoma, testis, and thyroid cancers. All of these are in stage IV—widely disseminated.

SS: Not much left. What patient comes to you whom you have to turn away?

JF: That's a tough call and it's really hard to do. If they have a brain tumor and their cognitive function is poor and they can't understand what we are offering, we have to turn them away. If they are having un-controlled seizures, we have to turn them away. If they have an inconti-nency problem and can't be in the infusion room with other patients, then we have to do other things. Sometimes we just have to put them on oral treatments and not do the IV.

SS: What if patients come in who have been horribly chemotherapied and radiated and they look like Holocaust survivors and they cannot eat? Can you treat them?

JF: We can do things to stimulate their appetite. Of course there are the marijuana pills, Marinol; there are progesterone capsules. There are things we can do. Our advanced cancer patients are often hormonally de-ficient and are experiencing adrenal burnout. This requires adrenal corti-cal hormonal support with bioidentical adrenal hormones. Oftentimes once their cancer starts going into remission, their appetite will come back. But a patient who has been on long-term radiation or chemo can have any-thing from chemo brain to painful neuropathy, cardiomyopathies, renal failure, liver failure, severe cytopenias, lung fibrosis, devastating fatigue, anorexia and wasting syndromes, osteoporosis, osteoarthritis, severe rashes from some of the targeted therapies, and even death. Many patients who have been treated with platinum-containing drugs are platinum toxic when tested by hair analysis. This fact goes unknown and untreated by most conventional oncologists.

Unfortunately, those are the long-term benefits of so-called conven-tional chemo, and we just don't see that with our alternative therapies.

SS: Is cancer manageable?

JF: Yes, it is. You can manage it, especially certain bone cancers, lym-phoma, Hodgkin's disease; breast cancer is very manageable . . . prostate cancer, certainly. Some of the cancers that are obviously more difficult to manage would be liver cancer, gallbladder, pancreas, but not impossible. We have had successes with all cancers.

SS: Now that I realize chemosensitivity tests exist, it feels uncon-scionable that chemotherapy would ever, ever be administered without testing first to find out if the chemo is even compatible with the specific cancer.

JF: If you came to our office and wanted chemo, we would absolutely send your blood to Germany or Greece, where they do chemosensitivity testing. They harvest the cancer cells out of your blood, break them down genetically, and then find which markers are compatible with treatment of your tumor. Then you get a report back in about a two-week period which will show the best drugs for your particular cancer, the intermittent drugs, and the drugs to stay away from that aren't going to be effective in any way in treating your specific cancer.

SS: Hallelujah. I've been waiting for someone to say this. I know there are two doctors in southern California that do this testing, Robert Nagourney and Larry Weisenthal.

JF: Yes, but they have to get tumor samples. And you can't always get tumor samples, especially if it's in the bone, lung, liver, or colon. That is why the German and Greek tests are so valuable because it's all done on whole blood.

Just as another example, I had another patient from Sacramento who six months ago had been on a heavy-duty chemo protocol called FOL-FOX (containing oxaliplatin, 5FU, and Avastin). We found out from the German chemosensitivity test that two out of the three of those drugs were completely ineffective against his cancer cells. I switched him over to a sensitive drug and he's now out playing golf three days a week and his liver has cleared up completely on recent follow-up scans.

SS: You must feel really good about what you're doing.

JF: It keeps me going.

SS: When I look at orthodox oncology, I think about those doctors who worked and studied so hard to learn how to treat this, and they must go home every day frustrated because of the dismal outcome.

JF: It is very rewarding and energizing to go to an alternative medicine meeting as opposed to conventional cancer meetings. Conventional cancer meetings are dismal. You listen to the talks and you see their survival rates are two to three months longer than before, and they are all so proud of that. They never mention a word about alternative treatments; they are afraid to mention any vitamin therapy or any supplements. It's just a terrible experience because you know they must know there is a better way.

SS: Do they ever make the connection between the cancer rate and what we are eating?

JF: Never. It's not a factor in mainstream cancer therapy. But it is extremely important. You can never underestimate the importance of diet in beating cancer. It's everything. For every cancer we have a group of supplements that are for prostate, breast, lung, colon, and rectal that we feel are most helpful for them. They take that little packet every day and they have that as the backbone of the basic supply of supplements.

SS: I would imagine it's important for a patient who chooses your protocol not to get careless.

JF: You know, cancer patients are the most compliant patients in the world. They are so dedicated to getting well, for the most part. They stop their bad behavior. Many of them will stop smoking, stop drinking, they will change their diet, they'll do anything—and they are very motivated to do the right thing because they want to get well.

SS: What do you want to say to people who are going to be diagnosed with cancer in the next few years, because we know there is an epidemic? How would you assuage their fears?

JF: I think the main thing is to take charge of their own health, just as you have done, Suzanne, and as many of my patients have done. Don't let the doctors dictate to you what has to be done. Seek second opinions, especially from alternative doctors, if you have the ability to do so. And think very hard about your lifestyle, your diet, your supplements, your exercise, and your personal stresses. Try to get your stress under control, and remember what I said earlier—that any improvement in quality of life is directly proportional to the improvement in your overall response.

So even if you don't respond completely to the treatment, if your disease is stable, it's never going to kill you. It can metamorphose into a chronic, livable condition where you basically live in a symbiosis with the cancer, and you learn to live with it and it does not dominate your life or kill you.

Those are the important things. Remember that the alternative therapies do not have all the toxicities of the unholy triad of surgery, radiation, and chemotherapy. You've got to remember that you must preserve your immune system and build it up. Learn that the body is self-healing if it has the right tools.

SS: Do you dream that one day alternative medicine will be an equal force and that insurance will pay for it?

JF: I dream about it, but I'm not yet real hopeful. I'm sorry. I wish I was more positive, but I just don't see it happening with the incipient national health program. The German health system at least allows it. So I would have to say that Germany is more enlightened. But we in the alternative world are having major successes, and people are starting to realize that cancer can be managed without taking the life force out of you. And that many, many patients who have embraced alternative cancer therapies are living long, happy, normal, healthy lives. That's what keeps me going and that's what keeps me feeling good about what I do.

SS: Thank you so much, and continued success.

DR. FORSYTHE'S PATIENTS IN THEIR OWN WORDS

I was diagnosed in April of 2008. I live in Oklahoma. I didn't want to treat my cancer in any orthodox way. I had a friend, a Ph.D. at Oklahoma University, and he treated me with essential oils, oil of oregano, and others. And really that's all I did, and I was fine until my mother died. It was so stressful, and that stress brought the cancer back. So I had heard about Dr. Forsythe and decided his treatment agreed with my philosophy—using the best from both worlds—so I went to his clinic and stayed for the first three weeks of February. At that time he gave me Salicinium. This was in two IV drips. We did this for three weeks and we also did fractionalized chemos, but when I went back to Oklahoma, no one wanted to do fractionalized chemos; they only wanted to do the regular chemo. In fact, my oncologist said, "It's either my way or the highway," and I said, "No, it's not. This is my body."

That oncologist kept pushing, and then she says, "Even if you do this, you have a 25 to 30 percent chance you are going to die." But I wouldn't budge. And then she said, with tears rolling down her face, "Without it you have a 95 percent chance you're going to die. You have stage IV breast cancer." But I said, "I want quality of life." I don't agree with poisons. Around this time we had those tornados that killed nine people, and the stress activated my cancer again. So I went back to Dr. Forsythe and decided I was going to stay until we got rid of this thing.

Now I'm doing real good. I take Salicinium and Poly-MVA, just four tablespoons of that twice a day, and of course my diet is real good. He also found that I have "leaky gut," meaning everything is just pouring out into my bloodstream; in fact, I had a doctor in Dallas tell me that I have the worst-looking blood he's ever seen, which is type A blood, real thick. You don't want to have thick blood. That's when I thought I had better do this German blood test, even though it was kind of expensive. But I thought, This is my life. I was worried about spending this money, and my husband said, "Quit worrying about me, and quit worrying about money. Just do what you have to do to take care of yourself." So that helped me with my burdens. Having a support like that helps a lot.

I have always been into natural medicine; we never use any kind of drug medicine at all. So this was just the natural way for me to go. I knew I had to kill this thing in me, but Dr. Forsythe's program was not so harsh. There were no terrible side effects. In fact, I felt good during my treatments. Since I changed my diet, my blood is not thick anymore; my allergies are gone; I don't have those terrible sinus headaches anymore.

I love Dr. Forsythe's clinic. I like his way of doing things, his manner; he makes me feel secure. My blood work is looking real good. I will come back for treatments for as long as it takes. I'm alive and feeling good and I have quality of life. I also believe in him. I believe I'm going to get well.

I love that man. He's been through the wringer but he just keeps on with his incredible work. He's a comfort. He cares. And in the medical field you rarely get that. And I have quality of life while I am managing my cancer.

—Sharon Hancock, stage IV breast cancer

I had or have prostate cancer, however you want to look at it; I was diagnosed in 1996, thirteen years ago. My PSA was 71.5—pretty high, not good. At this point it was stage IV, so I started to take Zoladex, Lupron, and Casodex. I am a veteran, so I was going to the veterans hospital over there and the doc said don't take any supplements or anything, but my PSA started to go up again.

Then I heard about Dr. Forsythe from a friend of mine, and he started treating me with low-dose chemo and homeopathics, like very large doses of vitamin D, 10,000 units a day, SAM-e, and a lot of other supplements.

Today my liver functions are fine and I'm doing well. I run a mile a day without the slightest struggle, and I am eighty years old. Yes, I run around with a lot of energy all the time. People tell me I look twenty years younger than my years. I need hormones and when I was on the Zoladex it blocked all hormone production. With Dr. Forsythe, he gets you off the drugs real fast. Only take them when the numbers go up and then the rest is management with supplements and diet.

Dr. Forsythe is very thoughtful and careful with his patients, making sure I don't feel pain whenever we do treatments. When I was in the veterans hospital they would stick a needle in my stomach, which was excruciating.

Dr. Forsythe understands supplements. My daughter is an M.D. and she takes supplements and says there is a place for them, and that alternative and traditional medicine should be working together and not fighting one another. Dr. Forsythe gets a lot of flak for his approach, but I'm living proof that you can live with and manage cancer and utilize the best of both worlds.

Remember, I had stage IV cancer—I should have been dead. If I had listened to my original M.D., there is no doubt in my mind that I would be

*dead. Dr. Forsythe has changed my life. My diet is great now because of him.
I eat the right kinds of food and I exercise. My wife fixes me a cocktail of
blackberries and yogurt, half of a pomegranate, orange juice, and wheat germ
every day. That's the only sugar I have, even though Dr. Forsythe warned me
to stay away from sugar because it feeds cancer.*

*Dr. Forsythe saved my life. I feel like I got a second shot and I also consider
him a personal friend. I don't consider myself cured; I consider myself as
someone who is managing their cancer. Sometimes I have to get one of those
hormone blockers when my PSA goes up, but it is only for a short time and
then things go back to normal. We are managing my cancer. But right now I
don't have any symptoms. People think I'm the fountain of youth. And I
don't know what you are doing, Suzanne, but from the look of the picture on
the front of your book, you look like you could win a beauty contest.*

—Miles Oliver, stage IV prostate cancer, diagnosed 1996

*I was diagnosed with large-cell carcinoma lung cancer, stage IV, which is
pretty much a death sentence. They gave me six months to a year to live, and
this was diagnosed at UC Davis. It was terrifying, frightening . . . very scary.
Then I happened to be watching TV and a show called* Health Watch, *and
there was Dr. Forsythe. He was talking about how they did low-dose
chemotherapy along with alternative medicine. This intrigued me, and I
called him. And the first words he said to me when I was in his office were
"You're going to do okay." This was just like the beginning of a new world.*

*At this point I had not had chemotherapy or radiation; frankly, they told
me at UC Davis to go home and live the best life I could with the time I had
left. They did say that if I took chemotherapy I would have a 10 percent
chance. But I knew that meant 10 percent of a bad quality of life. My
advantage was that I came to Dr. Forsythe with a clean body, not messed up
with chemicals and poison like so many other cancer patients.*

*The first thing Dr. Forsythe did was an infusion. It was his own formula
with multiple medicines in it. I took Iscador shots plus homeopathic shots
with lots of vitamin C, Bs, E, and flax oils and bioflavonoids plus three pills
and shark cartilage. They had me juice broccoli and anything else green. He
was making my body strong enough to fight this horrible disease. I did this
regimen for three weeks straight until my body was built up enough to
introduce me to low-dose chemotherapy. I did this for six years straight,
nonstop.*

*The drugs in low dose I was given to my now built-up, strong body were
Taxotere, Adriamycin, Paraplatin, Navelbine. The last two bring my sugar*

levels down as low as they can go before they inject you with chemo, because that cancer really likes sugar.

Today I take a fortifier, which is their immune booster, and Salacinium. And the vitamins and minerals and herbs that they prescribe for me. Plus they stress diet, which is very, very important. I know for a fact when I blow my diet, my tumor markers go high. When he tells me they are going up, I already know what I did—been eating ice cream and cakes and such. Remember, I had stage IV breast cancer. This is a matter of life or death for me. And so far I'm alive and feeling good; I feel normal. It's been nine years.

I trust Dr. Forsythe. I never questioned him. I told him whatever he felt he could do to help me I was willing to do, and I meant it.

I don't feel that my cancer is cured; I feel like I am managing my cancer, which is pretty exciting. If I continue my regimen and stay on my diet, I can manage this thing for a long, long time. It's exciting to know that I am in control. I was stage IV when they removed tumors as big as golf balls in the lungs. It had spread through my body and I was told I had six months to live. When I met Dr. Forsythe, it all just made more sense than the strong poisons the others were offering me. I wanted to live, I still had grandchildren I wanted to see, and thankfully, now that has come true. I am fifty-four years old, I was diagnosed at forty-five, and I know that I got this from household chemicals and the chemicals I used when I worked. But now I feel like I have gotten a second chance at life. I have two grandchildren, one seven, one eight, and I was able to see my son graduate from high school.

I feel special, I really do, because I was fortunate enough to live close by a doctor that was able to do this for me, and I feel this has saved my life. I have a normal life and a family I love, and I am with them.

—Marilyn Harrowsmith, stage IV lung cancer

Chapter 10

DR. JULIE TAGUCHI

Dr. Julie Taguchi is my personal oncologist. She is a mainstream doctor, so it might surprise you that I would have chosen to work with someone who is enmeshed in "standard of care." But Dr. Taguchi believes in the importance of honoring the wishes of the patient. My choice was to treat my breast cancer with bioidentical hormones and nutrition (after surgery and radiation), but I needed the guidance of a professional to monitor and test to be sure my body was responding. I am a part of a study she has conducted of women who have chosen to treat their cancer with bioidentical hormones rather than chemotherapy. For me this is the best decision I have ever made. Most of the other women in the study have done equally well, but as with all cases of cancer, there are no guarantees.

Dr. Taguchi is thorough, smart, and open. I love her as my doctor, and I'm sure you will be enlightened by her observations.

SS: Hi, Julie. You are my oncologist and we are good friends, but you are a mainstream oncologist who has been conducting a study of fifty-five women with breast cancer who have chosen to use bioidentical hormones as a means of preventing a cancer recurrence. I know I am feeling great—perfect, in fact; how are the rest of the women in your study doing?

JT: Please, before I answer that question, let me explain why I undertook this observational study. From 2002 until 2008, I have been observing women treated for breast cancer and ductal carcinoma in situ or "pre–breast cancer," who also have desired to take bioidentical compounded transdermal and pharmaceutical-grade estradiol and progesterone in the name of quality of life.

SS: Right, but this is unusual for a mainstream oncologist. That is my point. Why did you undertake this study?

JT: Because women with cancer are desiring quality of life and there is a theory that bioidentical hormones taken properly are protective.

My study includes over a hundred women in total, but fifty-five of them are on a unique, specific, compounded, physiological, rhythmic, cyclical transdermal protocol that has never been studied. This program differs by way of dose (more than traditionally prescribed compounded products) and schedule in the attempt to mimic a woman's reproductive cycle.

SS: What kind of cancer did these women have?

JT: These women had different types, stages, and treatments for breast cancer, but they all wanted to feel better or "feminine" for whatever time they had left on this planet. The average length of use is nearly four years now, and most women are doing well. However, to be accurate, there are a few who have had relapses or new breast cancers or other medical complications which may or may not be due to just hormones.

SS: Please explain.

JT: Okay . . . Let me share some details regarding what we call "serious adverse events." Three women with involved lymph nodes and estrogen-receptor-positive breast cancer at diagnosis progressed to stage IV or became metastatic at one, three, and four years, and all are alive and doing well now.

Two of the three were treated with chemo, two only with radiation, one with aromatase inhibitors for a year. Currently, all stopped the hormones, and only one of the three is on an antiestrogen pill.

SS: What happened?

JT: Three of the women developed new early estrogen-receptor-positive breast cancers at two and three years. The two new tumors that were discovered at two years were actually present at the time of their original breast cancers but only in hindsight were present on imaging. Two of these women are back on BHRT [bioidentical hormone replacement therapy] and the other on the estrogen inhibitor.

SS: Back on BHRT because of quality-of-life issues?

JT: Yes, they just feel terrible without them. One seventy-six-year-old woman with type 2 diabetes was on hormones for five years but since her treatment experienced an uncomplicated heart attack.

Another seventy-four-year-old woman was treated for stage 1 breast cancer, was on BHRT for six years, and survived a pulmonary embolism, or blood clot to the lung, of unclear etiology. We agreed to stop her BHRT, since we didn't know if there was a contribution. But three months later, after she was off BHRT and on blood thinners, she died suddenly.

SS: Was this related to BHRT or coincidental?

JT: Don't know. So in terms of breast cancer, within one and a half to four years of traditional treatment of some sort, there are six new or progressive tumors out of fifty-five women on this particular BHRT program.

SS: Six out of fifty-five is actually pretty impressive. The others are getting the protection and they get to feel good and "of life." I'm impressed.

JT: It is impressive. In my practice, there are women who have been on synthetic estradiol patches and oral progesterone and have also developed new breast cancers within two years.

There are women who have completed breast cancer treatment and never used HRT [hormone replacement therapy] and either progressed or come down with a new cancer, so you just don't know why some survive and why some don't.

SS: What about women who have had "standard of care" surgery, radiation, and chemotherapy?

JT: In this study there are women who have been treated with everything—bilateral mastectomies, chemotherapy, and radiation—who still progress to stage IV while taking an antiestrogen. No one guarantees that a treatment provides complete risk reduction.

SS: In your view, are bioidentical hormones protective?

JT: Can't say. We don't have enough data. Let me say this on prevention: the accepted conclusion about HRT (synthetic) is that there is increased risk of breast cancer as documented by the Women's Health Initiative [WHI]. The WHI studied postmenopausal women who either took a placebo or Premarin alone if they had a hysterectomy or Premarin and Provera, synthetic drugs with hormonelike effects, not real hormones nor a natural replacement. Provera, which is more androgenic and estrogenic than progestogenic, was given daily; therefore no menses occurred.

It's important to understand that it was the Premarin-plus-Provera group that was stopped early due to increased incidence of breast cancer at a rate of 0.4 percent per year of use.

The Premarin-alone group did *not* have an increased risk of breast cancer. Further evaluation by Dr. Chlebowski, one of the investigators, even showed a slight risk reduction in the Premarin group, or if women in the placebo group had taken estrogen in the past! So there seems to be a subset of women who benefited from estrogen.

SS: Really? Horse estrogen? A pregnant mare's urine? A horse's estrogen has no compatibility with a human female's estrogen. I find this remarkable, or maybe just luck. Why wouldn't we rather take bioidentical hormones, an exact replica of what we make in our own bodies? Why bother with synthetic? Also, women on Premarin aren't cycling; therefore they are not mimicking nature.

JT: The risk for breast cancer is really more complex than we can understand at this time. I suppose if you have breasts, you are at risk.

You can reduce your risk of breast cancer by several modes such as multiple pregnancies starting early (before age twenty-eight; age twenty is even better) and then breast-feeding that baby for years, not three months, which is our U.S. average. We now have proof that diet and exercise also play a role in prevention, yet some of the healthiest women who had children early have had breast cancer, like you, Suzanne. So how you metabolize your hormones and the other lifestyle/environmental / hormonal interactions must also have an influence.

An interesting role for estrogen is controlling some gene methylation. You will hear more about this in the near future, if not already. But put simply, as one ages, genes can get hypermethylated (too much methylation) and then turned off. You don't really want to turn off a gene that protects you from developing cancer!

SS: Interesting. Dr. Burzynski also talks about this—that we have cancer-protective genes that get turned off by certain factors: aging, lifestyle, poor dietary habits, not managing stress, and exposure to toxicity. His belief is that we can turn these genes back on by reversing these factors, i.e., changing diet, sleeping, avoiding chemicals, and taking detoxifying antioxidants to keep up with the exposure, and by all means replacing lost hormones with natural bioidentical hormones.

Let's get specific—can you tell me about a few of these women in your study and their individual success stories?

JT: Absolutely. I have seen some pretty amazing results with this program, which has made me appreciate and respect the power of hormones.

Let's call this patient I.R. She is now seventy-six, but when she was diagnosed she was sixty-six with stage II node-positive breast cancer and was treated with a lumpectomy, radiation, chemotherapy, and tamoxifen for three years and an aromatase inhibitor for two years. At the end of her treatment, she was in a wheelchair because she hurt too much to walk. She couldn't exercise, so she gained weight, which is not a good thing for women with breast cancer.

SS: Why? Because of the estrogenic effects from her fat tissue?

JT: Yes. And weight gain also made her unhappy, as it would anyone. She could no longer shop or participate in family activities and she lost her independence. She also was no longer sexual as a result of her treatment and missed that in her marriage. She understood that estrogen would help, as she had been on estrogen before her cancer diagnosis. She began this compounded hormone protocol, and six years later, her pain lessened so she could walk, her depression and hot flashes improved, and she and her husband resumed their sexual relationship. She is now a very happy woman! She is also the one who survived the heart attack.

SS: What I'm hearing is that she is alive and "of life." That is huge.

JT: Let's call this next one A.A. She was fifty when she was told she had several cancers. After a mastectomy and complete node removal, chemotherapy for eight sessions, radiation, and one year of aromatase inhibitor, she was bedridden with pain. She also had a sleep disorder and fibromyalgia, which were worse. She stopped the aromatase inhibitor and although she felt a little better, she wasn't living well. She started estrogen and progesterone, and later DHEA and testosterone were added. Her sleep study resulted in her being given a new drug, which greatly improved her sleep. One year after being in bed most of the day, she was a competitive ballroom dancer! She was still dealing with joint and body pains, so human growth hormone [HGH] was started, since her IGF-1 levels were very, very low. The HGH definitely added to her quality of life. Three months into the HGH, I found one very tiny tumor under her skin that turned out to be breast cancer. So typically, we'd stop all hormones and treat her with an antiestrogen after removing the tumor and radiating the area. Well, after many discussions with several physicians, we decided to stop the estrogen; she declined radiation and agreed to take tamoxifen along with her other hormones including DHEA and HGH. Currently she is in remission two years later and is still competing on a national level.

SS: When women are diagnosed with breast cancer, they are immediately told to stop all hormones. So these fifty-five women are in essence crossing a line, because "standard of care" does not recognize nonpatentable natural hormones. What made you decide to go in this direction?

JT: As I said, I am a mainstream oncologist, so I always recommend "standard of care" for a breast cancer diagnosis. However, if a woman is suffering despite all of the possible interventions, then estrogen and progesterone are the only treatment that will restore the symptoms from estrogen loss. There are some women who will not take the antiestrogens to reduce a risk of metastatic relapse, like yourself. It is also my single ladies who are very concerned about the changes in their bodies and still hope to attract a lifelong mate. These women know that being sexual or hormonal is important and are willing to take the chance or risk. After being an oncologist for over twenty years, I give recommendations and explain why we give the treatment program we prescribe. However, if a woman wants hormones for quality of life versus lowering a risk of relapse or a new cancer, then who am I to judge them and prevent them from that informed decision? Smoking and drinking cost health care millions of dollars, and tobacco and alcohol are very accessible. Try getting estrogen for a woman with breast cancer history. Good luck!

SS: Well, that needs to be changed. I also feel that belief is a huge component. I believe that hormones put back in my body in youthful optimal ranges are protective. Young women don't get cancer unless there is some genetic aberration or exposure to environmental toxicity. So I believe that my youthful hormones keep me protected, as though my brain believes I am reproductive again and therefore, biologically, important as a reproducer.

JT: And that is your right to believe that theory.

I like compounded hormones because they are given twice a day or pulsed, and the dose can be easily adjusted. Replacing hormones in the pattern of a reproductive female just makes plain biological sense, but I know there is no data for that. In my observation, I see that there is a dose-response relationship to hormone replacement. Women on physiologic doses of estrogen and progesterone, for example, seem to have much better bone densities, like you, Suzanne.

SS: It is pretty amazing that at sixty-two I have zero bone loss, and before I started on bioidenticals I was showing signs of bone loss. Osteopenia. But now that has been restored. I can do handstands and backbends like a contortionist. Pretty cool.

JT: It is pretty remarkable. Some women who had been on several medications, including bone restoration meds, were able to discontinue their use due to BHRT replacement. The woman back on hormones felt better and had the interest to be part of life and started to exercise, eat well, dress more feminine, and sleep better. The weight loss and exercise are also known to reduce the risk of breast cancer relapse.

SS: When I was on *Oprah*, it was said that compounding pharmacies were not licensed and had no oversight.

JT: There are clear, valid issues regarding compounding hormones, and I do share the concerns with the FDA. So any compounding pharmacy has been able to mix a product and label it estrogen, but there is no standard or minimum or best way to make it. No one checks to see if it is the right concentration or the right product. One pharmacy can make estradiol, but it will be a different product if ordered from another pharmacy. The cost might be different also. So in a way they are correct—there is no standardization yet.

SS: Is it coming?

JT: It takes perseverance. We don't know the best site or method of application. There are so many different delivery possibilities: oral troches, skin gels. There has not been a head-to-head study of the different methods of delivery, but we know that the body responds to them differently. More research is needed and will have to come from government-sponsored sources, as no one except the compounded pharmacy will profit.

SS: Well then, forget it. That's not going to happen. No patent, no profits, no studies. Guess we have to find the highest-quality compounding pharmacists. I list the ones I have had interaction with at the back of this book.

Hormones restore quality of life. When you are fighting breast cancer there is a lot of residual stress; for me, stopping hormones was not going to happen. I did not want to become symptomatic, and I also had the firm belief from my own research that hormones are cancer protective if taken in the right ratios. Do you believe correct hormone replacement is cancer protective?

JT: I agree that many hormones, not just estradiol, are required for managing stress. Estradiol is the Xanax and Prozac for women! Did you know that depression is the leading diagnosis in women ages forty to fifty when estrogen is falling? Antidepressants and antianxiolytics can definitely help with symptoms, but there are many unwanted side effects. There is nothing, however, that can take the place of estrogen if a woman needs it.

So yes, for women and men who have a cancer diagnosis, certainly hormones can help with quality of life, and I have concluded from reading, not from a clinical trial, that hormones are protective in many ways.

But the common thinking in mainstream medicine is that hormone replacement for women with breast cancer is still a no-no.

SS: But these fifty-five women seem to be proving otherwise. I guess time will tell. It is my belief. Do you take bioidentical hormones and why?

JT: Yes, I do take bioidentical hormones. Nearly ten years ago I was having problems with a chronic shoulder/neck/back pain issue and discovered my hormones were low. I realize now that my hormones were low as a result of the pain and not sleeping. It wasn't until I started the physiologic, rhythmic program that my physical status improved dramatically. I learned something!

SS: Do you think oncology will change as a result of this study?

JT: No changes should be made based on this observational study of fifty-five. However, I think it is important to realize that being on hormones after a breast cancer diagnosis does not mean a death sentence, like you were told.

SS: There is a war on cancer that we don't seem to be winning. Do you feel you are onto something, that correct hormone replacement might factor in as a safe choice for women with cancer?

JT: Yes, I actually think that hormones—all hormones we know about now—are important for optimal, not "normal," levels, as our test result range tells us. I think optimizing hormones as we age will improve quality of life and, therefore, our health.

SS: How important are nutrition and supplementation and exercise?

JT: About as important as breathing. What we put in our mouths and how we move our bodies are actions we can control. This should empower us to reduce our cancer risks. Our foods are not as nutritious as they once were, so some supplementation is helpful. For everyone I recommend at least 5 to 7 grams of omega-3 fish oil and 2,000 IU or more of vitamin D_3 depending on levels.

SS: Why are hormones so misunderstood?

JT: Well, the "evil" estrogen has had a bad rap! Medicine had highlighted estrogen as the "bad gal" for breast cancer, which stems from several places. As mentioned earlier, blocking estrogen will cause metastatic estrogen-receptor-positive breast cancer to regress, but only temporarily, and adding estrogen blockers after surgery will reduce the risk of relapse over time. So estrogen must be bad, right? Early studies show increased estrogen exposure as a risk for breast cancer. Early menses and late menopause are risks, but why? Early and multiple pregnancies reduce risk of breast cancer, and then breast-feeding will add to that risk reduction. But did you know that having your first full-term pregnancy after age forty is a higher risk factor than not having a pregnancy at all? So what and when events happen between menses and menopause matters. Medicine hasn't really picked up on that; it's not very politically correct to promote pregnancies in the early twenties. Then add this question: Why don't all women who have breasts have breast cancer if estrogen by itself causes cancer? Because there are so many other factors involved and we don't know them all yet. Progestins—drugs with hormonelike functions, not real progesterone—have been implicated in risk for breast cancer. Now also coming to light is the role of insulin and insulinlike growth factors, metabolic syndrome, and chronic inflammation as etiologies of breast cancer and other cancers. We know obese women have a higher rate of endometrial and breast cancer, for example.

Estrogen is a wonderful hormone in charge of so many important bodily functions other than the obvious sex-related duties: mood, sense of well-being, sleep, good skin and hair (a sign of health, not vanity), cognition, digestion, blood pressure control, and on and on.

SS: You are preaching to the choir with me. I am experiencing all those great benefits, and as a result I am enjoying a better quality of life than I did when I was making my own hormones as a young person. It has made aging a positive for me: a little wisdom, perspective, sexuality, a working brain, and strong bones. How cool is that?

Tell me, Julie—what do you dream about?

JT: That we do a better job of preventing cancer and then that we treat tumors with specific targeted therapy. That we in medicine evaluate and treat patients as a system, instead of a body part, and maximize patients' health utilizing information gathered from all over the world.

SS: Thanks so much, Julie. You are a great friend and doctor.

Knock It Out

- We have cancer-protective genes that get "turned off" by certain factors: aging, poor lifestyle and dietary habits, stress, and exposure to toxicity. By reversing these factors, i.e., maintaining a good diet, sleeping, avoiding chemicals, and taking detoxifying antioxidants to keep up with the exposure—and replacing lost hormones with natural bioidentical hormones—we may be able to turn these genes back on.

- How you metabolize your hormones and the other lifestyle, environmental, hormonal interactions have an influence on your breast cancer risk. You can reduce the risk by having multiple pregnancies starting at an early age (before twenty-eight; twenty is even better) and then breast-feeding that baby for years, not months.
- The accepted conclusion about HRT (synthetic) is that there is increased risk of breast cancer as documented by the Women's Health Initiative. It's important to understand that it was the Premarin and Provera group that was stopped early due to increased incidence of breast cancer at a rate of 0.4 percent per year of use. The Premarin-alone group did *not* demonstrate an increased risk of breast cancer.
- There are women who have been treated with everything (bilateral mastectomies, chemotherapy, and radiation) who still progress to stage IV while taking an antiestrogen. No one guarantees that a treatment provides complete risk reduction.
- If a woman is suffering despite all of the possible interventions, then estrogen and progesterone are the only treatments that will address the symptoms from estrogen loss. If a woman wants hormones for quality of life versus lowering a risk of relapse or a new cancer, then she should be able to make that informed decision.
- The FDA has valid concerns regarding compounding hormones. Any compounding pharmacy has been able to mix a product and label it estrogen, but there is no standardization. More research is needed and will have to come from government-sponsored sources.

PART III

Preventing Cancer Before It Starts

Once seen as a possibility, it can never be unseen.

—Forrest Fenn, author of ten books, art historian, and philosopher

A little knowledge (which is what we call ignorance) is, in fact, a dangerous thing. Almost everyone, at least in the industrialized world, knows that drinking water from a filthy pond or polluted lake can cause life-threatening diarrhea, but still only a few realize that holding on to resentment, anger and fear, or eating fast foods, chemical additives and artificial sweeteners is no less dangerous than drinking polluted water; it may just take a little longer to kill a person than tiny amoeba can.

—Andreas Moritz

Chapter 11

DR. RUSSELL BLAYLOCK

I interviewed Russell Blaylock in my last book, *Breakthrough*, but this man has so much to say I felt he needed to be heard a second time.

I first became aware of Dr. Blaylock when I read his book *Natural Strategies for Cancer Patients*. Now, this was unusual—an oncologist, brain surgeon, and neuroscientist writing a book about natural strategies. Before I even spoke with him I knew this was one special man. Dr. Blaylock attended Louisiana State University School of Medicine in New Orleans, and completed his internship and neurosurgical residency at the Medical University of South Carolina in Charleston. After twenty-six years of practicing neurosurgery, in addition to having a nutritional practice, he has recently chosen to devote his full attention to nutritional studies and research. His newsletter is *Blaylock Wellness Report* (www.blaylock report.com). His goal is to supply cancer patients and their families with the latest in nutritional methods to boost the immune system and fight cancer. Simple things such as food preparation can make a critical difference in the ability to overcome the dreaded disease. He shares with us his vast knowledge of cancer-protective foods and which cancer-killers are in which fruits and vegetables.

Dr. Blaylock understands cancer from the inside out and how cancer cells differ from normal cells. He is convinced that if people are armed with enough smart information, they will understand the vital role nutrition plays in controlling and even eliminating cancer. His insights will give you food for thought.

SS: So nice to speak with you again, Russell. Last time we spoke for *Breakthrough*, I remember being emotional at the end of our interview. Your passion about the state of health, and in particular the cancer epidemic, was very moving. I know you are frustrated (and I think *frustrated* is too mild a word) at the present approach to cancer. I know you also believe that prevention is being ignored by practitioners everywhere. Is it out of ignorance or laziness?

RB: Mostly ignorance. Cancer prevention has been an interest of mine since well before medical school, and the connection between nutrition and health. I've spent my life studying it and looking at this aspect of prevention.

Initially, I went through the same thing most medical doctors experience as a result of what we are taught. I thought chemotherapy was the answer, the cure. You know, if they could just find the right agent. But then slowly I began to realize that the current approach to cancer is an absolute failure and that we were lying to patients. We were telling them that when they have metastatic cancer, their only chance of survival is a combination of chemotherapy and radiation.

But we know that once cancer metastasizes, conventional treatment won't do anything.

Doctors secretly talk among themselves about palliation, meaning to treat partially but not be able to cure, and patients don't know what that means. But when they ask us, we say it means it will make them more comfortable without poisoning them.

Well, if that's the goal, just to make you feel more comfortable, then we have ways to make a patient a lot more comfortable.

SS: As in it's better to just live out your life and enjoy what you have left?

RB: Well, there are all kinds of ways to be more comfortable, but they just don't tell the patients that. They don't tell them, "We're not trying to cure you, because we can't cure you." If you ask the doctor to his face, "Can this cure me?" he will have to say, "No, but I can make you more comfortable. This may give you an extra couple of months."

But I can give a cancer patient nutrients and a bunch of vitamins, and if I do the right ones, they can live a very long time. That's how powerful nutrients can be.

SS: You mean, for most of the cancers that are a real concern to the world, the present treatments are virtually ineffective?

RB: For leukemia, they have had real success, and also with some bone cancers. But if you look at the major cancers, the real killers—like lung, breast, prostate—they've made no significant inroads in reducing mortality. Plus, they are overdiagnosing cancers, meaning they are diagnosing a lot of cancers that never would have spread in the first place because they are very slow-moving and invading.

For instance, DCIS [ductile carcinoma in situ] breast cancer—in most cases this never metastasizes, never invades. And if you didn't know you had it, you could just go on living a normal life span.

SS: You mean mastectomies have been unnecessary for those women who have had DCIS?

RB: For the vast majority, yes. This is a big discussion among oncologists. You see it in their journals. They are overdiagnosing both prostate and breast cancers because we know if you look at a woman age fifty, about 40 to 45 percent of them will have breast cancer cells in their ducts. Most of them will never get breast cancer, or at least it won't spread. The same thing is true with male prostate cancer. You look at the majority of men age seventy, almost 70 percent of them have prostate cancer cells. If you don't look, far fewer than that will ever develop prostate cancer, maybe 2 or 3 percent, and these won't be aggressive prostate cancers.

SS: You are saying that if we didn't go through all this aggressive diagnosis of cancer, we would never have known these cancers existed, and the cancer rate would be much lower?

RB: Correct. By overdiagnosing, they improve their statistics. It makes it look like the war on cancer has made headway, when in truth they haven't made any headway. And then these poor patients go through all this hell, when, in fact, they had a prostate cancer that never would have escaped the prostate gland and never caused any problems. But now they've gone through this horrible surgery, radiation, ruined their bowel, ruined their bladder, and they have complications associated with it. All for a cancer that never would have caused them any problems.

SS: Why are they doing this?

RB: They're just not looking at the right things. Part of it is they are making a lot of money. Once these things get popular as diagnostic tests—like mammograms, for instance, which all the hospitals use—and you've got doctors who specialize in this technology, then all these things become big moneymakers. And then it feeds on itself.

> *There is evidence that mammograms are not really that diagnostic and may be inducing breast cancer, particularly in highly sensitive women. But so much money is being made, and so much money has been invested in these units in hospitals, that no one wants to admit the truth.*

The defenders come out and say mammograms are the greatest thing ever, and other physicians say if we don't have early diagnosis, we don't have anything. As an oncologist, I think to myself, Why? You can't cure it. Your chemotherapy is ineffective. And radiation doesn't work so well. So all they can talk about is early diagnosis.

But what these tests are telling us is that the diagnostics are really not that accurate, and they are causing a lot of women to have chemo and radiation for no reason at all. This is a big discussion in oncology journals, but the public never hears about it.

SS: I've heard that with the amount of radiation a woman receives with mammograms, if she started out at forty with no cancer, by the time she was fifty she would have increased her chances for cancer by radiation exposure by 30 percent. Is that true?

RB: Yes. The most conservative estimate is 1 percent per year. Another estimate is 3 percent a year. Some radiologists say it's even higher than that. But there is also a subgroup of women who have a strong family history of breast cancer, and their rates are infinitely higher than that. The reason they have a high risk factor is that they can't repair their DNA very well. They have BRCA1 and BRCA2 gene mutations, which is the gene that repairs DNA when it's damaged by radiation. For these women the same dosage of radiation given to women without the BRCA gene causes much more damage. It's probably equivalent to three, four, or five times the amount of radiation. For women with BRCA1 and BRCA2, mammograms can induce not only cancer but also a very aggressive cancer.

I've spoken to a number of women whose sisters didn't survive. They did the routine yearly mammograms, but because of strong family history they developed a very aggressive cancer and died within a year, and it was a type of cancer that was unresponsive to anything.

When you look at experimental studies with animals in which the researchers damage their DNA repair ability and radiate them, they develop very deadly, aggressive cancers. To me it doesn't make sense that we know this, and no one is talking about it.

SS: And women have yearly mammograms innocently, trusting, unaware of any danger.

RB: Yes, they don't want to talk about it because they know that person should never have gotten a mammogram in the first place, and these are precisely the women we are telling to get mammograms every six months.

SS: And women logically think that if they have a family history they should be diligent about mammograms.

RB: Right, because people don't understand radiation biology and most doctors don't understand radiation biology. But this is certainly known to the radiation oncologists.

SS: Does radiation work sometimes for the treatment of cancers?

RB: There are some cancers that are extremely rapidly dividing that are sensitive to radiation even in lower doses, and if the cancer is not widely metastasized, you can eradicate it. So it has some place.

SS: What kind of cancers are those?

RB: Hematologic cancers are sensitive to radiation, like myelomas and some liver tumors that are rapidly growing. Any rapidly growing tumor is radiosensitive. But the problem is if they are rapidly growing they also metastasize earlier, and they escape the radiation. The bad part is that the radiation is known to induce cancer, so then you worry if it is going to induce cancer in some other tissue, and that is always a concern.

With pregnant women just a couple of doses of pelvic X-ray will increase the risk of leukemia in their offspring dramatically, because that baby has been exposed to the radiation. We know at certain critical periods of life we dramatically increase the chances of cancer, and we know that a pregnant woman is much more sensitive to radiation effects than when not pregnant.

SS: Why is that?

RB: Progesterone increases your radiation sensitivity.

SS: And I've heard that the whole idea of smashing a woman's breasts between the plates of the mammography machine can also be damaging. Is that correct?

RB: This is something I knew long ago, that no one ever talked about either. We were taught in medical school if a person has a tumor—say, a woman with a lump in her breast—you shouldn't feel that lump except when you initially examine it, because every time they squash it, the cells are pushed out into the lymphatic system and also the blood vessels, and you are more likely to cause metastases. So yes, there is a real concern about this, but they never tell this to women. And women don't know what the doctors are saying among themselves.

Another secret among oncologists that women don't know is that some women who have fibrocystic disease in their breasts are told that they need a mammogram once a year for sure. Problem is, when a breast is dense, you can't see very well. So the radiologist tells them the breast is too dense, and to make an accurate determination, they should return in six months. So they return in six months, get another mammogram, and then they say the same thing.

SS: Why don't they tell us?

RB: Because of the fear of being sued for misdiagnosis of a cancer in a breast that cannot be read. But my question is, if the breast is that dense, why do it in the first place if you know you can't read it? You'd feel it a lot sooner than you'd ever see it on the radiograph. The other thing is some women have small breasts. You can feel everything in a small breast.

If I were a woman I'd never have a mammogram.

I mean, if you feel a lump, then have it biopsied, then you would know for sure if it was cancer or not. And you wouldn't get all that radiation and the smashing of the breast.

SS: So, connecting the dots, in mainstream oncology there's no effective treatment for BRCA1 or BRCA2; chemotherapy is not working; mammograms exacerbate potential cancers and give you a higher risk that you might get cancer because of exposure. So what *do* we do?

RB: The best thing is to get screened with an MRI. That gives you a lot more as a diagnostic picture. Now, they complain that the picture is so clear that they can make mistakes, but you are going to make mistakes on any kind of radiological examination because it's never 100 percent. But the clearest vision of the breast is with the MRI scan. Thermogram is also good because we know tumors are hot and benign lesions tend to be cool.

SS: But what is a woman to do if through MRI or thermogram she does find cancer?

RB: If it were me, I would say I'm not having chemotherapy, and I'm not having radiation. I would let them surgically remove the tumor with a simple lumpectomy and then I would take care of the rest nutritionally.

SS: Okay, now we're getting somewhere. What would that program be?

RB: We know that a combination of nutrients has a far better chance of controlling cancer than anything conventional medicine has to offer. It's in the journals, found in the guidelines, the government medical peer-reviewed journals. But the problem is that physicians don't read those articles; they don't know what to do with them. They are trained in medicine, radiation, and surgery, so they don't have a clue how to put together a program for patients that says, "If you put this combination together it is one of the most powerful inhibitors to breast cancer anyone has ever known."

If you look at the molecular action of flavonoid combinations and vitamin combinations, it's all been worked out down to the exact cell signaling method—what happens in the cell, why it only affects cancer cells, and why it doesn't affect normal cells. The beauty of flavonoid combination treatment is that it protects normal cells and kills and suppresses cancer cells. It's very selective. This is information oncologists have always claimed they have looked for, but chemo drugs are not selective at all. They damage every kind of cell, normal cells and cancer cells. There's no selectivity.

SS: So once again, it always comes back to nutrition.

RB: The final theory of cancer causation is that what is causing most of the disease is chronic inflammation. All cancer is caused by chronic inflammation. The number one link to cancer is aging. If we look at who gets the most cancers, it's people who are older, and that's why cancer before age forty in women and men is a very, very low risk. It's only after age fifty that it becomes a disease of concern, and at sixty and seventy it increases a lot faster.

SS: What is the difference between older people and younger people relative to contracting cancer? Why are they at such risk?

RB: Number one, as you get older you undergo immune suppression because of the aging process, and because of the high intake of omega-6 fats—corn oil, sunflower oil, safflower oil, peanut oils. We know that vaccinations, particularly if they contain mercury [as a preservative], are an immune suppressant. They are exposed to a lot of types of toxins. And older people are nutrient depleted. We know that the cause of age-related immune suppression is nutrient deficiency, even a single nutrient deficiency. You can take all the nutrients and miss one of the critical nutrients and your immune system doesn't work. So immune suppression associated with age is a leading cause, and then just nutrient depletion itself. We know that if you make animals chronically deficient in folic acid, they have a very high cancer incidence; same in humans. Humans who are chronically folic acid deficient develop a high increase in their risk of developing cancers of various types.

SS: What foods have folic acid?

RB: Most folic acid is found in leafy green vegetables, particularly broccoli, Brussels sprouts, kale. Also cauliflower.

We also know that a lifetime accumulation of toxins stays in your body. They did a study on Bill Moyers to see how many toxins he had in him—as in industrial pesticides and herbicides—and he had eighty-four different residues in him at any one time.

SS: So does this accumulation of toxic residues cause DNA damage?

RB: Yes, the older you get the more DNA damage you get, and many of these toxins produce enormous numbers of free radicals, which damage DNA. As you get older you have more trouble repairing your DNA, so if you are age seventy-five or eighty, your ability to repair DNA is just a fraction of what it was when you were forty or even fifty. And that puts you at extremely high risk.

SS: Is aging simply an acceleration of inflammation?

RB: Yes. By the time you are in your sixties, the amount of inflammation in your body is considerable. By the time you are seventy or eighty, it's astronomical. This constant inflammation in the body is damaging your DNA and setting the stage for cancer development.

In one study, they looked at people who had cancer and found out that about 69 percent of them had identifiable chronic disease fifteen years or more before they developed their cancer. If you look at other studies, 70 to 75 percent had chronic inflammatory diseases before they developed their cancer. So yes, the strongest link to cancer is chronic inflammation.

SS: What about glutathione? Do we continue to make it in our bodies? Because this is protective against inflammation, right?

RB: It's like nothing lasts, Suzanne. As we age we have fewer antioxidant defenses like glutathione, so we can't defend ourselves against these free radicals that are increased. As we get older we have lower melatonin levels, and now it's known that melatonin is an anticancer substance, not just for the brain but for the entire body. So if your melatonin levels have decreased, you are at greater risk for cancer.

SS: That's important to know. So many people think melatonin is simply to sleep better.

RB: One of the real biggies is as you get older you become severely depleted in vitamin D_3, and if I had to pick just one vitamin that would be the most powerful cancer preventer and inhibitor of established cancers, it would be vitamin D_3. The elderly stay indoors; they're cold most of the time, so they wear long sleeves. They avoid the sun, they wear hats. And so they begin to get severely vitamin D_3 deficient, which puts them at enormous risk of developing cancer—and some of the worst cancers, like glioblastoma, which is a very malignant brain tumor. Studies found that if you gave people with this type of cancer large doses of vitamin D_3

they lived about five times longer than with even the best medical treatment they could get. So it has a powerful influence, and unfortunately the elderly are severely depleted.

Exposure to MSG is a powerful inducer of free radicals that last for a lifetime and have been connected to powerful stimulation of cancer growth. Glutamate receptors on tumors are now being shown to be a major stimulator of tumor invasion and spread. The problem is that people eat a lot of omega-6 fats, which not only produce immune suppression but also are a major promoter of inflammation. Americans consume about fifty times more omega-6 fats than they should for normal health, so they're highly inflamed just from their diets, and they have very low omega-3 fat intake, which reduces inflammation.

So you look at all of those things combined for older people, it's no wonder they're at the highest risk of developing cancer, or higher than anyone age forty.

SS: So it's aging, bad oils, diet sodas, packaged foods, lack of sun, lack of vitamin D3, and chemicals in our food and environment—all of which have contributed to what is now an epidemic, right?

RB: Absolutely, because most of these things are getting worse. They tell people to stay out of the sun because they will get cancer, with no thought that when you lower vitamin D3 you are dramatically increasing your cancer risk. Yet if they develop cancer, the cancer is more likely to go out of control because they are vitamin D3 deficient.

SS: So if we develop a tumor but we are eating right and we're avoiding bad oils and chemical food and glutamates, it's very likely that the tumor will just stay nicely tucked away?

RB: Exactly. You see, the one thing that's known in oncology that the general public doesn't know is that tumors can change their characteristics based on these factors.

> *With good nutrition, a tumor will become very benign in its behavior.*

In labs, the animal will live much longer. But if you take the same animal and give it a bad diet and toxins, the tumor will change its characteristics and become highly aggressive, highly invasive, and kill the animal very quickly.

SS: Let's talk about sugar.

RB: I really find it appalling that some of the biggest cancer centers in the world tell their patients to eat sugars: pies, cakes, even cheesecake and birthday cake. They tell them this so that they don't lose weight. All these things are filled with MSG and sugar. Well, this is crazy, because cancer is fueled by sugar. It can't use other things to grow as do other cells. If you take animals in a lab with cancer and feed them sugar, they die sooner. They should be telling their patients not to eat sugar and aspartame, and to avoid chemicals. They need to be on a sugar-free diet. No artificial sweeteners.

SS: I have heard that many oncologists have candy in their offices for their patients.

RB: Feeding cancer patients sugar is really a cause for malpractice, because if you feed a cancer patient sugar, they are going to die faster.

SS: What's wrong with our medical schools? Why aren't they teaching what we need to know?

RB: The problem with medical centers is two things. One, the medical centers get most of their funding or large blocks of their funding from pharmaceutical companies, and these companies produce all the major manufacturing chemotherapeutic agents and other drugs used in cancer patients. When you give millions of dollars, tens of millions of dollars, to universities such as Harvard or Yale or Columbia or Duke, you're not going to have physicians who are dependent on pharmaceutical money criticizing chemotherapy. They'll lose their grants and the president of the university will tell them, "We're at risk of losing tens of millions of dollars." If they continue, they risk being let go by the university.

Researchers and doctors in big universities actually depend on these grants both from government and from the private institutions for their survival. Who gives the grants? The pharmaceutical companies. Who controls the grants the government gives? The pharmaceutical companies. So both the government and the pharmaceutical companies are making billions of dollars off the improper treatment of cancers.

The medical student goes to medical school all excited because he's told it's the greatest medical school in the world, and then they start teaching him about all the drugs. This student pays no attention to biochemistry—medical students hate biochemistry, think it's a waste of time. They can't wait to start learning how to deal with drugs, radiation, diagnostic tests, and chemotherapy. Basic sciences are just a lot of nonsense. The only basic science they know is how a drug works. As a result, our medical students are poorly educated and they don't even realize it. They are ignoring a mass of knowledge, which is truly unfortunate. Now we have huge knowledge of plant extracts, flavonoids, vitamins, and minerals, and it is so extensive. The science is so well demonstrated, there's just no excuse for not using it in everyday cancer patients.

SS: What would you give a cancer patient?

RB: Turmeric, one of the most powerful cancer inhibitors. It's just enormously powerful, and it's even more powerful when you combine it with these other things, because you have synergistic and additive power to control cells. This is the difference between nutrition and chemotherapy. Chemotherapy targets one or two enzymes in the cancer cells or a process in the cancer cells. The cancer adapts quickly and bypasses that blockage and goes on growing. Flavonoids and other plant-based nutrients attack the cancer cells and don't attack the normal cells. So nutritional therapies attack twenty, thirty, fifty, a hundred different sites, where the chemotherapy might attack it at two sites.

SS: Is this what you call a natural approach to cancer?

RB: Right. Natural is where the cancer cell is incapable of overcoming that blockage, and that's why it works so much better. The cancer cells don't develop resistance.

SS: Tell me about the multidrug resistance I have heard about in cancer.

RB: Oh, this is one of the big secrets in oncology. Multidrug resistance happens when you give chemotherapeutic agents to a patient and a great number of the cancer cells will become resistant to the chemotherapy, meaning it won't work even the least bit. And once it develops this multidrug resistance, it resists every chemotherapeutic agent from then on. This means the cancer is not only not sensitive to the agent, but also it grows much faster because these chemotherapeutic agents produce enormous inflammation and free radical generation in the entire body, which is what stimulates the growth of cancer. It makes the cancer invade a lot more and metastasize, and shortens the patient's life span. But in our research we have found that a number of natural supplements will reverse multidrug resistors.

SS: Like what?

RB: For instance, indol-3-carbinol, found in broccoli. And like I said, turmeric and flavonoids.

SS: Do they want to find a cure for cancer? Because it seems to me if this was something that those in the cancer arena really wanted, it would have happened. It appears to be such a failure.

RB: The problem is that it has gotten to be such big business. If we found the cure to cancer, there would be a terrible economic impact. Hospitals would have to get rid of all their mammogram units; they would get rid of a lot of the CT scanners and MRI scanners. Oncologists would be out of their jobs; radiology units would close. The impact would be hundreds and hundreds of billions of dollars. The pharmaceutical companies would lose major revenues. The impact would be enormous, and that is what keeps research from following a course that would lead to truly curing patients.

SS: I've seen a number of celebrities of late on television who've done chemo and radiation and who look great and healthy. And then my daughter-in-law recently told me about her girlfriend diagnosed with breast cancer nine years ago, who also had a couple of rounds of chemo and radiation as well as after-care drugs and seems to be living a normal life. Are these women well? Did chemo work?

RB: The answer lies in the fact that in many cases of chemo following breast cancer surgery, the cancer itself was of a very low malignancy, meaning that it has a low risk of metastasizing. It is the spread of a cancer that kills. Many of these patients would have survived and done well even without chemo and post-op radiation. There is a big controversy among cancer specialists concerning overdiagnosing breast and prostate cancers. The idea is that most breast cancers are in situ cancers and would never develop into full-blown invasive cancers. Also, even in the case of some invasive cancers we know that their ability to invade and kill varies considerably. Some are highly invasive and fast-growing and will kill over a very short period, while others grow very slowly, are very slow to metastasize, and can recur decades after they are declared cured. It used to be thought that if patients survived five years without signs of recurrence of their tumor, they were cured forever. We now know, especially for breast cancers, they are recurring after even ten years. Studies have also shown that cancer cells are found circulating in the blood of 50 percent of breast cancer survivors five years after they are supposedly cured. So many, such as the woman nine years free of cancer, are still at risk.

As for their appearance of being "well," recent studies have shown that chemotherapy produces brain damage in a substantial number of people undergoing it. This can manifest as depression, memory loss, and difficulty thinking clearly. They also suffer from fatiguability and other systemic effects. We also know that the chemo damages the DNA in all cells of their bodies, especially those cells that divide the fastest—such as bone marrow cells, cells lining the gut, and liver cells. What most oncologists never want to talk about is that people taking chemo and/or radiation treatments are at an increased risk of a second malignancy not related to their first one. That is, women who have post-op chemo are at risk of developing leukemia/lymphoma or even thyroid cancer. They are also at a greater risk of developing one of the neurodegenerative diseases, such as Alzheimer's disease.

A woman on tamoxifen is at a much greater risk of developing uterine cancer, and the effectiveness of tamoxifen in preventing breast cancer recurrence is in question, especially for black women. There are a number of studies that show tamoxifen increases breast cancer risk in black women. So, while the women you speak of may seem to be "well," it is very early in their course of treatment, and later in their lives they may pay a heavy price for the chemo and radiation treatments.

As far as chemo working, it depends on your definition of *working*. For cancers that have already metastasized, which includes a great number of cancer cases, chemotherapy and/or radiation therapy is ineffective and there is growing evidence that it may actually reduce survival times; that is, it is killing the patients earlier. Chemo can make a great number of cancers temporarily shrink, but then the cancer becomes resistant to not only that particular cancer chemotherapy but also to all forms of chemotherapy— as I discussed earlier, it's called multidrug resistance. This makes the patient die faster, because the chemo damages their immune system as well as body resistance to cellular and organ stress. Suppression of immunity, all agree, speeds the growth and invasion of all cancers. It gets rather involved, but new studies have shown that chemo causes the tumors to shrink temporarily by killing the low-grade malignant cells and has no effect on the cells generating the cancer—the cancer stem cells. This is why when the cancer recurs it grows with a vengeance.

It is also important to emphasize again that a great number of studies reported in prestigious journals demonstrate that flavonoids, as well as special vitamin-mineral mixtures, can powerfully suppress cancer development, growth, and invasion of a great number of cancers. There is compelling evidence that a nutritional approach to post-op treatment of breast cancer far exceeds in safety and effectiveness any regimen of chemotherapy and/or radiation treatments.

SS: I know you don't take patients anymore, but if you had a patient in front of you who wanted to change their life and start today on a program to prevent cancer, what would you tell them to eat?

RB: I would tell them to avoid red meat if they are at high risk for cancer.

SS: Why?

RB: Because if you are at high risk for cancer, red meat is high in iron, particularly the most absorbable form of iron we know of. Iron is a major carcinogen because it triggers massive amounts of free radicals and inflammation. If you take mice and have them breathe iron dust, a high percentage of them develop lung cancer. Children with leukemia with high levels of iron in their system have a much higher death rate. Iron plays a big part in mortality, growth, and aggressiveness of tumors. So if you are at high risk of cancer, you should avoid it. Don't let meat burn; don't let it get charred, because it produces carcinogenic chemicals that are potent. Now, if you just love red meat, then be sure you eat it with vegetables, and they will dramatically reduce the iron absorption.

Avoid omega-6 oils. Use extra-virgin olive oil or coconut oil. Don't cook at high heat because heat oxidizes the oil and ruins it. Put turmeric in your olive oil and it won't oxidize.

SS: What other foods protect us from cancer?

RB: Berries are very important: blueberries, raspberries, blackberries. I would take the densest vegetables, which I mention in my book, and put them in a blender and drink at least ten to twelve ounces a day, preferably with a meal. As I've said, flavonoids are extremely powerful cancer inhibitors of all kinds. They also prevent iron absorption.

Also, drink purified water. Don't drink fluoridated water, chlorinated water, or distilled water. But if you do drink distilled water, add a little magnesium citrate or magnesium malate to a gallon of water and that should be your main drink.

Red wine is good for the antioxidants, but not to excess. A couple of glasses a day is good and it relaxes you. And it prevents cancer. Avoid sugar, avoid artificial sweeteners. Avoid anything with MSG or any kind of excitotoxic chemicals and glutamates, as they have been found to be an enormously powerful stimulant for cancer growth and especially cancer invasion. Many tumors grow fast, like melanomas and certain types of breast cancer, ovarian cancer, pancreatic cancer—all are very glutamate sensitive.

SS: Explain glutamates, please.

RB: Glutamate is an amino acid called glutamic acid, and it is one of the most abundant neurotransmitters in the brain, but its concentration outside the brain cells needs to be very carefully controlled because of its toxicity. Glutamates are excitotoxins, or chemicals that are harmful to the brain, and are found in processed foods and have many names, such as hydrolyzed protein or hydrolyzed vegetable protein, soy protein or soy protein concentrates, soy isolates, MSG, caseinate, autolyzed yeast enzymes and autolyzed yeast extract, and "natural flavoring."

SS: Soy is always surprising. Explain why soy is bad.

RB: The soy industry spent millions of dollars putting out stories that soy is the miracle food. What they don't tell people is soy has one of the highest concentrations of manganese.

Avoid all soy foods. Soy products have a very high concentration of fluoride and a very high concentration of glutamate. Studies show that if you feed soy to animals that have breast cancer, it makes the cancer grow faster. We know that manganese, fluoride, and glutamate are terrible brain toxins, and in my neuroscience journal it shows that giving soy formula to children is associated with Parkinson's, because of the manganese. Women have been lulled into thinking that eating and drinking all this soy is good for them, but it is loaded with all this manganese, which is a powerful brain toxin and has been shown to cause brain atrophy.

> *A study done in Hawaii showed that people who consumed the greatest amount of soy products had the greatest brain atrophies and dementia.*

SS: How ironic. Women are told pretty much at every juncture that soy is breast cancer protective. They always point to the women of Japan and their lower rates of breast cancer and say, "It's the soy."

RB: Soy has been shown to be a powerful aromatase stimulator. What that means is aromatase is an enzyme that converts testosterone into estrogen, and we know that breast cancers produce a lot of aromatase, and things that stimulate a breast cancer also stimulate aromatase. Almost all flavonoids, like curcumin, inhibit aromatase, and that's one of the ways they prevent breast cancer. Soy massively increases aromatase, so that's a reason not to consume soy.

The other thing is that most soy is genetically modified. Genetically modified foods have shown increased evidence that they induce sterility. So young women who are consuming it may find they are having trouble getting pregnant. That's another reason not to consume a lot of soy products.

SS: Well, as always, Russell, you are a font of information. I just have one last thing I'd like you to answer. If you were talking to a group of medical students about to become oncologists, what would you say to them?

RB: I would tell them to question all paradigms, not to accept it at face value. To start thinking for themselves, to look at the literature. If you are going to be an oncologist, you should understand cancer biology inside and out. If you understand cancer biology, you should look at what is known about the nutrients, what they do to alter the cancer process. Don't just memorize the latest combination of drugs.

I would tell them never to use the words *evidence-based medicine* because that is the biggest con job in the history of the world. That is a term used to imply that traditional medical practices use evidence-based medicine and everything outside of that does not. Evidence-based medicine makes it impossible to recommend anything alternative, as though alternative medicine has no evidence.

I would tell them to think about the compromise and conflict of interests of medical schools being funded by pharmaceutical companies. And I would tell them to look to nutrition for their answers.

SS: Thank you, Russell. As always, it has been an honor.

Knock It Out

- Unlike traditional cancer treatment, which damages all cells, flavonoid combination treatment protects normal cells and kills and suppresses cancer cells. With good nutrition, a tumor can become very benign in its behavior.
- Avoid red meat if you are at high risk for cancer, as it is high in absorbable iron, a major carcinogen that can trigger massive amounts of free radicals and inflammation. If you love red meat, eating it with vegetables will dramatically reduce iron absorption. You should never let it get charred, because doing so produces potent carcinogenic chemicals.
- Don't consume sugar or artificial sweeteners, MSG, or any kind of excitotoxic chemicals and glutamates. These have been found to be enormously powerful stimulants for cancer growth and invasion.
- Natural folic acid (found in leafy green vegetables, particularly broccoli, Brussels sprouts, and kale, as well as cauliflower) boosts the body's natural defenses against cancer.
- Vitamin D_3 is the most powerful vitamin in preventing new cancer and inhibiting established cancers.
- Cut back on omega-6 fats and increase omega-3 fat intake to reduce inflammation. Use extra-virgin olive oil or coconut oil, and don't cook with oil at high heat, which oxidizes the oil. Putting turmeric in your olive oil keeps it from oxidizing.
- Drink purified water. Avoid water that's fluoridated, chlorinated, or distilled, whenever possible. If you do drink distilled water, add a little magnesium citrate or magnesium malate.
- Drinking red wine is good for the antioxidants, but don't drink to excess.

Chapter 12

BURTON GOLDBERG

I believe we must use the best from both worlds.

—Burton Goldberg

Burton Goldberg is not a doctor but a passionate layperson who has devoted his life to finding the answer to cancer. Among his many projects, he
funded, supervised, edited, and published *Alternative Medicine: The Definitive Guide*, which has become the bible for alternative medicine for
laypeople and practitioners everywhere. If you need to know something
about the alternative world or whom to go to, you will find it in this mag-
nificent book.

Burton Goldberg says there are two systems of health care that exist in
the United States today: conventional Western medicine and alternative
medicine. The first is the world of the American Medical Association,
medical doctors who rely on drugs and surgery to treat disease symptoms,
and who inadvertently align themselves with the multibillion-dollar
pharmaceutical industry. Conventional medicine, he says, is superb in
dealing with acute medical conditions and traumatic injury. But, he says,
there is no question that alternative medicine works better for just about
everything else, especially for chronic degenerative diseases such as cancer, heart disease, and rheumatoid arthritis, and for more common ail-
ments such as asthma, gastrointestinal disorders, and headaches.

He says alternative medicine is more cost-effective in the long term, because it emphasizes prevention and goes after causes rather than symptoms. Alternative methods work by assisting the body to heal itself. They don't trap people on a merry-go-round that begins with one drug and requires them to take another to compensate for the side effects the first one causes. Burton Goldberg is disillusioned that our government ignores well-established alternative medicine treatments and does not allocate federal funds to study them.

Since being diagnosed with prostate cancer several years ago, Burton Goldberg has devoted his life to researching the causes of cancer and also educating the public about alternative treatments. He has produced several DVDs on the subject; especially of note is *Cancer Conquest*, which presents the best of conventional and alternative medicine, and *Greed*, which talks about the robbing of America's health. He believes cancer can be managed by integrating conventional cancer treatment, including low-dose chemotherapy, with alternative medicine, which combines cutting-edge natural treatments and building up the body nutritionally. For those of you who are fearful of using nothing but alternative treatments, you will find this interview of particular interest. He is a passionate and fascinating man. At eighty-two, he defies aging and has the vitality, vigor, and good looks of a fifty-year-old. He walks his talk. And it is impressive.

SS: Good day, Burton. You have seventeen books to your name, all of which are incredible, important, and life-changing, but I think your most amazing effort is *Alternative Medicine: The Definitive Guide*. Every time I walk into the office of one of "my kind" of doctors, I see your book sitting on their coffee tables. Why did you undertake a project of such magnitude? Most alternative doctors tell me it's their bible.

BG: I am a consultant and my work is to guide people and patients to the right doctors to facilitate the reversal of this dreaded disease of cancer. So yes, putting together the guide was like putting the entire alternative school under one roof, and was quite a project. I wanted it to be put in a language that the public could understand. I didn't really do this project for doctors. I also have another book coming out called *How to Thrive or Survive in a Toxic World*, which is about what causes cancer.

SS: Well, let's get into it, then. How do you prevent getting cancer?

BG: Frankly, it's almost impossible. Our food supply is not the identical food supply we used to have at the turn of the century. In 1900, cancer was maybe the sixth most common cause of death; by next year they predict it will be number one. It will have surpassed heart disease. Of course there is a genetic element, but that's only about 5 percent, and experts are trying to lay off the epidemic on genes, but that is nonsense. They are saying that because they just don't know how else to explain the pandemic.

It's clearly about the food we are eating; it's about the chemicals in our environment. It's the environmental toxicity. We've been exposed to thousands of chemicals that haven't been on the planet before a hundred years ago. The body has twenty-five-thousand-year-old genetics and doesn't really have a mechanism for getting rid of a lot of these chemicals—toxins, plastics, hydrocarbons, and pesticides—that we now have in our bodies. We do not have a tool for this. As a result, there develops an accumulation of these toxins—including that we have styrene and phthalates from Styrofoam and plastic bottles. Plasticizers are in the food wraps, plastic water bottles, new car smell, amongst other things . . . that's phthalates.

Cancer is an epidemic and it boils down to a mixture of poisons in the environment and poisons in our food, coupled with genetics. But how do you explain that many, many women are getting breast cancer with no family history of breast cancer? It's obviously toxicity from pharmaceuticals, technology, and the environment.

We also have a tremendous amount of radioactive fallout, and viruses are out of control, along with pesticides and herbicides, which are xeno-estrogens. An overload in estrogen results not only in breast cancer and prostate cancer, but also brings you out of your equilibrium with your progesterone, testosterone, and estrogen. If you are not in balance hormonally, then there is a great chance that you will develop a tumor.

There are many, many causes of cancer, and it's a multifaceted activity that goes through years and years of changes in the body. We are not eating properly, nor are we aware of the damage caused by eating chemical-laden foods, plus we have tremendous amounts of stress in our lives. So you see, there are a multitude of factors that play a role in why we are getting cancer in these unprecedented amounts. But know this—many of these things you can regulate yourself.

SS: I guess that's the whole point here. We have to understand that if we are going to consume chemicals, live with chemicals, and breathe chemicals, we are asking for it. It's not an accident to get cancer. If we allow our stress to run unchecked, if we don't value sleep and get enough of it, then the consequences are ours.

BG: But we have not educated the public. People do not know or understand the consequences of toxicity, so they continue to eat poisoned food loaded with chemicals, with no nutritional value, which is like not eating at all . . . yet the toxins are creating disease with each breath or bite they take.

We are being poisoned to death, and we're being starved to death in the land of plenty.

SS: I agree. I call it the slow poisoning of us. The chemicals have crept up on us. We didn't realize, but now, little by little, one by one, some of us are starting to wake up. Unfortunately, most people are not aware that there is this silent enemy out there, and everyone is deaf and asleep and they don't see it coming.

BG: Yes, and as a result our immune systems are down. We are living in a pressure cooker; the economic conditions are such that our emotions are affected and so are our hormones. I know this because I did a documentary on depression and another one on addiction. Hormones play a role in depression, as you know, Suzanne, and very few doctors pay attention to women's hormones.

Then there are food allergies and food intolerances, which is how I got started in this field. It was because of a very sick little girl who I brought to a doctor in Connecticut who no longer practices, and I watched him put people in and out of depression just by giving them food substances. She was so sick because she was hypoglycemic, but it took this alternative doctor to get to the bottom of her problems. Allergies play a big role in health; for instance, some people eat wheat and they fall under the table.

SS: Yes, my daughter had a severe allergy to eggs, and we never put it together. We thought she was just really tired. We never connected the dots that every time she ate eggs she would pass out and fall asleep for a couple of hours. She was gaining weight and no one could figure out why. She was eating salads and eggs so she wouldn't get fat, and then we found out that it was the eggs that were the problem. She was allergic. It took years to find that answer.

My husband is severely gluten intolerant. We didn't connect those dots, either; a plate of pasta and he was out like a light. I had guests recently. We all went out for lunch, and they had cupcakes. An hour later they were sound asleep on the couch. Food affects us, but we have not been trained to listen to our bodies. If you eat something and you bloat afterward, have indigestion, acid reflux, or pass out, that's your body talking—screaming, in some cases.

BG: Now the problem with these food intolerances is that after a while the body stops working correctly; it can't absorb the nutrients anymore, from the gut being disturbed for so long. Now you've got trouble.

No absorption of nutrients, no nutrition, and you starve to death, even though you are eating. Starvation leads to disease. Food intolerances clearly affect those who fall into this category.

Then we have the other outrage—the inappropriate use of antibiotics in farmed fish, in beef, in chicken, and hormones being put into the animals.

SS: Why do they give the animals hormones?

BG: To make them big and fat so they can make more money. There are estrogenic effects from all the hormones that affect us negatively. And another big problem is genetically modified foods (GMO), but the government isn't paying attention to it. There are no studies on what is going on with GMO food and its negative effects. They don't want us to know because it will affect business. Then factor into the puzzle of our national poor health all the additives, such as high-fructose corn syrup, in virtually everything. So blend it all together and you realize we've created this milieu of disease.

I'll say it again—we're being starved to death and poisoned, right here in the land of plenty.

SS: How did this happen?

BG: It happened because of greed. It begins with politics, and in order to change things there has to be campaign reform. You want to know how to prevent cancer? Make the government agencies aware of what causes cancer, so they can change our food supply and our eating habits and stop poisoning America. Campaign reform is the only way this change can happen, because the money and big business that support our politicians and government officials are the reason these things stay in power.

SS: The food manufacturers are not going to tell us their food is making us sick.

BG: We need a huge call to action. We need to understand that we have to drink bottled water without chemicals. Water that comes in plastic has phthalates in it, and this is a cause of the high spike in breast cancer and prostate cancer.

In Israel, they did a study on breast cancer and found that the hormones, antibiotics, pesticides, and herbicides used on dairy cows affected women dangerously, so they forbade the use of pesticides and herbicides and all those chemical substances they had been putting into dairy cows, and as a result the female breast cancer rate plummeted in ten years.

At Hartford Hospital they did toxicology on samples of women's breast tissue and found that inside their tumors was arsenic, DDT, and PCPs. So this is what's happening and we the people are the losers. It's impossible to get studies done because there is an entire cabal against finding out the causation of cancer.

SS: Why? Why can't we find the answer? Why aren't there studies?

BG: Because of the fear of not getting funding for research. Holistic physicians know the causes of cancer, but the industry ignores causation because of the greed of politics . . . so instead they allow the public to be poisoned, protecting industry instead of us, the people.

SS: What new therapies do you find particularly exciting?

BG: I am very enthused about the work of Dr. Munoz in Tijuana, Mexico. He uses immune therapies, which are the use of substances, biological and synthetic, that will enhance the immune system and direct a response of our immune system to attack and destroy cancer cells. It is called dendritic cell therapy, and it is a very impressive vaccine, an autologous vaccine. *Autologous* means that we need to take blood samples from the patient, culture it in the lab, and from there we administer it to the patient. Dendritic cells are part of our immune system, but they only produce a small amount of immunity; they don't really know they are in the body, they don't know what their function is, even though they are produced in the body.

Dr. Munoz's work is to culture these cells and from there train them outside of the body—grow them, mature them, and then train them to tag and attack the cancer cells in the patient. When they tag the cancer cells, they start to send signals to macrophages, T cells, and natural killer cells to come and help them destroy the cancer cells, and it's amazing what happens. You can see the activity of these cells in the microscope. If you take a blood sample from the patient and give them the dendritic vaccine and start to track those dendritic cells, you can see the activity.

SS: What kind of results is he getting?

BG: Out of twenty patients he has nineteen patients responding "excellently" to this therapy. He has at least six full remission patients, and the other thirteen are considered stable, between stable and partial remission. He is seeing this in the first seven to ten days after he applies the dendritic cells. Miraculously, the patients start to feel better so quickly, their symptoms become less aggressive, pain starts to subside, and they start to eat better. Dr. Munoz had one patient with prostate cancer whose PSA at the beginning of treatment was 800, with bone metastasis, spreading to all the vertebrae, the ribs, hips, legs, plus this man was in severe pain. After the treatment, and within one month, his PSA was 0.89, the pain was completely gone, and the bone scans showed a 60 percent improvement for all the bone lesions.

As a consultant, when someone comes to me looking for the appropriate doctor and treatment and if they have a stage IV cancer, I always send them to Dr. Munoz. He's got a great understanding of this disease and uses the vaccines but also enzymes, like Wobenzym, which takes away the shield that cancer cells develop against any antagonist. Dendritic cell therapy trains your immune system to attack your cancer.

Many vaccines are available from integrative medicine, but they are ignored by conventional cancer therapy. Most sick people have to have their nutrition delivered by IV. It's far more effective because they can metabolize it this way.

Dr. Marty Dayton is a brilliant doctor out of Florida and he's done research on the need for nutrition concurrent with chemotherapy. Nutrition is everything. We have to understand where the poisons are coming from; when we open a can of beer or soda or water we don't realize it's lined with bisphenol A, a chemical poison. We think we can take in all these poisons and not get ill? What are we thinking?

Conventional medicine will tell you nutrition isn't all that important; in fact, they say it's antagonistic to chemotherapy to feed nutrition to chemotherapy patients. But nutrition is crucial for sick people. When using chemo, it is imperative to properly nourish the patient, as ultimately it is your immune system that will save you. This is integrative. Conventional therapy says that nutrition is counterproductive and offsets chemo's efficacy. Well, they are totally wrong, and consequently patients are being starved to death in a land of plenty.

SS: What do you think of conventional cancer treatment, i.e., chemotherapy?

BG: The way chemo is practiced in this country is medieval. It is cookbook medicine. You must treat the person who has the cancer, not the cancer or tumor alone. It requires a systemic lifestyle change and detoxification.

When I did my book in 1997, I didn't believe in chemo because at that time (and still today) the success rate using chemo alone after five years was a dismal 2.5 percent. With the sophisticated testing now done in Germany, doctors can target cancer cells with low-dose chemotherapy (as little as 10 to 20 percent) and insulin potentiation therapy [IPT] used in conjunction with full-body hyperthermia, which can have amazing results.

The theory behind insulin potentiation therapy is that cancer grows on sugar. Insulin is used like a Trojan horse to carry chemo or other natural substances into the cancer cells, thereby using less toxic amounts with greater efficacy.

SS: Explain to me the new cutting-edge, integrative cancer treatments. For instance, what is Poly-MVA?

BG: Poly-MVA is alpha-lipoic acid with palladium. It is an over-the-counter, natural chemotherapeutic agent. And its usefulness depends on the stage of the cancer, the virulence of the cancer, and the compliance of the patient, the mental state of the patient. It has multiple factors, all of which come in, but number one is the maestro—in other words, the doctor who is handling it. And there are very few doctors who understand this therapy and know how to do it.

Poly-MVA is a very interesting therapy. I was in Texas at a conference on cancer and I met a guy who was on Poly-MVA—which, incidentally, Dr. Forsythe administers within his protocol and does it very well. Anyway, this guy had multiple myeloma, which is a severe blood/bone cancer, a terrible cancer which cracks up the bones, and sadly, conventional medicine has had zero success with it.

So the oncologist gave this man three months to live, and naturally he was depressed. His wife was reading Dr. Stephen Sinatra's newsletter where he was talking about multiple myeloma and said an effective treatment for this disease is Poly-MVA treatment. So he tried the therapy and three months later he went back to his original oncologist and his doctor said, "Guess what? You don't have multiple myeloma."

SS: If this is such an effective treatment, why isn't it mainstream?

BG: No one is going to spend millions researching something you can buy over the counter.

SS: What is hydrazine sulfate?

BG: Hydrazine sulfate is a chemical produced for industry and is sold over the counter, and it has had great success with cancer. It is used to stop cancers from producing lactic acid, which turbocharges cancer cells. Hydrazine sulfate is much maligned by the cancer industry but is very effective against brain and all other cancers. It is very inexpensive. But because it competes with extremely expensive chemo drugs, its efficacy is played down. There is so much deceit exercised by the cancer establishment; hydrazine sulfate was discovered by Dr. Joseph Gold and is primarily an anti-cachexia agent, which keeps the body, for lack of a better description, from "eating itself," as so often happens in the last stages of chemotherapy treatments. A lot of testing has been done on this in Russia by the Petrov Institute in St. Petersburg. [If you want more information about this, go to www.burtongoldberg.com.]

To fight cancer requires a strong body. Some beneficial treatments Burton Goldberg has come across to build up the body and strengthen it are:

- *Ondamed machine.* A German biofeedback device that finds the blockage in the patient—whether it be mental or physical—and relieves it, putting the body back into homeostasis. I own this machine and use it to determine areas of weakness in my body so I am able to do what is necessary to strengthen.
- *Asyrus devices.* Also known as electric-dermal screening. It is a testing device using resonance (quantum physics) to measure organ efficacy and determine what products will mediate homeostasis.
- *BioFocus.* For this promising blood test, they ship the patient's blood to Germany to determine the DNA of the patient's cancer cells, to find which chemo or natural substance will target the primary and floating cancer cells throughout the body.
- *Whole-body hyperthermia.* A sophisticated, computerized heat regulation that allows cancer-killing medications to penetrate cancer cells.
- *Iscador.* An extract of the mistletoe plant that has been used for centuries for cancer remission. Builds up the immune system.
- *Autologous vaccines.* Vaccines made from the patient's own blood.

SS: I have used Iscador and had many Ondamed treatments. In fact, I attribute my ability to recover from the trauma I wrote about at the beginning of this book to this device. It rebalanced my energies and allowed my body to recover from the emotional and physical trauma.

BG: The primary cancer is not the killer—it is the disseminated cells that mutate. We are looking for cancer in the wrong place, and that is why some integrative doctors are having an 80 percent success rate with end-stage cancers using these effective treatments I have mentioned. This is integrative medicine: using the best that orthodox and alternative medicines have to offer in conjunction with each other.

SS: What about diet? How important is diet relative to cancer prevention?

BG: It is imperative relative to prevention not to eat foods that turn into sugar, like pasta, bread, rice, potatoes. Cancer thrives on sugar.

SS: I'm happy to hear you say that. My series of Somersize weight-loss books subscribed to that theory. It's the insulin connection. Avoiding foods the body turns to sugar is not only cancer protective but also a great way to lose weight permanently.

What drives you, Burton Goldberg? You certainly have passion.

BG: What drives me is being incensed at the insensitive political situation that allows so much horror and illness to occur. Everybody's sick—your grandfather has a problem, your grandmother has a problem, your kids have a problem, attention deficit is out of control. What drives me is the passion to right a wrong.

What I have learned over the last thirty years on the causes of cancer is that cancer can be successfully reversed. Once you have cancer you have to stay on top of it; you can never give up. Treatment has to be specific to your cancer, and there are tests that are available today that will target your cancer cells, either with chemotherapy used interactively or with natural substances. This will be the difference between success and failure. I'm a consultant, and I'm available to guide anyone who wants my services to help identify a practitioner or therapy to treat this dreaded disease. I can be contacted at burton@burtongoldberg.com. I am giving away my film *Cancer Conquest*, on this subject, for free on the Internet.

SS: Thank you. We all thank you, Burton.

STEM CELLS AND CANCER

According to Dr. Robin Smith of the NeoStem company, there are the cancer protective possibilities of having one's own stem cells banked: Currently, there are preclinical studies demonstrating that gene therapy combined with one's own stem cells increases the ability of the immune cells derived from those stem cells to kill tumor cells. When the stem cells become immune cells, a very high percentage of these immune cells recognize the tumor cells and can kill them.

If you have cancer and you have your stem cells banked, it may be possible to regenerate organs damaged (from radiation therapy and chemotherapy) with autologous (your own) stem cells. Stem cells could theoretically be used to repair the heart muscle and regenerate new muscle cells if they are injured from chemotherapy.

Information on NeoStem is at the back of this book.

Chapter 13

DAVID SCHMIDT

The first time I met David Schmidt of LifeWave, LLC, he was trying to convince me that his nanotechnology energy patches were something from which I could benefit. I didn't really believe him at first, so he set out to prove it to me. He asked, "Where are you weakest?" I told him that when I used free weights I would fatigue after five or six reps doing flies. He said, "Okay, do your six flies." After six reps or so it became difficult. Then he said, "Wait two minutes and then put on the LifeWave patches." I did, and after thirty reps (effortlessly, I might add) I stopped because I had to work the next morning, and was afraid I would be sore. (I wasn't, by the way.)

I wear the LifeWave nanotechnology patch of glutathione every single day, to detoxify my body from the chemical assault that bombards all of us on a daily basis. I use the energy patches regularly, and the pain patches for an occasional headache or lower back pain from a yoga session that might have been too exuberant. I love these patches. They are nondrug and do the job perfectly. I couldn't be without them, and David Schmidt is a genius for creating them.

But it is his knowledge of why they work and how the body heals, plus his understanding of our inner workings down to a cellular level, that is most impressive. He is one of those rare people in the universe graced with extraordinary intellect as well as the ability to create a product for mankind that is nontoxic and remarkable in its ability to turn our health around.

David was formally educated in management information systems and biology at Pace University in Pleasantville, New York. He went on to specialize in energy production technologies for both military and commercial applications. He developed new methods for producing hydrogen and oxygen and constructed metal combustion engines. He also designed emergency oxygen systems for General Dynamics and the U.S. Navy, and was invited to participate in the navy's next-generation minisub program.

His background in biology helps him to explain how individual human cells operate and why we need to care for each and every cell in our bodies as a means of preventing cancer and other disease. If the human body is made up of cells reproducing, then taking care of each and every cell is crucial to sustaining life.

SS: Hello, David. So nice to speak with you again. Let's talk about glutathione and the role glutathione plays in preventing cancer.

DS: Great. Glutathione is the body's master antioxidant. What I've found in my travels is that glutathione is really not well known or understood in the United States amongst the public; however, outside the United States, especially in Asia, the role of glutathione in improving health and improving immune function is more readily understood and accepted. Because of marketing efforts in the United States, people are familiar with vitamins A, C, and E and their important role as antioxidants, but as it turns out, our bodies manufacture the most important antioxidant, and that antioxidant is glutathione.

SS: Is it true that around age forty, forty-five, our production of glutathione decreases? And does it also decline through toxicity and stress?

DS: Yes on both. With age, glutathione does decrease. But with respect to cancer, it is also generally well known that certain types of cancer will increase in incidence as we age. So one of the suspicions amongst researchers is the question, Is there a correlation between the decrease of glutathione levels and the increase in the incidence of cancer?

Many researchers have come to the conclusion that there is a relationship between the two. One of the things we know about glutathione is its role as an antioxidant, and that it helps to support the immune system. Our immune system protects us from disease, and one of the ways disease attacks our bodies is through the production of free radicals. This is why supplementation with antioxidants is so important, because it will help to neutralize these free radicals and protect our cells from damage.

SS: What diseases can result from a lack of glutathione?

DS: It's very well known that in certain types of medical disorders we see a depletion of glutathione, and this would include Parkinson's and also arthritis.

SS: And is toxicity a factor in declining levels?

DS: Yes. We know that there are pathways in the liver for detoxification of tissue or detoxification of carcinogenic materials. We also find correspondingly high levels of glutathione in the liver and in every cell of the body—that's how important glutathione is to health. But there is certainly a link to the removal of toxins and the body's glutathione levels. Let's use mercury as an example. Mercury by itself is not considered a carcinogenic material. However, there are organic compounds that are derivatives of mercury, such as mercury chloride, which are carcinogenic. It is very well known that glutathione is a chelating agent, which is responsible for moving toxic materials like mercury out of our bodies. When it comes to cancer there is also quite a bit of documentation that glutathione will in fact remove cancer-causing material from the body. One example is aflatoxins, which are produced from fungus, and then there are amines, which are produced from overcooking food. The list is quite long on what is known about what glutathione will remove from the body in terms of materials that are known to cause cancer. We have a clinical and scientific database establishing materials that are known to cause cancer, and that these same materials can be eliminated from the body through glutathione. As I just said, glutathione will actually bind to the cancer-causing materials in a process called chelation, but there are a number of biochemicals that are involved. Glutathione will attach itself to this cancer-causing material and help push it out of the body.

SS: Specifically, what are these materials?

DS: Aflatoxins, which as I said are produced by fungi. Overcooking, as in charred food; the technical name for that is heterocyclic amines. People don't take this seriously, but there is scientific research which has shown that charred food can cause the production of tumors in the liver, stomach, small intestine, large intestine, skin, and oral cavities. So this is something we should be concerned about.

SS: Do we continue to pump out a little glutathione forever, or do we get to a point where we are not making it at all anymore?

DS: I speak around the world at conferences and I try to take very complex subjects and simplify them. So in simplistic terms, everything starts and stops in the body with energy production and communication. It's just not possible for our bodies to do what they need to do without energy; it's also not possible for the cells to do what they do without communicating. So understand: as we age, the amount of energy our cells manufacture decreases. Also, the communications system of our bodies declines in integrity as we age, so when we look at most every abnormal, diseased state—viral infection, bacterial infection, cancer—it is associated with abnormal energy production and cell communication.

Cancer cells have a very, very high energy metabolism, much higher than that of a normal healthy cell. Cancer cells do not communicate with their environment as does healthy tissue. A disease state is a state in which the energy metabolism of the cell is different than a normal healthy cell, and the communication system is also different than a normal healthy cell.

SS: So how does glutathione fit into this scenario?

DS: If we first understand that the general energy production of the cell decreases as we age, then one of the things that is going to decline is glutathione production, and everything else the cell does, which could be tissue repair or hormone production. As a result of aging, we have decreased energy production and an associated decline in glutathione. What this means is that the cell simply doesn't have as much energy to do as many things.

SS: And this is why older people are often "out of gas"?

DS: Right.

SS: Why is there cancer?

DS: My personal belief is it's because of all the toxins in the environment. I read a study recently that when taking a sampling of two hundred people, all two hundred had toxins in their bodies.

SS: No matter what, even eating organic food and living a healthy lifestyle?

DS: Unfortunately yes, because we are breathing in toxins. So unless we are breathing through some sort of filter mask, which isn't practical, we will be getting toxins in our bodies through the air we breathe, from the water, artificial ingredients, preservatives, dyes, and cancer-causing materials in food which leach in from their packaging. The alarming news is that the average number of toxins in the human body is about 100.

SS: Like what? Pesticides, insecticides, radioactive substances?

DS: Yes, they accumulate in our fatty tissue.

SS: This is devastating because we know we are under the greatest environmental assault in the history of mankind. So if we are declining in glutathione, which is a defense against toxicity, it seems to me that your glutathione patches are coming in at the right moment in time. Could they be an answer?

DS: How about if we flip that around and look at it another way? You are asking a great question, but what if the reason our glutathione levels are declining is because of the toxins? So what does glutathione do in our bodies, anyway? We've already talked about how glutathione is the master antioxidant, we've talked about how glutathione will leach mercury from the body, but there is also a connection with how glutathione supports energy production in the body.

It can protect the eyes from macular degeneration, the lungs, and the brain. Glutathione will support the immune system, and it's found in very high concentrations in the liver, so it is liver protective. Glutathione also has a role in diabetic therapy, and in Europe glutathione is administered in conjunction with controlling and stabilizing blood sugar levels. So we see the enormous scope of benefits from the role that glutathione plays in our bodies. If glutathione levels are declining with age, or if we find disease states that are associated with low glutathione levels, maybe what is happening, as many doctors suspect, is that the toxins in the environment are causing the depleted levels of glutathione, therefore weakening our immune systems and making us more susceptible to cancer.

SS: I was thinking the other day, what is the tipping point for cancer? When we live with chemicals in our food, chemicals in our household cleaners, chemicals in the air, chemicals in the water, and the overuse of pharmaceutical drugs, and then add in diet soda, bug killers, and all the rest of the seemingly benign poisons we consume or live with on a daily basis, what is that last drop or pill that makes the cup runneth over, when the liver says: "I give up—I can't protect you anymore"? Because I think that is what is happening. This is the point of no return where the epidemic has been launched.

Is your glutathione patch, "the little engine that could," is it enough? Or is this the best you can come up with, but along with it we also have to clean up our lives?

DS: The more someone can do to protect their health, the better. Our message is always the importance of hydration. Most people do not drink enough water each day, and it is vital in terms of our energy production and also in keeping the lymphatic system clean. For me, glutathione is the most powerful antioxidant that I supplement with, and it turns out that our glutathione patch is the most effective way of elevating glutathione levels.

SS: Tell me, exactly how does a carcinogenic substance, a toxin, create cancer in the body?

DS: This is called chemical carcinogenesis, meaning there is a foreign substance, a chemical, and it will cause or induce a state of cancer in the body. Our bodies are composed of different functions with electrons. We get electrons from the sun, from our food—as a matter of fact, the whole process of energy production from food really boils down to our bodies' chemical system pulling electrons out of the food and then circulating these electrons throughout our bodies. That's the source of energy.

What happens with chemicals that cause cancer is they attack the body and try to steal electrons. Another name for this is radical, so when we have toxins in our bodies, some are natural, some are unnatural, and they are called free radicals; in the case of cancer-causing chemicals they try to attack certain portions of the body's cells.

Since the 1960s it has been documented in scientific literature that glutathione is one of the antioxidants that will bind to sites on the cell and protect the cell from damage by cancer-causing materials. We now have significant evidence over the past fifty years that shows and proves that glutathione will help prevent people from getting cancer; there is a link between depleted levels of glutathione and someone's susceptibility to cancer.

There is another part of this that is very exciting: if we can keep our glutathione levels elevated, we can keep our antioxidant supply elevated and hopefully keep our bodies away from harmful chemicals and harmful toxins.

SS: David, do you think this will ever become mainstream? I mean, I wear a glutathione patch every day and my feeling is "Why not?" If it detoxes me and protects me from the daily bombardment of pollution and chemicals which can lead to cancer, why wouldn't I do it? It doesn't cost much; it's painless and takes about a nanosecond to put on.

DS: I believe eventually this will become mainstream. What I have seen is that while most people are interested in being healthy, they are not very proactive about doing things like going on regular detox programs, because perhaps they don't see the benefit to it. So it's about educating people, and your books do that, Suzanne.

SS: I hope so. I think all of your patches play a role in cancer prevention—sleep patches, energy patches, glutathione patches, carnosine patches, pain patches. Can you explain?

DS: What our patches do is create a state of harmony or balance in the body. It is very well known that diseased states have abnormal energy production, abnormal cell communication. Our patches balance the electrical system of the body, so we are able to improve the health and integrity of the cells in the body. We can help ward off and prevent disease because disease occurs when the body is not in balance.

SS: Do you love what you do?

DS: I do, Suzanne, because every day I get to see people who have life-changing experiences with our products, and I can't think of anything more rewarding than that.

SS: And it's all without drugs.

DS: All without drugs. It is part of an overall approach. Dr. Steve Haltiwanger and I are very passionate about helping educate people to drink more water, eat right, supplement with antioxidants, and exercise regularly, and our patches are part of an overall health and wellness program. As a result, we see some very, very dramatic changes in people's health once they start using them.

Right now there is a very interesting scientific debate about how glutathione can help to treat cancer. The debate has one side saying that supplementing with glutathione is a means to remove the cause of cancer, and then you will see the body heal itself and the person recover from cancer. The other side of the debate comes from the pharmaceutical companies claiming they will administer a drug which will deplete the body's levels of glutathione. The reason for this is, when they administer a chemotherapeutic drug, they want the drug to be able to destroy the cancer cells, and some forms of cancer use glutathione (ironically) to protect themselves from damage. The thinking is that they want to administer a drug that will lower the body's glutathione levels and that will actually make the drug more effective at killing the cancer cell. Then there's a third side of the debate that says we'll administer glutathione first, and then we'll introduce the drug, and the drug will kill the cancer, and because the person has an elevated level of glutathione, it will pull the toxic by-products from the chemotherapy out of the body, and it will also help protect the healthy cells from damage.

SS: So where do you stand on all of this very confusing information?

DS: I like that there is quite a bit happening in the conventional allopathic medical community on ways to use glutathione to protect healthy cells from damage during chemotherapy, and as a method of leaching toxic by-products from the body during chemotherapy to make chemotherapy safer.

SS: It would be nice if alternative and conventional could cross over, like a figure eight. There's a place for both, and for those who do choose chemotherapy, to have a way of detoxing the body afterward through glutathione makes perfect sense to me.

DS: What I would say is what I said when we started this discussion: the human body is in a perfect state when it is in balance. And glutathione is the body's master antioxidant, which is found in every cell in the body for a very important reason, and that is to protect the body from damage. So the more we can understand about the role that glutathione plays in keeping our antioxidant system charged, the better. A real simple way to think about this is that this is our first line of defense in protecting ourselves from damage and helping to prevent states of disease like cancer.

SS: Thank you, David. I appreciate your time and insights very much, as always.

Knock It Out

- Glutathione is the body's master antioxidant, and it protects against cancer by supporting the body's immune system, neutralizing free radicals, and moving cancer-causing toxins out of the body. Glutathione production diminishes with age, but you can supplement with it.
- Drinking enough water each day is vital in terms of the body's energy production, and also in keeping the lymphatic system clean. Increased energy production means cells are able to produce more glutathione as well, and the body's cells are better able to communicate, reducing the risk of disease.

Chapter 14

DR. JONATHAN WRIGHT

There is no cancer that has not been survived by someone, regardless of how far advanced it was. If even one person has succeeded in healing his cancer, there must be a mechanism for it, just as there is a mechanism for creating cancer.

–Andreas Moritz

Hormones ... the backbone of health and quality of life.

As explained by Dr. Burzynski, we have cancer-protective genes in our bodies, like light switches. As we decline in hormonal production, these switches are turned off: by eating badly, by not managing stress, by consuming and living with chemicals, and by the aging process itself. In order to reinstate these cancer-protective genes, we need to reinstate the hormones to perfect balance. Then the brain perceives that all is well. If we are also following a healthy lifestyle, then the cancer in all of us is kept at bay.

The next interview with Dr. Wright will explain in depth the enormous cancer-protective components of hormone replacement. When I was diagnosed with breast cancer, I personally chose, after much research, to forgo the traditional cancer treatment of chemotherapy. I did have a lumpectomy and radiation, but I would not make the same decision regarding radiation today. That is my personal feeling, not advice. Also, I restored myself to perfect hormonal balance and decided to take nutrition seriously, as in *my life depends on it*. I have been cancer free for nine years to date.

I have never recommended that anyone do as I did. I am merely suggesting that you look into and understand true hormone replacement for quality of life and as a cancer protection device. I am not speaking of synthetic, dangerous so-called hormones such as Premarin, Provera, or Prempro. The Women's Health Initiative in 2002 stopped an eight-year study at a little over five years, declaring that "it would be better for women to take nothing at all than to take these dangerous, harmful, and sometimes fatal hormones." The report was speaking of synthetic hormones. The headlines declared, "Hormone replacement is dangerous and even fatal." Well, what woman in her right mind would continue taking anything with that declaration? So as a result, women stopped taking their synthetic hormones. And guess what? Breast cancer rates plummeted.

Unfortunately women then started viewing hormones as the enemy due to a lack of understanding by mainstream medicine of the protective nature of real hormone replacement (bioidentical hormones). Unfortunately as a result of loss of hormones, many women began to experience a diminished quality of life: no sex drive, inability to sleep, weight gain, bloating, body itches, mood swings, hot flashes, and memory loss. Women were expected to tough it out or take a myriad of pharmaceutical drugs for depression, sleep, and anxiety. Men are offered Viagra for loss of libido, but nothing of a similar nature exists for women. Guess it's not considered important.

Fortunately, women do have an opportunity to regain their sexuality, and that answer comes from the replacement of bioidentical hormones. BHRT, as you will read, is not only cancer protective, but also restores quality of life.

But today, without the protection of real hormone replacement, breast cancer rates are rising once again to frightening levels, one out of every eight women. Scientific studies suggest that bioidentical progesterone and estriol offer protection against breast cancer, but no one has connected the dots. Synthetics were chemicals and the chemicals were responsible for raising breast cancer rates. Dr. Wright and Dr. Julie Taguchi both feel that correct bioidentical hormone replacement is *protective* against cancer. Studies also suggest that this type of hormone replacement is related to favorable gene expression—explained by Dr. Burzynski as turning off genetic switches that enable cells to propagate out of control.

Men suffer from hormonal loss, too. They have the same cancer-protective switches that get turned off by the same lifestyle habits and toxicity. With bioidentical hormone replacement, men can maintain their edge. They can protect their hearts and, best of all, protect and prevent cancer, especially prostate cancer.

It is the theory of Jonathan Wright, an esteemed, Western-trained doctor (as well as Dr. Taguchi), that hormones replaced in perfect ratios will prevent breast cancer and all other cancers, provided the patient is compliant with good diet, stress management, and detoxification.

SS: Hello, Jonathan. It is so nice to interview you again—you always have so much to say, and your profound understanding of the hormonal system and hormone replacement is what I want to discuss with you today. In keeping with the ideas of this book, I would like you to tell us why it is that hormones protect us from cancer and why, as we age and decline in hormones, we need to replace the missing hormones in order to protect us from getting cancer.

JW: Thanks again, Suzanne, for this opportunity.

Let's start with the hormone DHEA. This hormone has the broadest application against cancers of all sorts because DHEA is a key hormone in regulating an important enzyme involved in the pathway that feeds energy to cancers.

In the nineteenth century, it was discovered that cancers operate by *anaerobic* metabolism, meaning operating without oxygen. The majority of metabolism in the human body is *aerobic*, with oxygen. You've heard of aerobic exercise, with increased oxygen use?

SS: Yes, absolutely.

JW: Uniquely, cancers operate with only anaerobic metabolism, meaning they cannot operate with oxygen. It actually kills the cells. There is one major pathway of anaerobic metabolism that feeds energy to cancers, and cancers must rely on that pathway to survive. If that pathway is slowed down or choked off or down-regulated, then a newly developing cancer can't draw as much energy. More cancers die in the early stages on their own because they don't get energy.

DHEA down-regulates that major pathway by its effect on the enzyme G6PD [glucose-6-phosphate dehydrogenase], which helps feed anaerobic energy to cancers. Populations who genetically have weak G6PD have been found to have a lot less cancer.

SS: You mean because this enzyme is weak in these people their pathway is automatically down-regulated because their bodies can't produce as much energy anaerobically, so cancers have a harder time even getting started, as well as a harder time growing if they do get started?

JW: Right. So if we keep our DHEA at Jack Benny levels—he said he was perpetually thirty-nine, or maybe even age thirty or so—the pathway that can feed anaerobic energy to the cancer will not be as active, and more cancers will die earlier.

SS: How do you know this? What studies or experiments have been done to prove this?

JW: Almost all research proving this point has been done in animals, because it involves deliberately giving them carcinogens. One such study divided animals into two groups. One group had DHEA in their animal chow, and the other half did not.

All the animals were then given the same amount of carcinogen in the same exact dose. In the group that got DHEA, 15 percent or so got cancer. That's a significant percentage, but in the group that did not get DHEA, over 50 percent developed cancer.

SS: That is quite significant.

JW: It's very probable that this down-regulation by DHEA of anaerobic energy fed to the cancer in the experimental animals is why they developed less cancer.

Similar animal studies have had similar results. We can conclude from all of them that DHEA can reduce our risk of cancers by putting a brake on feeding them anaerobic energy. Of course, we cannot say it totally eliminates the risk of cancer, but it does significantly reduce the risk.

Giving people carcinogens in experiments of course isn't done, so there are no human studies done the same way. But as I mentioned before, there are substantial populations of people, usually living in malaria-ridden areas, who have genetically weak G6PD enzymes—this actually is a partial protection against dying of malaria—and it's well established that they get significantly fewer cancers of all sorts.

SS: So DHEA is protective and preventative against cancer.

JW: Very protective, but for best results it must be used in a cream form so it can be transported through skin or mucous membranes and is delivered directly into the bloodstream, and from there to each and every cell in the body without being changed first by our livers. When we swallow DHEA (or any other natural steroid hormone such as estrogen or testosterone) it goes to the liver first, not the rest of our body cells, and the liver's basic job with steroid hormones is to alter them by conjugation with other molecules, like hanging a baggage routing tag on them, mostly so they can then be routed for disposal and excretion.

When we use DHEA in the cream form, only a little bit of DHEA is altered by the liver with every complete circulation of the blood, so more DHEA molecules survive for our other cells—skin, muscle, bone, brain, all of them—to use them before they're "thrown away."

SS: So if we swallow DHEA or another hormone, does a lot of it go to waste?

JW: Literally. And not only that, but sometimes they also cause trouble. That's very well established with estrogens. If we swallow estrogens—even bioidentical ones—they raise our risk of blood clots, affect our cholesterol levels adversely, and even increase risk of certain cancers. If we rub them on, that doesn't happen. There's considerable research on that point.

It always makes sense to copy nature as closely as possible in medicine—it's always safer, and usually more effective, too—and this is just another good example.

SS: So let's move on to estrogens. How do estrogens protect against cancer? Because we women are always being warned that excessive estrogen is a setup for cancer.

JW: Actually, estrogen can protect against breast cancer in many ways. In the 1960s, Professor Henry Lemon discovered a very interesting thing: Women were more likely to be long-term breast cancer survivors after the surgical removal of their tumors if they had *more* estriol in their urine specimens than estrone and estradiol. Conversely, if they had *less* estriol than estrone and estradiol, they were much less likely to be long-term cancer survivors.

SS: Well, that would be my scenario. My body does not make the very specific type of estrogen called estriol very efficiently at all, as you discovered, and I developed breast cancer.

JW: Yes, but now you've protected yourself by replacing the missing estriol in your body on a daily basis. So you've consciously provided your own protection, while most women's bodies do it automatically.

There was a very large study of estriol's relationship to breast cancer funded by the Department of Defense. Approximately fifteen thousand women enrolled in the Kaiser Permanente health system in Oakland volunteered during their first pregnancies in the late 1960s and early 1970s. They had specimens taken and measured for various things, including particularly estriol. Nothing further was done until the late 1990s, approximately thirty-five years later.

Pregnant women were picked because more estriol is made during pregnancy than at any other times of life. It's also been observed that women who make the most estriol during their pregnancies produce the most estriol throughout their regular menstrual cycles.

When the statistics were compiled approximately thirty-five years later, it was found that the women who had the highest amounts of estriol during their first pregnancies had more than 50 percent fewer breast cancers during that time, and the women with the lowest amounts of estriol had the most breast cancers during those approximately thirty-five years.

SS: So estriol is key and we can measure it through urine testing. It is vitally important that estriol is replaced in the proper amounts for cancer protection.

JW: Yes. Estriol by itself is a weak estrogen, but in the presence of another estrogen such as estradiol it becomes an anticarcinogen. This is definitely a good thing.

SS: My understanding is that textbooks refer to three "classical estrogens": estradiol, estrone, and estriol. And you are saying that for lower cancer risk, there needs to be the correct ratio of estriol to estradiol and estrone. You need to have more estriol than the other two and then it becomes cancer protective.

JW: Exactly! While estradiol is the most potent estrogen, and it's more responsible at puberty for most of the development of breasts and hips and other nice things that help make ladies, it is also procarcinogenic. But in the presence of estriol, much of estradiol's procarcinogenic effect is blocked. Estriol does that with other estrogens also.

SS: But if estriol is a weak estrogen how does it have the strength to be an anticarcinogen?

JW: By occupying the estrogen receptor sites, just sitting there, so not as much estradiol can get through. Some estradiol still gets through anyway, of course, just not as much. So if there is a lot of estriol—more estriol than estradiol and estrone, which is also a procarcinogen—it can do its job and protect against cancer.

SS: If estriol is so important, then why did Wyeth file a "citizen's petition" with the FDA to stop the sale of estriol by compounding pharmacies, and why was the FDA, in conjunction with pharmaceutical companies, instrumental in trying to make this happen?

JW: Because horse estrogens or estrogens sold by patent medicine companies, including Wyeth, do not contain estriol.

SS: So they want to take away a big advantage of presently prescribed bioidentical estrogens—cancer-risk reduction with estriol—because women will buy the pharmaceutical products.

JW: You got it. When you have more estriol occupying the receptor sites than the procarcinogenic estrogens, then they haven't much of a chance of causing cancer.

SS: This is fantastic information, important information. Women need to know this.

JW: Since you mentioned your situation, may I discuss it a bit more?

SS: Sure.

JW: You found out, unfortunately, that even though you were taking a good-size quantity of estradiol, when you did the twenty-four-hour urine test—considered the gold standard for steroid hormone testing—your body wasn't transforming much estradiol into estriol. Your estrone (also metabolized from estradiol) was significantly higher than your estriol. This is not good. Most women's bodies metabolize most of their estrone into estriol but your body was not doing that.

SS: So I was set up for another cancer.

JW: Your risk was definitely higher. So we added extra estriol to your estrogen regimen and compensated for your body's faulty metabolism—in your case probably a genetic problem—and made your overall estrogen replacement protective.

SS: And now I have another layer of protection against breast cancer.

JW: Yes, this was so important for you! I'm glad we got that checked.

SS: I thank you for finding that—it most probably saved my life.

JW: At the very least it increased your odds of not getting another cancer. And thank you for sharing your story so other women can check themselves, too. I hope to do all I can for you and for everybody else I am working with.

Another thing women should know is that iodine stimulates the metabolism of estradiol and estrone into estriol. I've worked with many, many women who had test results like yours to start with. The large majority have been premenopausal women with fibrocystic breast disease. The outright cure for both fibrocystic breast disease as well as raising estriol levels internally without taking estriol from the outside in nearly all cases is just using sufficient iodine or iodide.

SS: That would have been me. I had fibrocystic disease in my premenopausal years. I also experienced childhood abuse, which I think is a significant factor in breast cancer. So, putting these factors together, I was kind of marked, and I guess a lot of women are, but this is why what you are saying is so important. Women reading this are going to connect the dots for themselves, and maybe save their lives as a result.

I use Lugol's iodine orally, but if I get breast pain I put it right on the breast for a while until it calms down. I guess it flares up from stress when the estradiol/estriol quotient gets messed up.

Why is iodine such a big protector against breast cancer?

JW: According to researchers, it directly stimulates the formation of iodolipids—fats combined with iodine—in the breast. Iodolipids kill many types of breast cancer cells: bang, dead! Iodine also promotes the formation of more estriol, which is protective against cancer formation in the first place.

SS: I imagine you are going to say that iodine supplementation should be done under the auspices of your doctor, right?

JW: Absolutely, because if we take too much it can inhibit our thyroid glands and we don't want to do that. Iodine is key but there are some technical points about iodine and iodide use, so it's best to work with a physician skilled and knowledgeable about natural and nutritional medicine and bioidentical hormones for this problem.

SS: On my urine test report there are some more estrogens called 2-hydroxyestrogens and 16-hydroxyestrogens. You are always very concerned with these numbers. Please explain why.

JW: If a premenopausal woman's body is producing more 2-hydroxy-estrogens than 16-hydroxyestrogens, her breast cancer risk is less. This is good. But, if it's the other way around, her breast cancer risk is higher.

SS: How do we keep these two—2 and 16—in the right order?

JW: By eating broccoli, cabbage, cauliflower, Brussels sprouts, bok choy, and other brassica vegetables. They contain compounds that shunt the metabolism of estrone toward the 2-hydroxy, which is more anticarcinogenic, and away from the 16-hydroxy, which is procarcinogenic.

SS: How many servings a week of these vegetables?

JW: Three or more servings a week will reduce breast cancer risk and, incidentally, will also reduce prostate cancer risk for men. A research team reported that if a man's body is producing too much 16-hydroxy, he actually has a greater risk of prostate cancer also.

SS: Can you get the benefits of these vegetables in a supplement form, such as indole-3-carbinol?

JW: Yes. Indole-3-carbinol [I3C] and DIM, a supplement, are actually very concentrated forms of the natural active ingredients in brassica vegetables. Some people prefer supplements, and some physicians recommend that any woman using bioidentical hormones should automatically take DIM or indole-3-carbinol.

SS: I take these supplements even though I consume huge amounts of vegetables daily. But is it possible to take too much DIM and I3C?

JW: Yes, because too much of either will raise the 2/16 ratio too high—too much 2-hydroxy, not enough 16-hydroxy. A high ratio will increase risk of osteoporosis.

SS: Can you eat too much broccoli, too?

JW: That would be almost impossible! This warning applies to sup-

plementation. Don't take I3C or DIM without checking your 2/16 ratio;
if it's too high, research shows it raises your risk for osteoporosis.

SS: How can we tell if it's too much?

JW: You can tell by taking a specific 2/16 urine test, or the twenty-
four-hour urine test, which gives much more information. Either test can
spot if a woman is taking too much DIM or I3C. But if a woman is getting too little iodine or iodide for her body to metabolize estrogen properly, it will show exactly the same pattern of estrogen metabolites, so it's
best to work with a skilled physician.

SS: So if the 2/16 ratio is too low, it's higher cancer risk, and if it's too
high, it's osteoporosis risk.

JW: Right.

SS: Women have three "classical" estrogens plus many others and men
have estrogens also.

JW: That's right. One of these many other estrogens is called
4-hydroxyestrogen. It is a very potent precursor of further metabolites
that are very procarcinogenic. Dr. Henry Lemon did his estriol research at
the University of Nebraska decades ago, and now at that same university
Dr. Ercole Cavalieri has published many papers on the carcinogenicity of
4-hydroxyestrogen.

While the 2/16 hydroxyestrogens are evaluated as a ratio, 4-hydroxy-
estrogen is evaluated by itself. The higher it goes, the greater the cancer
risk.

SS: So what does one do about this?

JW: At present, 4-hydroxyestrogen can only be evaluated on the
twenty-four-hour urine test. If it is higher than desirable, work with a
physician who understands how to alter estrogen metabolism safely with
botanicals and other techniques to shunt your metabolism away from
4-hydroxyestrogen.

Another very important estrogen metabolite—again, only checkable at
present with the twenty-four-hour urine test—is an exceptionally potent
anticarcinogenic estrogen called 2-methoxyestrogen, which is totally natural and made in every woman's body. The pharmaceutical companies
also realized this is anticancer so they decided to try for approval by the
FDA.

They changed the name of their product from 2-methoxyestradiol to
Panzem. In their research, they had women (and men, too) swallow it,
which is totally wrong, as it's well known that swallowed estrogens cause
more tendency to blood clotting and inflammation.

The patent medicine company which renamed 2-methoxyestradiol as Panzem was giving it in dosages as high as 1,000 milligrams daily, which is more than a thousand times as much as is usually found in anyone's body. And this can raise our risk of blood clotting, inflammation, and other problems caused by overwhelming the liver with estrogens of any sort.

But Panzem (2-methoxyestradiol in disguise) is showing positive effects, and it should, because 2-methoxyestradiol is cancer protective. Even some pancreatic cancers are showing improvement, and pancreatic cancer is one of the toughest to treat. Some breast cancers are improving, as are prostate cancers, cervical cancers, endometrial cancers, lung cancers, osteosarcomas, and other cancers.

Unfortunately, by not copying nature—giving enormous quantities of this bioidentical hormone [renamed] and having people swallow it—side effects are showing up, and some individuals stop taking it even though it's helping against their cancers. One of the side effects is nausea and vomiting.

SS: But if it is helping in certain cancers, is it worth the risk?

JW: Sure, but why not give it by nature's route—which is not the gastrointestinal tract—in smaller quantities and see what happens? In fact, Mayo Clinic researchers sort of gave it that way—they used injections instead of having patients swallow it. And surprise! They reported it was effective at lower quantities.

Think about this. Our bodies make 2-methoxyestradiol. Why not make more of our own, internally, and prevent problems as much as possible? It takes much less of anything to prevent a problem, but much more of anything to treat a problem once it has occurred. 2-methoxyestradiol is a methylated estrogen. The enzyme that does the methylation is called COMT, catechol-O-methyltransferase. It transfers the methyl groups to the estrogen and it comes out as 2-methoxyestradiol.

SS: Okay, but I don't know why we care about this.

JW: Because that same enzyme, COMT, helps activate adrenaline when we are under stress by adding more methyl groups. If COMT is kept busy methylating adrenaline, it can't methylate as much estrogen, so our own internal production of 2-methoxyestradiol goes down. Since our own internal 2-methoxyestradiol helps prevent cancer, this is one of the reasons why prolonged stress opens us up to more cancers, especially for premenopausal women. We believe, although it's not yet proven, that stress also affects women on hormone replacement in the same way, that if they are under prolonged stress and their 2-methoxy levels go down (because all those methyl groups are going over to adrenaline), women enduring prolonged stress will have less cancer-fighting potential being made internally.

SS: So let me go over this again: 2-methoxyestradiol is a very potent anticancer hormone that our bodies make, so potent, in fact, that the drug companies want in on it even though it is a nonpatentable substance because it comes from nature. A drug company took 2-methoxyestradiol and changed the name to Panzem so it sounds like a drug, even though it's 100 percent natural. Since they can't patent it, they're counting on the FDA to prevent or eliminate any competition from compounding pharmacies.

It's being administered in huge dosages, a thousand times more than the body ever made, to fight cancers, and it is being given orally, which is dangerous because when taken orally even bioidentical estrogens can create damage in the liver, create blood clots, and drive up inflammation in the body. So it won't do as much good or be as safe as if it were given in a way closer to the way nature uses to circulate it into our bodies, which isn't through our GI tracts and then past our livers first.

You are saying if the FDA would get out of the way of natural medicine, women and men could take 2-methoxyestradiol from a compounded pharmacy in its natural form in a cream base. It could be rubbed on to be received transdermally and it could provide huge anticancer functions.

Why is the FDA in our way? Why are they involved?

JW: If the FDA is successful at preventing compounding pharmacists from compounding nature's own bioidentical hormones, then the patent medicine companies will be the only ones who are approved to sell this stuff. If no one else is allowed to sell these hormones, then patent medicine companies still have an "exclusive"—as if they had a patent on nature—and they would be able to make enormous profits, which is the whole point with patent medicine companies.

SS: And the fact that people will have blood clots and inflammation, which is dangerous to their health and lives, by taking such big dosages, and that they are throwing up, is not an issue with them.

JW: Right. These huge doses are not good for people, and it is not good for those of us who want to go natural or alternative.

SS: I am constantly astounded that big business and government in our great country has such a hold over our abilities to treat our bodies the way we choose. I don't want their drugs unless absolutely necessary. I want to live a natural life. Where does someone like me get the treatment I desire?

JW: You have to go around and find out the information for yourself, as you do, Suzanne. You have to do your own research and read between the lines when attacks come out, like this latest *Newsweek* article attacking you and Oprah for featuring bioidentical hormones.

SS: Yes, you are right, and it is true. So let's go back to hormones and their cancer-protective advantages.

JW: Okay. The subject was stress reduction so our bodies can make more cancer-fighting 2-methoxyestradiol. We can also take safe, natural supplements from natural food stores to help our bodies manufacture 2-methoxyestradiol. This includes supplements with the word *methyl* or *meth* in them, such as methylcobalamin, which is a particular form of vitamin B_{12}; methylfolate, a more active form of folic acid; and S-adenosylmethionine, also called SAM-e. Those three supplements will help our bodies increase our own anticancer 2-methoxyestradiol.

> *Another research paper showed that even in very tiny amounts, 2-methoxyestradiol inhibits the growth of uterine fibroid cells. So not only is it cancer inhibiting, it also inhibits benign abnormal growth.*

SS: This is fantastic information. B_{12} injections and SAM-e increase cancer protection. Women are having such problems with fibroid growth . . . and as a result the remedy is to do total hysterectomies. And you and I both know that women are never the same after a total hysterectomy unless they are fortunate enough to find a doctor who knows how to restore them hormonally—which rarely happens.

JW: Most doctors don't understand how to work with human chemistry using bioidentical substances and substances found in nature. In a couple of generations we are going to look back and say, "Oh my, why weren't we teaching this in medical schools?"

Most doctors don't study how to manipulate normal body chemistry safely and effectively with molecules natural to the body, so they would not have a clue about 2-methoxyestradiol and its anticancer effect, but there are many research papers about it.

SS: Well, while we are at it, why isn't this being taught in medical schools?

JW: Because medical schools teach about body chemistry, but when it's time to teach how to work with body chemistry to treat illness, medical schools switch away from using chemicals naturally made in our bodies or introduced from nature—which our bodies are adapted to, with some exceptions, of course—and start teaching what to do about illness with patent medicines.

By law, patent medicines can't be naturally occurring. The vast majority of them have never, ever been in human bodies. So how can we expect them to work as well as molecules that belong there? Besides, as our bodies aren't designed to use the molecules of patent medicines, they always have adverse effects. Natural molecules can and do have adverse effects, too, but they're many, many fewer than patent medicine molecules.

SS: What else should we know about hormones and cancer protection?

JW: There is a testosterone-metabolizing enzyme called 5-alpha reductase and the patent medicine companies are all over that one. They've made patent medications including Proscar and Propecia that inhibit 5-alpha reductase, and research has found that inhibiting 5-alpha reductase could lower a man's risk of prostate cancer. But there's a potential problem with doing that.

Here's the natural pathway of metabolism: testosterone can turn into dihydrotestosterone (DHT). The enzyme that helps do that is 5-alpha reductase. DHT is an even more potent version of testosterone than testosterone itself and is thought to be procarcinogenic.

An article in the *New England Journal of Medicine* pointed out that after testosterone turns into DHT, DHT is then metabolized into androstenediol, which is actually anticarcinogenic. So what's important is the balance between the procarcinogenic DHT and the anticarcinogenic androstenediol, not just the amount of either one alone. It's a very similar situation to the ratio between procarcinogenic estrone and estradiol and the anticarcinogenic estriol that we covered earlier.

SS: So if a man has more androstenediol than he has DHT, that man is less likely to get cancer from the procarcinogenic DHT because of a properly balanced ratio?

JW: Correct. We can do twenty-four-hour urine tests that check the DHT and the androstenediol and we can also check blood tests. But if a man is taking either Proscar or Propecia or another 5-alpha-reductase inhibitor, the lab report will show it. DHT will be significantly reduced. If that were the only effect of these patent medicines, we could say there's no question that they reduce cancer risk, so—as some urologists have written—every man should use them. Unfortunately, sometimes these drugs lower androstenediol even more than they lower DHT, which gives an improperly balanced ratio—too little anticarcinogenic androstenediol, even though procarcinogenic DHT has been lowered, and that increases cancer risk.

This was pointed out by the *New England Journal of Medicine* article, that too much inhibition of 5-alpha reductase with Proscar and Propecia might inhibit androstenediol, resulting in the wrong balance.

There was actually a study called the Prostate Cancer Prevention Trial that illustrated this hazard. Men were asked to take one of the 5-alpha reductase inhibitors or a placebo in a double-blind, randomized, controlled study over a number of years. In the placebo group, 24.4 percent of the men ended up getting prostate cancer. In the group that took the patent medicine 5-alpha-reductase inhibitors, 18 percent ended up with cancer. That is significantly less. But if you read this prostate trial completely, it turns out that amongst the 24.4 percent of the men in the placebo group who got prostate cancer, only 22 percent of the cancers were highly aggressive. But in the men who were taking the patent medicine 5-alpha-reductase inhibitors, 37 percent of their cancers were highly aggressive. Highly aggressive means more likely to be deadly.

SS: So that's why we never heard of the Prostate Cancer Prevention Trial.

JW: Right! Can you imagine the ad saying, "Take my patent medicine because you'll get less cancer, but if you do get cancer, you are more likely to die"? I don't think they want to say that.

But of course there's debate. Just last year, some researchers in the United States said that their reevaluation of the research didn't come to the same conclusions, and wrote that all men should take a patent medicine 5-alpha-reductase inhibitor to reduce their risk of prostate cancer. But a very prestigious review from the United Kingdom—the *Cochrane Database of Systematic Reviews*—concluded that there just isn't enough information about the effects of these patent medications on prostate cancer deaths.

SS: What about men taking the supplement saw palmetto? Isn't that a 5-alpha-reductase inhibitor?

JW: Yes, it is. Saw palmetto can be used as a 5-alpha-reductase inhibitor for men whose 5-alpha-reductase enzyme is overactive. And it works, but even though it's natural and less hazardous than patent medicines, it's still important to check both DHT and androstenediol if you're taking saw palmetto for years and years.

But before a man reaches for the saw palmetto, he should know that both supplemental zinc and some fatty acids—especially gamma-linolenic acid (GLA)—can inhibit 5-alpha reductase, too, and should be tried first, because they are both essential to life, and saw palmetto isn't.

SS: Why is that important?

JW: If our bodies need an essential nutrient for one purpose, it's very likely our bodies need it for many other purposes, too, including many we don't even know about. If a man needs zinc to modulate his testosterone metabolism, he may need it for his vision, his hearing, or something else. But if he uses saw palmetto instead, it won't help these other areas.

But one thing we all need to understand: even though bioidentical hormones are much safer than patent medicine versions of hormones, there's no such thing as perfect safety. The best we can do is minimize our risk. That's why very careful follow-up testing is so important.

SS: So you are saying there is no surefire protection that will absolutely, positively prevent cancer? Are you saying that cancer is deadly and sometimes it kills in spite of everything one does to minimize risk?

JW: It's important to state that fact. Even premenopausal women or men can develop hormone-related cancer from time to time, and these are people who are still manufacturing their own hormones and they *are* bioidentical because they are internally produced. So no, we cannot eliminate the risk totally, particularly in today's world with all the toxic chemicals out there. But at least we can minimize the risk by getting a comprehensive test that shows not only your levels of hormones—as in "Is it too much, or is it too little, or is it just right?"—but also checks all these points of metabolism of hormones, whether they're made internally or taken as bioidentical hormones from the outside. If hormones are not metabolizing properly, there is something that can be done nearly every time: a vitamin, a mineral, an herb, or something natural that will stimulate normal metabolism or inhibit abnormal metabolism.

SS: What about men whose bodies turn their testosterone into too much estrogen? I don't think men understand this, but whenever I see a man with breasts and a big belly, I usually presume that it might be that too much of his testosterone has turned into estrogen. This is a dangerous scenario for men, isn't it?

JW: Yes it is . . . too much or the wrong kind of estrogen can be a cancer setup for a man's prostate gland.

SS: Besides the visible effect of too much estrogen in a man—including breasts, big belly, high voice, sagging shoulders, lack of energy, lack of vitality, inability to achieve potent erections—all can indicate that the ratio of estrogen to testosterone is off and causing symptoms.

You see, this is where women are different: if we were experiencing equivalent symptoms, we would be at the doctor's office immediately. Men will just accept these symptoms as normal and give in.

JW: If too much estrogen for a man is the problem, he can easily pick this up with a twenty-four-hour urine test because the urine test can show estriol and other estrogens that a blood test can't.

If a man finds higher estrogen levels than normal and relatively low testosterone levels, he shouldn't push testosterone replacement until he works to correct the reasons why too much of his testosterone is turning into estrogen. This is one of several ways to reduce cancer risk, too.

If a man sticks to the program—which involves diet change and several supplements—he can lower his estrogens and more safely use testosterone supplementation. He can get to feeling so much better, he gets his energy back, and if he works on his health seriously, he can achieve his optimal self.

SS: Has anyone ever gotten cancer from using bioidenticals?

JW: I can't say there is research on this; in fact, there's virtually none. But I can tell you that I started prescribing bioidentical hormones in the early 1980s. Until now, 2009, I have talked to exactly one woman who came back and said, "I started taking bioidenticals and I ended up with cancer," but I think she had some other problems behind it. Her cancer was diagnosed almost exactly three months after she started taking the bioidenticals. But because of the size of her cancer there is no way it could have grown that fast in that amount of time.

SS: What is the relationship of progesterone to cancer?

JW: Progesterone is generally considered to be anticarcinogenic. It does reduce a woman's risk of cancer if one is taking bioidentical estrogen. Testosterone (in woman-size quantities) reduces a woman's risk, too, as does melatonin. But progesterone is the major protector in this group.

SS: What do you mean, "major protector"?

JW: If a woman is using bioidentical hormones, she should be using a pattern that includes estrogen, progesterone, DHEA, melatonin, and likely testosterone and a little bit of thyroid.

Men using bioidentical testosterone should likely be using DHEA, melatonin, and a little bit of thyroid, too.

SS: Should women be using estrogen in a cycling pattern? Mimicking nature, just like when we were making a cycle naturally?

JW: It's always safest to mimic nature. It's a bit of work getting older—we've all heard that before—but if you pay attention and do this work, it can give you a longer, healthier, more active life.

SS: Let me tell you, it's not work—it takes me about fifteen minutes a day to do my routine and about $85 a month for hormones, and for this I get to live a more youthful, happier, higher quality of life.

I get attacked for doing this by journalists incorrectly saying I am doing this to *look* youthful. I can never refute this because it draws more attention to it, but my objective is not about looking younger, although I find that to be a nice side effect. My objective for doing this is to keep my insides young and working at optimal levels as a means of disease prevention. I do not want to be sick again ever.

JW: Absolutely! Fool all those people out there who are saying you are a quack.

One more bit of information: Dr. Guy Abraham, who has led the revolution in iodine use, reminded us that a *Journal of the American Medical Association* article in the 1970s reported that women who take thyroid and do not take iodine had precisely twice the risk of cancer as those women who take thyroid and iodine. And on its own, iodine (not iodide) protects a woman against breast cancer. Two groups of researchers have reported that iodine actually helps kill some breast cancer cell lines.

SS: Well, then that's another area where I am protected. I take thyroid and iodine and iodide thanks to you.

JW: And it should be all three: thyroid, iodine, and iodide. Women who want to take advantage of iodine's protective effects against breast cancer should check with a physician skilled and knowledgeable in natural and nutritional medicine and, if possible, knowledgeable in bioidentical hormones, too.

SS: Iodide also helps with acid reflux—a manifestation they don't tell you about when undergoing radiation.

One last question. The last time we were together you mentioned that Dr. Bill Cham, who wrote a book called *The Eggplant Cancer Cure*, actually has come up with a nontoxic cream that kills skin cancer. Tell me about that.

JW: Yes, Dr. Cham has found substances that can penetrate and kill skin cancer cells, but can't penetrate normal skin cells. So normal skin cells are untouched and unhurt while the skin cancer cells die.

SS: We're talking basal cell carcinoma and squamous cell carcinoma, right?

JW: Correct. You can read all about it in his book, and you can order his cream from our dispensary at the Tahoma Clinic.

SS: I used his cream Curaderm on a skin cancer on my leg that according to my doctor "needed to be cut out," and after a month of application, the skin cancer disappeared. I'll be sure to put this information in the back of the book.

What keeps you going?

JW: My major goal is for our children—and for sure everybody's grandchildren—to have the freedom to choose any type of health care they would like. Whether it is patent medicine or natural medicine, it doesn't matter, if there is a choice—freedom—to choose without persecution or prosecution by any government interference, without FDA raids or harassment, without even much criticism.

Academic debate is fine, it'll go on forever, but the kind of criticism I am specifically talking about comes from people who are given the power to harass and even arrest those who are taking care of their health in ways they don't happen to like.

We are told we are fighting for freedom overseas, but what we need to do—in my opinion, of course—is to bring the army, navy, and marines home to help restore health care freedom along with the many other freedoms we are supposed to have if we follow the Constitution of these United States of America as was intended by the Founding Fathers of our republic.

SS: Well, it does amaze me that we do not have that freedom in this country. Kind of boggles the mind.

JW: Because this is not at all what was intended by the Founding Fathers, nor what they wrote in the Constitution. It is also amazing that our Congress has allowed the growth of giant bureaucracies, giant government agencies, most of them federal, which are allowed to promulgate regulations without any congressional oversight. Those agencies then turn into judge, jury, and, in fact, executioner—no separation of powers. While they don't actually cut off anybody's head, they do impose enormous fines, they destroy businesses, and they can do all that by administrative process.

SS: A number of doctors in my book, yourself included, have been persecuted.

JW: Imagine how many more innovative physicians we would have doing safe, natural therapies if they weren't simply so intimidated by what they have seen happen to so many of these doctors. Dr. Burzynski is the best—or the worst—example of intimidation, however you'd like to look at that.

SS: And with Dr. Forsythe, for him with the FDA guns drawn, it was like the Wild West. Hopefully this book will continue to educate my readers about the realities of true health, what is available, and the spin that big business puts on this type of approach to health. I always say, if we all felt as good as those of us on full bioidentical hormone replacement, no one would need all their drugs, and that is what this is all about. We are not the customer they want. Big business would prefer we are in a constant state of degradation and needing many of their drugs to get us through the day.

Thank you for your insights, Jonathan. Bioidentical hormones are cancer protective, and now you have educated my readers so that they can take advantage of your knowledge for a healthier and longer life with quality and cancer protection. I appreciate you.

JW: Thank you for all you are doing, Suzanne.

Knock It Out

- DHEA is a key hormone in regulating an important enzyme involved in the pathway that feeds energy to cancers. By keeping DHEA at the right level, we can make the pathway less active, so more cancer cells die sooner. DHEA must be used in a cream form, so it can be transported through skin or mucous membranes straight into the bloodstream.

- Estriol by itself is a weak estrogen, but in the presence of another estrogen such as estradiol it becomes an anticarcinogen, making it important for cancer protection. If you are not making enough estriol, then you should replace it in the proper amounts to reduce your cancer risk.

- Iodine stimulates the metabolism of estradiol and estrone into estriol, increasing your cancer protection. In many premenopausal women with fibrocystic breast disease, the outright cure for this is getting sufficient iodine (working with your physician); you can either rub it directly on the breast or swallow it in less severe cases. It has also been reported that women who take thyroid, but not iodine, have twice the risk of cancer as those women who take both thyroid and iodine.

- It's important to have the right balance of 2-hydroxyestrogen and 16-hydroxyestrogen. In premenopausal women, if there is more 2-hydroxyestrogen than 16-hydroxyestrogen, breast cancer risk is less. If it's the other way around, more 16 than 2, breast cancer risk is greater. Eating three or more servings a week of broccoli, cabbage, Brussels sprouts, bok choy, and other cruciferous vegetables helps keep the right balance. You can also get the benefits of these vegetables in a supplement form such as indole-3-carbinol.

- 2-methoxyestradiol is a very potent anticancer hormone that the body can manufacture. According to research, 2-methoxyestradiol can also inhibit the growth of fibroid cells in the uterus.

Chapter 15

DR. STEPHEN SINATRA

Cancer is but one of the many ways the body tries to change the way you see and treat yourself, including your body. This inevitably brings up the subject of spiritual health, which plays at least as important a role in cancer as physical and emotional reasons do.

—Andreas Moritz

Speaking with Stephen Sinatra, M.D., F.A.C.C., F.A.C.N., was an absolute pleasure. Soft-spoken and with a heart of gold coupled with an extraordinary intellect, he has the capacity to forever change the way doctors interact with their patients, for the better.

He is a board-certified cardiologist, certified bioenergetic psychotherapist, and certified antiaging specialist. He is a fellow of the American College of Cardiology and former chief of cardiology at Manchester Memorial Hospital, where he was director of education. He is also assistant clinical professor of medicine at the University of Connecticut School of Medicine.

An overachiever for sure, his more than forty years of experience in helping patients prevent disease through the integration of conventional medicine and complementary nutritional and psychological therapies have provided a whole new approach to wellness and healing. He works with his patients through encouragement, much like an athletic coach, confirming to his patients that they can do it. It's a huge part of healing that is often overlooked or ignored.

If you or a loved one is wrestling with a serious disease like cancer, or any other disease, you will truly gain new insights into your own innate abilities to heal yourself by reading this interview with Dr. Sinatra.

Dr. Sinatra has written eight books, including *The CoenzymeQ10 Phenomenon; Heartbreak and Heart Disease;* and *Lower Your Blood Pressure in Eight Weeks.* He is the editor of a monthly newsletter called *HeartSense.*

SS: Thank you for your time, Dr. Sinatra. Your philosophy as explained in your books resonates with the way I try to live my life. The power of belief and the power of your thinking ties in beautifully with this project about preventing and curing cancer. Can you elaborate?

SINATRA: Well, belief is the most important element. Attention and belief. I stumbled upon this maybe five, ten years ago as the most important aspect of healing. In my history as a cardiologist, I see people with devastating disease, I've resuscitated dozens and dozens of people from sudden death, I've taken care of hundreds of patients with myocardial infarction, heart attacks, and I've pronounced many people dead in the middle of the night. I've spent lots of time with dying people, had many death experiences with people. And what I learned after practicing medicine for almost forty years is that with any illness, I don't care if it's cancer or heart disease or severe crippling arthritis, the most important thing I can instill into the patient is the belief that he or she can get well.

Once a doctor instills that confidence, the patient takes part in it. Then there's a dance that goes on. It's a marvelous dance because then it is the patient's intention to get well and not be a victim of the illness. This is where a lot of oncologists really destroy people, by saying, "Well, you have six months to live," or, worse, "You'd better get your things in order." You see, once that is said, it wipes out everything.

As a doctor, you have to instill in them a belief that they will get well, and convince them of this fact so they truly believe it. And then they will get well. Once belief is established, that's 50 percent of the battle. Then comes the easy stuff—working on the physical body.

SS: Is it because you've instilled in these people an emotional and spiritual path that they are taking it in?

SINATRA: Yes. Have you ever read Bruce Lipton's book *The Biology of Belief?*

SS: Yes, I have. It seems he is saying essentially the same thing.

SINATRA: Yes, that if your intention and belief are strong enough, you can change your DNA. Look at cancer. Cancer is DNA gone wild, an aberrant DNA gone off on its own course, which has changed other DNA, meaning the cells have changed. I understand that people get cancer for a variety of reasons, but basically there is now a change in the DNA, and *you* have the power to change your DNA by believing you can achieve wellness. Paracelsus was a physician in the Middle Ages who used to say that a doctor guides a patient on their track, and that a doctor doesn't heal, only nature heals. He was right. Physicians can put people on the right track or the wrong track.

SS: That's an interesting approach. So a doctor is really more like a nurse—guiding, helping, but not healing?

SINATRA: Right. The doctor just coaches the patient while instilling intention and belief in the patient. I don't care what the illness is—when the patient has the right intention, trust occurs and nature then takes its course.

When I see patients in the office, I look them in the eye and tell them they are going to get well. I touch them physically and try to transfer my positive energy to them. That's the joy of medicine, when the patient takes it in. I've had many a patient with end-stage heart failure say, "Do you think I'll be here in six months?" And I say, "Absolutely, you will be here," and the truth is they will be.

SS: You are an extraordinary and evolved person and doctor. Let me tell you about me for a second as an example of what you are saying. I am an extremely upbeat person. So when my house burned down and I stood and looked at the smoldering rubble, and all the ashes, and everything was gone, I remember hearing myself, barely audible, still saying, "I am going to learn something great from this." And when I was misdiagnosed with lung cancer, I said to the doctor, "You are wrong." And it turned out she was. You see, I had that belief.

But last November an episode occurred that I write about at the beginning of this book, and although I am an upbeat person, a person who always sees the glass as half full, I have to say that after six days and six doctors telling me I had inoperable metastatic cancer and that the only thing I could do was accept full-body chemotherapy or get my things in order, it wore me down. The constant assertions of these doctors did me in; the message got into my cells, where I accepted that I was going to die.

I found myself thinking of who would get what, and what I was going to say to my children to prepare them for a life without me. I was extremely sad—unbelievable sadness. And the emotional recovery from the horrible misdiagnosis for me was very, very long and it was very difficult to turn things around on a cellular level.

So what I am trying to say is, you are one in a million. I don't think this kind of philosophy is happening in mainstream medicine. I think most people being given a cancer diagnosis shut down. In my case, my acceptance finally came to the overwhelming evidence that was presented to me daily by "professionals" that my CAT scan showed full-body cancer. I don't care how positive you are—at some point, you give in: "How can I be right when they are all saying the contrary?"

That is what we are fighting, how to teach other doctors to adopt this positiveness, rather than saying there's only one way. No one ever said, "Visualize yourself better, Suzanne, you can do it." Instead, I was presented with a death sentence. It's very, very, very debilitating.

SINATRA: Yes, I agree, and you said it beautifully. Because even you, being very evolved, when the envelope was pushed to the maximum, where even your cells questioned whether you were going to live or die, even you at some point questioned. People will resonate with that struggle. But you never gave up hope.

When I lecture to doctors, I say, "Look, as a physician, I have seen people turn around who were in comas for weeks, when loved ones and doctors wanted to pull the plug and I would say, 'Don't pull the plug.' I have had patients transferred to my hospital who were deemed terminal, where I would treat them differently, and they would recover and walk out of the hospital. In fact, there was a patient who was on CNN with me after seven doctors had certified her as dead."

This woman was seventy-five years old. She had gotten a new carpet in her home which was full of formaldehyde, and she developed pneumonia and was admitted to the hospital. The only other time she had ever been in a hospital was when she gave birth. To make a long story short, she developed GI bleeding, went into respiratory failure, developed renal failure, and had swelling of the brain and bacteria in her blood. She had seven specialists working on her and they all wanted to pull the plug. Her son was a biochemist who did a lot of work on CoQ_{10}. He called me up and asked me if I would take her in as a transfer. He said, "At least with you she would have a fighting chance." He was crying. I was worried that the ambulance ride would do her in, and that the artery pressure would be impossible, so I told him I would take her but I couldn't be held responsible if she left the world in the ambulance.

The reason I tell you this is that as a physician, I always believe, as Yogi Berra said, "It's not over till it's over." There was still a chance, you know, until there is a flat line, and I felt against all odds she might make it. When I took this woman into our hospital the head nurse was very angry at me, furious, and I said, "Look, if this were your mother, wouldn't you want to do anything, anything to save her?" She said, "No, because there is no hope." I asked for another nurse and was able to bring back the same one who took care of my own mother, a nurse with a lot of love in her, the kind who takes care from her heart.

We gave this woman CoQ_{10} and magnesium, plus IV vitamins, and she started to blink her eyes in three days. Seventeen days later she walked out of the hospital under her own power and lived another seven years. I tell you this because physicians are so quick to pull the plug, yet all I did was treat her nutritionally and energetically.

Even if patients have terminal metastatic cancer, I feel that if they are still breathing on their own, there is hope. I'm teaching this to doctors.

SS: It's quite interesting that you are a cardiologist and a psychoanalyst—a combination of professional skill plus the ability to embrace the human condition. It almost seems like this is the way it should be.

SINATRA: I did five years of training after medical school, three in internal medicine, two in cardiology, and I took my boards in 1977. I was seeing a lot of sudden death when I was a resident around the time the Vietnam War was winding down. I realized that stress and illness were big factors, because I was doing angiograms on thirty-five-year-old men, many of them had Ph.D.'s and were engineers, and I was seeing a lot of stress with their hearts.

Many of these young men were losing jobs around this time because the war was winding down and Pratt and Whitney and Colt firearms was a big part of our economy. That's when I realized that the mind-body connection was so enormous when it comes to heart disease, and that is when I realized I needed to learn about cardiology from the neck up. I enrolled myself in a two-year Gestalt psychotherapy program based on Fritz Perl's work. One of the books on the reading list was *Bioenergetics* by Dr. Alexander Lowen.

> *Bioenergetic therapy is about resolving blocks and tension in the body through emotional release work and exercises that release energy in the body.*

The years I spent in that psychotherapy training program were harder than going to medical school. You had to do about two hundred hours of personal therapy on yourself and fifty hours of supervision.

SS: Don't you think this makes you a better doctor? That your approach to wellness entails body, mind, and spirit? To me, what's missing in doctoring today, amongst other things, is taking in the person as an individual: what he's been through and what he needs to work through in order to handle whatever disease might manifest.

SINATRA: You got it, absolutely got it. All the patient wants is to be seen. In other words, they want you to understand their suffering, their terrible journey, how they are feeling in their bodies. They want you to touch them. Doctors today don't even look at their patients, they're writing as they talk to them. Doctors rarely truly *examine* patients anymore, and basically what today's doctors do instead is write prescriptions. We've gotten away from real doctoring and it's become all about pharmaceutical drugs, computers, and diagnosis.

SS: When I was a kid the doctor would come to your house and listen to your heart and lungs, and would touch your body, and feel for your temperature and place his hands on you. And it would be in its way very healing, calming.

SINATRA: Yes, and that no longer happens. Medicine has become too mechanized. It has lost its personal touch; it's all about insurance and money. My mission is to spend the next twenty years teaching medical students, naturopathic students, as well as doctors and even older doctors, so that they understand the value of treating patients as individuals. Show them how to give energy and healing through compassion and healing touch.

SS: What a noble thing to do for the next twenty years. I realize my experience I describe at the beginning of this book was sent to me for a reason. I had to see it firsthand, yet the ER experience in its way was extraordinary.

ER docs and nurses are very nurturing and protective. Even though I was at death's door, literally out of breath, their confidence reassured me. The ER doc kept yelling at me to "breathe, breathe!" I lived because of them; they saved my life. It was once I got into the "system" upstairs in the hospital that the indifference and arrogance of modern medicine reared its ugly head. The oncologist was actually angry because he had declared that I was riddled with cancer and it turned out to be incorrect, and I presume he felt stupid. No compassion, no tenderness. I'm sitting there having had to look at my impending death, with my neck cut open from surgery, and he wasn't able to say a kind word or put his hand on my shoulder. If that is what is going on, then it's a disaster.

SINATRA: You are correct. Going back to the seventy-five-year-old woman with the seven doctors where they said to pull the plug, that's a story I use often to teach doctors that you never give up until it's over. Unless a patient is severely brain-dead and you see a flat line on the brain and there is absolutely no hope, you don't give up. She lived another seven years and clearly lived. She had a library of over three thousand books; she invited me to her home for dinner, and her son was there, and she told me a story that made me cry. She was dismayed that after she left the hospital—it was now three months later—not one of those doctors ever called her to tell her how happy they were she was alive. But that's the way it is. Not one of them ever called me either and said, "Good job." Not one of them.

SS: They were probably embarrassed. Ego. It's easier to be silent; certainly not as healing, but it is an easier out.

SINATRA: Let me tell you a story about me. When my son was dying—

SS: What do you mean dying? Did he die?

SINATRA: No, thank God, he didn't, but I was terrified for two years. I brought him to over a hundred doctors, everyone from friends at Yale to the Mayo Clinic. I brought him to alternative doctors and the doctors in my circles. He had an unexplained illness, an illness of this millennium; we think the problem was an extension of his work on Wall Street and that he got electrically polluted from cellular phones. I mean, he always had a cell phone in each ear, and worked in a sea of computers, six feet of computers actually, like a horseshoe around him. His GI tract shut down, his hormones shut down, and his pituitary was out; also, his temperature went down to 95 degrees. I was giving him IV vitamin C from my kitchen, and eventually put a catheter in his heart. I tried everything. I flew him to Dallas to see a specialist, flew him all over the place, anything, anyone who might be able to help him.

Eventually conventional medicine pulled him back. We did total parenteral nutrition, but during this time he went down to eighty-five pounds and spent forty-two days in the hospital. I slept there night after night, and then one day he said to me, "Dad, I'm thinking dark thoughts." That was a bottom for me. In retrospect, my son has taught me more about illness than anyone or anything or any patient I have ever treated. I knew the tide was turning when one day he said to me, "Dad, I can cure this, I can survive." And he became very spiritual. He was on the other side, praying all the time.

The reason I tell you this is because I developed a really bad pulmonary infection during this time. It was a dark night—my son was still in the hospital and he had no blood pressure, salmonella in his blood, and I thought it was over. As a result, I developed asthma and a pulmonary infection. I went to one of my go-to docs and he said, "The lung is the organ of grief. Don't treat your infection." I said, "What do you mean?" He said, "Look, when the lung develops bacteria or fungus or TB, it's going to end up as cancer. When people have grief, they get cancer of the lung." I sat there stunned. I knew I was in such a weakened state from all the grief, all this terror of losing my child, and it had never dawned on me that it could manifest as cancer. So he said to me again, "Don't treat the infection, treat the grief." That's when I went to Ryke Geerd Hamer's work. He said when people get lung cancer it's because of grief, and a classic example is Dana Reeve [Christopher Reeve's wife]. She developed lung cancer because she lost her husband. She never smoked; it was the shock of suddenly losing someone she loved that much, and instead of developing breast cancer, which is a slower entity, with lung cancer you can go quickly. She wanted to go with him, so from shock and grief she developed lung cancer.

I don't know why things are placed in our paths. You had this fungus in November, but you were not supposed to die. This was placed in your path for a reason. You've had a lot of opportunities to leave, but you are here. You have a mission.

SS: I see that reasoning. I have come to grips with that. I believe that is why I can't find any anger at my misdiagnosis, just the knowledge that it happens to so many and people need to know there are options, choices. That it's not over even if they tell you it's over.

SINATRA: And now your life is going to be on a higher vibration. I always tell doctors, "Follow your intuition, think it through. Don't worry about the diagnosis. Follow your inner voice."

Illness gives us an opportunity to dig into our emotional and spiritual self. That's why I became a bioenergetic psychotherapist, because I realized that illness can be looked at as an opportunity. If you can reframe that to patients and say, "Look, this is placed in your path for a reason," and if they take it in and believe it, then they grow, and that growth and the energy from it, that in itself cures them.

SS: I agree with that. I was able to take myself from this "episode," as I call it, and recover.

As I listen to you, I think having training in psychoanalysis should be a requirement for being a cardiologist. I mean, you are dealing with the heart, the heart of a person, and you are dealing with life and death on a daily basis.

SINATRA: It's very important to just see the patients. That's all they want.

Patients come in with their cancer and they are angry—cancer patients are often very angry—and anger is a good force. Bernie Siegel, my old colleague in cancer who used to lecture with me all the time, would say that one of the best ways for patients to survive cancer is to fight back, to get into their shadow, get into their dark side, and I wholeheartedly agree.

Now, having said that, a lot of patients will come into my office and they'll say to me, "You know, you're not doing a good job. I'm not getting better. I'm still sick." They come on with this anger force. Before I understood, I would get defensive and say, "I'm doing the best I can." Well, that just heightens the fire and heightens the exchange and then you're into an argument. But after all of my training and therapy I changed my approach. I would say now, "Jill, I'm so sorry that you are suffering and I feel for you." I will say these words again and again. Remember what I said before: all patients want to be seen and to have their struggle acknowledged. Once the patients get that you see their struggle, they bond with you, and that is so important. So now I say it: "I'm sorry you are so sick" or "I am sorry that you are suffering and I will work harder, and we will find an answer." A doctor has to speak in positives. If a doctor puts out negative energy, the patients will take it in unconsciously.

SS: This is a crucial thing to teach to other doctors and to influence the new young healers. And you have to mean it. Then you know that you are on the same team. You're not opposing forces. I was reading your book *Heartbreak and Heart Disease* about the shadow, the dark side, about normal patterns of healing. Can you explain that?

SINATRA: Normal patterns of healing?

SS: You said that unfortunately in our society, "normal" is frequently not healthy, and it just may have been our "normal" patterns of feeling, thought, and behavior that brought us to this physical crisis point. You said we are born with a natural capacity to release emotions as soon as they arise.

SINATRA: Right, like when a baby comes into the world and is very flexible and pliable. They haven't developed attitudes or beliefs, but they do have feelings. A baby cries because the only way a baby can really communicate is by crying. Unfortunately, so many children hear the words "Stop crying or we'll give you something to cry about." But you need to understand that basically feelings never lie . . . they never lie.

SS: Okay, feelings never lie.

SINATRA: As psychoanalysts, we used to always tell patients to honor their feelings. Here's an example. The patient says, "I'm feeling sad." We don't tell them to edit the feeling and say, "Oh, I shouldn't be sad. I've got this great marriage, I have all this money, but I'm sad. I've got heartbreak. I want to cry." We would just tell them to cry. In other words, the feeling is the truth. That's the truth in the body. So the most important thing about having sadness, for example, is to experience it, even anger. Not rage—I mean, people are killed in fits of rage, and it's a very destructive emotion. But anger can be healing, especially with a cancer patient who can turn anger into a mobilizing force.

In any illness I would encourage feelings of sadness and anger. Sadness is a very healing emotion, because in order to heal the heartbreak of heart disease—and I firmly believe one of the biggest risk factors in heart disease is heartbreak—we need to cry.

Crying is the most healing of emotions because when you go into deep sobbing, not only does it alleviate tension in your vocal cords, in your lungs, in your diaphragm, and in your heart, but also the tears themselves are healing. Tears contain endorphins, and these are healing chemicals.

Whenever you cry, you are healing the body. In 1982 I did a workshop in my hospital with forty-four men and women with and without heart disease. I did this because I wanted to show the emotional impact of release work on biochemicals that are put out in your blood like adrenaline, epinephrine, and serum cortisol, and then we measured the by-products in the urine. This was an incredible workshop. There was a lot of anger and every other emotion I could think of, and after three days, as you can imagine, we all really bonded. What I learned was that women who networked during the workshop, who hugged one another, who cried with one another, who allowed their anger to come out, they had very low levels of stress breakdown products in the urine. And none of them had heart disease.

When men said things like "I'm fine" but had their arms across their chests, who didn't cry, who didn't get angry, who were macho, their codes showed enormous levels of stress hormones, of cortisol and adrenaline. Suzanne, for the first time in my life back in 1982, I realized that men who don't cry get heart disease. After that revelation I spent the next ten years learning how to cry. That's when I went into bioenergetic psychotherapy. Even as a high school and college athlete, I never cried. I thought not crying was really the way to be until I realized that, my God, I am setting myself up for heart disease by not crying.

SS: Changing gears a little, from middle age on, life becomes very difficult for women. They decline in hormones, lose their sex drive, and in many cases lose their youth and beauty, and unfortunately today's society is obsessed with youth and beauty. They feel "invisible," "sexless," "put out to pasture." So when these women develop breast cancer, the love that is showered on them is unbelievable. It comes from every direction. Even people who used not to like them suddenly feel sorry for them. For many women this is the most attention they have ever gotten in their lives.

SINATRA: So they're getting something out of the illness. They are getting a lot of love and lots of tenderness. They are getting something the body was starving for. And this is why sometimes we create our own illness. In cancer, especially breast cancer, it's about preservation of the nest. Now when she takes this to her heart, to her nest, to her chest, to her femininity, and her safety is threatened, sure, a woman could develop breast cancer—absolutely. That's why every woman who has breast cancer needs to look at the emotional conflict in her life. That's Hamer's work in Germany.

As a psychoanalyst, I believe that every cancer has some form of internal conflict going on, whether it's on the conscious level or the unconscious level. Remember, Suzanne, our unconscious drives are more powerful than our conscious drives. When a patient says to me, "I went to a movie and it made me cry," but then they say, "I have no sadness," well, that's their conscious opinion, but the body always tells the truth.

When the body gets sick, it is giving a message that it is out of balance, it's out of alignment physically, spiritually, and emotionally. So as doctors, when patients are sick, we need to tell them that they are out of balance somehow, and figure out what it is and how to get the balance back.

Emotions are the most powerful aspect of creating illness, but also in taking away illness. Whatever gave the illness was a powerful, deep-seated emotion, but it can be taken away by renavigating that emotion into healing.

There is a simplicity in this approach that is too often diminished because it isn't based on surgery or pharmaceuticals, which absolutely have their place. But compassion and caring and attention and touch are the healing tools of nature. They work. I've seen it time and time again: the power of the mind, body, and spirit.

When my patients contract catastrophic disease, it's like the old Chinese saying, "There's always opportunity in crisis." You must find the good. You must find the lesson and then you will heal.

SS: Thank you for this beautiful insight. I think what you are saying is a big part of the cancer puzzle, and I feel as though a large arm has just been put around both me and my readers and we are comforted. Thank you, Stephen.

Knock It Out

- Attention and belief are the most important elements in self-healing. Believing you can get well is 50 percent of the battle. You have the power to change your DNA by believing you can achieve wellness.
- Seek a doctor who believes you will get better, one who is willing to treat you as an individual, and one who operates by the philosophy "It's not over till it's over." Unless there is absolutely no hope, you don't give up.
- Illness gives us an opportunity to dig into our emotional and spiritual self and treat the source of the pollution that's causing the body to be sick.
- One of the best ways for patients to survive cancer is to use anger to fight back.
- All feelings should be honored as truths in the body.

Chapter 16

DR. MICHAEL GALITZER

Michael Galitzer is my personal Western-trained, integrative antiaging doctor. He understands it all: how to balance hormones, how to strengthen the weakest glands and organs, how to strengthen the body to prepare it for fighting cancer or tolerating conventional therapies, and how to prevent getting cancer in the first place through lifestyle and dietary changes coupled with antiaging therapies. He provides this at his office in Santa Monica, California.

Most of all, he is a compassionate and caring man. He has brilliant instincts and is a proponent of the triad that body, mind, and spirit all work together toward the goal of optimal health and happiness. He has been one of my great teachers.

SS: Hello, Michael. Let's talk about your approach to treating people with cancer.

MG: Okay, Suzanne, let's start with a basic premise: cancer is a disease of the whole body and a tumor is just a symptom of the disease. So basically you've got to treat the whole body; you can't just treat the cancerous tumor and try to kill it or eradicate it with chemo without supporting the whole body. We all have cancer cells in our bodies and that's important for people to understand, but you need about a billion cancer cells to get to the lump or bump stage, which is why a tumor takes years to develop. When traditional medicine diagnoses a tumor—whether it be by mammogram, MRI, or a CAT scan—whatever the diagnosis, it is important to understand that you have time. It is not necessary to start therapy the next day.

SS: As patients, we don't know this. My two cancer experiences both had a rushed element to them, as in "Let's start treatment tomorrow."

MG: Right, but a lump or a bump is an indicator that your body is now extremely toxic. Plus just the experience of being diagnosed with cancer will set a person's immune system back enormously. This is the point when the building-up process has to begin. The patient needs to eat better, take nutrition seriously, and try to only eat organic. And then I would start the detoxification process. The stronger a patient gets, the more likely he is to do well with the therapy given in terms of surgery, chemotherapy, and radiation.

Most cancer patients are depressed and frightened at the possibility of dying. Then on top of that they are given treatments that usually weaken the body. Unfortunately, this combination is a recipe for disaster. When they come to me in this condition, I ask them to take a deep breath. Go find a doctor who does integrative medicine, build up their bodies for four to six weeks with me, and then choose whatever treatment resonates best with them.

SS: Are you a proponent of integrative medicine only, or are you open to patients like me who want to do everything alternative? And just to put you on the spot, who do you think has the better shot?

MG: Who has the better shot? [Laughs] You always do this to me. Okay. We've talked about this in previous interviews. What's more important—the belief of the patient or the belief of the doctor? I think it's the belief of the patient, and as a doctor, you must respect that. If the patient believes chemo is going to help, then most likely it will. The placebo effect works one-third of the time, and the placebo is basically belief overriding biology. I always say to people, "If you can believe it, you can achieve it; if you can see it, you can be it." I truly believe the first key is to respect the belief of the patient.

SS: That's refreshing. Having your doctor work with you is so very helpful. I've spent so much time fighting with doctors, because I want to do everything natural if I can, and their resistance and, worse, mockery make for a contentious experience. Finding alternative Western doctors such as yourself has been a godsend for me.

MG: I work with patients however they choose. For instance, for the past twenty years, I've supported people who have chosen chemo, and many sail through it pretty well. Chemo when coupled with integrative medicine is going to allow most patients to feel safe, and that alone is healing. Then there are patients like you, who see chemo as the poison devil.

SS: I do. The whole idea of putting chemical poisoning inside my body is not, and never will be, an option. That thinking alone on my part means that I would not accept this treatment as a healing cure for me. I would see it as a foreign enemy, trying to kill rather than cure.

MG: That is your belief and you have to go with that belief and do what resonates for you.

I really believe we have all the tools to support any patient doing any sort of allopathic or alternative treatment. Again, one of the key elements of healing is to build that patient up first and then support the patient every day—not only before but after they go through chemo and radiation. My approach is to honor the patient's belief system and then support the patient all the way along the road.

SS: I agree with that, but I have to say in learning about cancer and writing this book there just do not seem to be that many cancers that respond to chemotherapy. And also they are not doing chemosensitivity tests in this country. It just feels like it's off track.

MG: The most off-track aspect is that patients who elect to do these treatments don't see integrative doctors. Their oncologists usually say that what doctors such as myself do won't help. One of my best friends had kidney cancer and went to see the head guy at UCLA, who told him not to bother with homeopathy, nutrition, or vitamin supplements. He said, "None of it works." So my friend just did chemotherapy for four or five months and did very poorly—total body degradation.

SS: To me this is a perfect example. If you don't bother to empower yourself with information and do the research, and just listen to the doctor in front of you, you most likely won't do well or you will die.

One of the problems with chemotherapy is that it doesn't kill the cancer stem cells, and that is something everybody is missing, both conventional medicine and integrative medicine.

MG: The drug companies are very aware of this and they're trying to develop ways to kill these stem cells, but I'm not quite sure that approach will be that successful. So yes, Suzanne, I do agree with you that there have been very few cancers that have been treated successfully with chemo; leukemias in kids, testicular cancer, Hodgkin's, and some other lymphomas are the ones that might respond to chemo.

Bottom line: conventional medicine believes that it is about killing the bad guys and once we kill all the bad guys you're fine. But is it? Isn't it about having a healthy body? What you're saying, Suzanne, is that there is no way the present protocol of surgery, chemotherapy, and radiation is going to result in a healthy body. And if you do this without first strengthening the body, I would agree.

SS: What I have learned writing this book is that cancer appears to be manageable, that we can live with cancer whether the approach is integrative or alternative. So, specifically, what does building up actually mean?

MG: Okay, let's first talk about what causes cancer. We need to define what cancer is before we can actually treat it whichever way the patient desires.

Toxicity accumulates over time, whether it be nutritional toxicity, emotional, physical, mercury-induced, or environmental. These toxins deplete respiratory enzymes so these cells can no longer utilize oxygen.

Healthy cells utilize oxygen to create energy. But with cancer, instead of utilizing oxygen, cancer cells revert to a primitive way of creating energy by fermenting sugar. Once you ferment sugar, you create lactic acid, which makes the acidic condition of the body even worse. Now you have both acids and toxicity, which increase total body acidity through fermentation. This was discovered in the twenties by Otto Warburg. He's a German doctor who won a Nobel Prize.

SS: Is the not getting enough, or getting no, oxygen to the cells what is called anaerobic metabolism? Dr. Wright talks about this.

MG: Absolutely. You got it. Anaerobic metabolism is occurring. So what do you do at this point? You want to limit sugar intake; this is vitally important. No sugar for any cancer patient. Number two, you must increase the oxygen supply to the cell.

SS: How do you do that?

MG: We know the more toxic you are, the thicker your blood, and all cancer patients have thick blood. Cancer patients have enormous amounts of toxicity, and they have very thick blood. As a doctor, I know you've got to thin the blood, and you do this with garlic, ginkgo, enzymes, and a natural blood thinner called nattokinase. The thinner the blood (like red wine as opposed to ketchup), the more nutrients and oxygen can get to the cells.

Exercise is crucial. In the 1950s, a lady by the name of Joanne Budwig who was a German biochemist discovered that if you combined cottage cheese with flaxseed oil in the diet (a unique combination), you could increase oxygen supply to the cells.

The Budwig diet has been a mainstay in a lot of therapies that have not been talked about, but you can look it up on the Internet, and there's a lot of valuable information there about the Budwig diet.

SS: What exactly is it?

MG: It's pretty simple. It's two-thirds of a cup of cottage cheese plus six tablespoons of flaxseed oil. You mix them together and then you can put them in a blender with berries or nuts. No peanuts.

SS: How often would one take this?

MG: Once a day, divided into two doses. For maintenance you can take half of that amount. It's a very easy thing to do.

SS: Okay. I always need to know, what does this do? Why do I want to eat this?

MG: This combo gets to the cell membrane, increases the oxygen level in the cell and can also cause increased cellular energy production. It's all about getting energy production into the cell. Alkaline water will reduce the total acidity, which is a little bit of the job, but the best way to reduce total body acidity is to get the cells to make more ATP. Once the cells make more energy, the acidity of the body goes down.

SS: Cottage cheese and flaxseed oil appeals to me. I get it. But it's as "out there" as coffee enemas in terms of mainstream reaction to alternative treatments. Cottage cheese and flaxseed oil will be laughed at just as coffee enemas are laughed at. Why is there such a disparity between what you guys are doing and what the orthodox docs are doing?

MG: All doctors want to help people, whoever they are, and whatever therapies they are administering, they truly believe in those therapies. Doctors, number one, are very bright people. Number two, they're often very conservative people. And number three, frequently their basic assumption is, if it wasn't taught to me in medical school, or it's not presented to me at conferences, it doesn't exist.

There's an old saying, "If you're not up on it, you're down on it." So I think, as an oncologist, you're so overwhelmed with the amount of information, the amount of patients that you have to deal with, plus the new information that is presented to you at conferences, that really there's no time and no room to learn anything else. And I think that is a flaw in the medical system.

SS: What do you mean?

MG: The flaw is in not presenting the alternative way as an option or a choice. Currently, the medical system is a study of disease. We're taught how to treat disease. And unfortunately with a traditional approach, people either become diseases or are diseases in progress. It's not a health model; medicine sees disease on one end, health on the other end.

So it goes like this. If you can't sleep, you don't have a disease. If you've got night sweats, you don't have a disease. And this is the model all med students are taught. As a disease model in terms of cancer, it's "kill the bad guys."

SS: Burton Goldberg talked about hyperthermia as a treatment for cancer. Do you support that, and what exactly is it?

MG: Hyperthermia is an innovative treatment for cancer. It involves increasing the body temperature so as to use fever to kill the bad cells. Cancer cells are more susceptible to heat, and temperatures of 104, 105 degrees will actually kill them. In Germany, they're using low levels of chemotherapy and radiation along with hyperthermia because at that point of high body temperature, you don't need as much chemotherapy, and that's a big thing.

When I was an intern, I could rotate through the subspecialties at the hospital and my last subspecialty was cancer. I found that every cancer patient had a body temperature of about 94, 95, when normally it should be 98.6. This was consistent. Putting things together, I realized that if everyone with cancer has a low body temperature, then maybe high body temperature would prevent cancer. I was twenty-six and trying to figure this out, and I was so enthusiastic I wrote an article and sent it to the *New England Journal of Medicine*.

Dr. Issels, a German doctor, found that when he created fevers in cancer patients or when they got an infection with a high fever, they would survive. In fact, the cancer disappeared. Then he looked at people who had very high fevers in childhood, and he found that those whose temperatures got up to 105, never got cancer. This has always been one of the treatment modalities in cancer patients, whether the patient choses natural treatments or radiation, because it is known that the higher your body temperature is, the healthier you are.

As doctors, we are very interested in blood pressure and pulse, but we've forgotten to take body temperatures on our patients. We've got patients at 95 degrees versus 98 degrees, and we have to see that as a sign that something has gone amiss and that the patients with low temperatures may have a systemic disease.

We've known for years there have been spontaneous remissions in people with cancer, so it only makes sense that these are the people who should be studied. Yet no one has looked at these cases at all. Think about it—if there are spontaneous remissions in cancer patients, obviously the body has some way of producing something that takes care of the cancer. So the big question is, what can we do to deal with this situation naturally?

Clearly the answer is to build up the body, and the antiaging approach uses the same methods to strengthen the body. And as we know these same methods will prevent the development of cancer.

Dr. Gary Gordon, whom you know pretty well, Suzanne, came up with a program called FIGHT as a way of preventing cancer and preventing all illnesses. *F* is for fruits and their importance in your diet, plus you also eliminate coffee, Coca-Cola, alcohol, and cigarettes. And it's important to understand that we eat too much in this country, as most people in industrialized countries do.

SS: Some people require protein and animal fats. I believe I am one of them, but I do think that eating organic food and avoiding chemicals at all costs would certainly be cancer preventative.

MG: Absolutely, but in this country we eat too much animal protein, and too much animal protein causes too much cellular acidity. Then on top of it we don't consume enough fruits and vegetables. So nutrition and supplements are vital.

I is for infections. We're all carrying a huge load of bugs. Whether you call it candida or chronic viral syndromes, there are just too many infections going on. One great source of infections is teeth, particularly root canals. Dr. Rau at the Paracelsus clinic in Switzerland found that in one hundred breast cancer patients, ninety-six of them had a root canal in the molar tooth.

SS: Interesting. I had root canals on my right side, which is where I had breast cancer.

MG: Right, ninety-six out of one hundred people with breast cancer had root canals, a source of chronic infection in the root. When you try to clean it out, there are so many canals that it's almost impossible, and consequently it often represents a potential problem. Some of these canals still have bugs in them, which can go through the rest of the body. Now, Dr. Issels, who was the father of integrated cancer therapy in the fifties and sixties, had remarkable success with terminal cancer patients—in fact, so remarkable that about 70 percent of his patients survived and did well. Here is what is interesting, though. He found that tonsils swelled up in his cancer patients every time he drained the infections in the teeth, and when he did tonsillectomies on these people they did much, much better. Tonsillectomies were laughed at, but you remember when we were kids we all got tonsillectomies, and on a certain level he found, relative to the treatment of cancer, that by removing the tonsils it eliminated a source of chronic infection.

Another therapy that integrated medicine utilizes is to reduce the viral load with intravenous vitamin C. Some people also do intravenous hydrogen peroxide; others irradiate their blood or do ultraviolet radiations for the blood. These are all natural treatments and are very, very effective in killing viruses.

SS: I know that these treatments are very popular in Germany. In fact, I feel the Germans are way ahead of us relative to alternative medicine, and it's because their government supports it.

MG: But in this country, as we've talked about, this treatment is a no-no. A couple of states are open to it a little, like Arizona and Nevada, but it's illegal in California and probably the rest of the country. Too bad, because it does kill viruses and yeast organisms in the body.

The next one is the G in FIGHT. G is for geopathic stress.

SS: What is geopathic stress?

MG: It's a frequency called the Schuman frequency, which is a nourishing frequency that comes out of the crust of the earth at 7.82 Hz, which is the frequency of alpha waves in the brain. People always talk about being in the alpha state in terms of meditation, and the 7.82 Hz frequency is a nourishing frequency in the earth that's been found to not only support life but enhance it. Unfortunately, these electromagnetic frequencies are way off 7.82 Hz.

SS: What causes this?

MG: Well, for instance, there are Curry lines that come out of the atmosphere that can affect people by going through their homes, especially homes that are built over underground water. Or having your home too close to high-power lines can stress the body. Cell phones stress the body. So geopathic stress is a major stressor or cancer trigger.

There are things you can do to balance and minimize exposure. Your bedroom should be the quietest place in your house, especially when you sleep. You don't want to have your head anywhere near a computer that's on. You also want to eliminate all electromagnetic stress as much as possible.

The *H* in FIGHT is for hormones. You've got to have balanced hormones. You know that better than anyone, Suzanne. All these cancer patients are completely depleted of hormones, whether it be adrenal hormones, thyroid hormones, bioidentical progesterone, estrogen, or testosterone. They've got to optimize hormonal output. Also, a lot of these cancer patients have too much insulin (a major hormone) because they're eating too much sugar. So it's important to increase estrogen, progesterone, testosterone when indicated, and definitely maximize adrenal output, then replace cortisol and DHEA at the same time you're maximizing thyroid output.

T is for toxins: mercury toxins from the teeth, mercury in tuna and swordfish, mercury in the atmosphere from coal burning, and then there are winds that blow from China which consequently blow a lot of that mercury from Chinese industrial coal production over the West Coast to California. They also found that 10 to 20 percent of the population in New York City has highly elevated levels of mercury. So mercury is a key toxin. The other heavy metals that are toxic are cadmium and lead. We've talked about your exposure, Suzanne, in the Las Vegas casinos years ago to the secondhand cigarette smoke you inhaled while you were performing. And we found you had high levels of cadmium in your urine twenty years later. This is how pervasive toxic poisoning can be, and it is affecting all of us.

SS: I remember being so shocked by this, because I never smoked.

MG: Right—it was all from secondhand exposure. We are also exposed to enormous amounts of pesticides, which have an affinity for the pancreas, and the pancreas creates digestive enzymes, which I will explain the significance of in a bit.

So there you have FIGHT. Now I've added more to it. And I call it FIGHT EM. Because I think that emotional and mental states have got to be looked at.

I see you, Suzanne, attending the antiaging conferences in Las Vegas, the American Academy of Anti-Aging Medicine [A4M], where the latest advancements in alternative medicine are discussed. I also go to the American College for Advancement in Medicine [ACAM], and these are not only alternative but also integrated doctors. So I have to say I am always surprised that no one talks about the emotional and mental states in relation to health or in relation to treating disease. And obviously it's never talked about in traditional medicine.

SS: I think it is a crucial element of healing. Dr. Stephen Sinatra discusses this extensively in his interview in this book, the power of intention and belief.

MG: Right, and in terms of a person's emotions it is crucial that we live our lives with purpose, passion, and gratitude. Granted, when you're feeling terrible and you have cancer, it's a little difficult to get passionate when you don't have the energy. But I try to tell people, "Do what you love, help others, and healing will follow."

Then you've got to take care of your body. You've got to look at your body as a Ferrari, and Ferraris need high-octane gasoline. So basically you must be very selective about what you put into your body in terms of food.

We all need to find exercise programs that we enjoy, and exercise regularly. Make fun and relaxation a daily priority. Learn to love yourself, and once you learn to forgive yourself, it's easy to forgive others. Find your inner peace and don't let go of it. You'll make decisions that give you the greatest peace of mind.

More important, connect with your higher source as often as you can. You can call it a guide or inner guides or higher self, but tap into it. And that's the value of meditation, because this inner you is always a source of knowledge, inspiration, and guidance. Involve yourself in cleaning up the environment, and it will help cleanse you emotionally. Once you decide that someone up there is your friend, everything else flows a lot easier.

Going barefoot in the grass is very, very important. Taking hikes, walks on the beach . . . all these things connect you to nature. The emotional, mental aspect has got to be addressed in terms of the concept of FIGHT EM. The antiaging approach is both preventative and has a huge role in the treatment of cancer.

There is a quote from Gandhi that says, "First they ignore you, then they laugh at you, then they fight, then you win." I think this applies to you, Suzanne: first they paid no attention to you, then they started laughing at you, now they're fighting you and writing articles about you, and soon you're about to win.

SS: Thank you, but I think it applies to all of us in the alternative world, and it's the essence of passion—you can't walk away once you have seen the light.

It doesn't seem, though, that this approach is being taught in medical school at all. Today's students are taught allopathic medicine as though this is all that exists. Do you think there's a shot that alternative medicine will ever get big enough, important enough, and financially set to where studies can be done on nonpatentable medicine? Do you think the value of nutrition, and cancer being viewed as a manageable disease, will ever have acceptance and legitimacy?

MG: This is a huge problem, because there is no incentive for any drug company to fund these kinds of studies that basically look at nutraceuticals.

So how do we change this consciousness? How do you get more people or more doctors to start thinking the way you think or the way I think? At ACAM, we try to get medical students involved by reaching out to them and inviting them to our conferences. We let them come for free to expose them to our possibilities for healing. Show them our approach. You're not going to be able to change the approach of many of the older doctors who are set in their ways, as you might be able to do with young doctors.

As far as doing studies, the only way to do an integrated study is to work together with mainstream and alternative, present them with our successes, and show how integrating the two modalities is better for everyone. We'll show that we can get great results, and this allows orthodox doctors to sell their chemotherapy, and everyone wins, but mainly the patient wins.

SS: Even as you say this, it feels a long way off. But it sounds like a great starting point to invite medical students who are not yet locked into their thinking. That thrills me. This is the first idea I have heard that has the potential to effect change: get the young minds and maybe there's a shot.

MG: We need to teach reducing toxicity, which is not taught in traditional medical schools. And a very crucial step in reducing toxicity is drainage.

SS: How do you do that and why?

MG: We want to neutralize and eliminate toxins in the body, and the key organs to do that are the liver, kidneys, and the lymphatic system. For the liver we want everybody to take a fresh lemon every morning, cut it in half, squeeze the juice out of both halves, pour it into six to eight ounces of water. Drink that down.

We want people to have healthy water. For years I've been studying water. The elements of water that make it good are a pH that's slightly alkaline and lots of electrons, because electrons are energy. You don't want the water to be distilled, because distilled water is dead water; it doesn't have any minerals. At the same time you don't want lots of minerals in water, but you want some.

Vegetables have got to be consumed two, three, four times a day for liver health: carrots, beets, zucchini, squash, artichoke.

The lymphatic system needs to be stimulated. You can use a trampo line or rebounder, or if you're going to a gym use the elliptical machine, a jump rope, anything that bounces, because that causes the lymphatic system to be stimulated. Deep breathing also helps the lymphatic system.

Colonics can be helpful. Most cancer patients are toxic. You've got to have bowel movements every day. If you're not, colonics can be very helpful. Skin brushing can be helpful.

This is all about getting your drainage systems working efficiently. If the liver, kidney, and lymph systems aren't working, you can't pull toxins out of the tissues, because they go from the tissues to the blood to the liver, kidney, lymph system. Kind of like a bowel movement in a toilet bowl that won't flush. Drainage is first, detoxification second.

Detoxification: saunas, homeopathy, herbs, juice fasts, chelation (where you pull heavy metals out of the body again). You're pulling them out of the tissues, into the blood, and out through the liver, kidney, lymph system. To do this I use intravenous vitamin C.

Number one, clean the liver, stimulate the liver.

Number two, stimulate the immune system.

Intravenous vitamin C is used in a couple of different ways. The National Institutes of Health have proven that intravenous vitamin C will produce high enough blood levels to actually kill cancer cells.

We frequently use 50,000 milligrams of vitamin C intravenously over the course of an hour. Some people go up to 75,000 or 100,000. To the vitamin C we also add vitamin K_3 orally to the C in a ratio of 100 to 1. So if it's 50,000 milligrams of C intravenously it will be 500 milligrams of K_3 early, while you're getting the vitamin C. That seems to enhance the effect. If you're getting chemotherapy which kills cancer cells, then we'll reduce the vitamin C to 25,000 milligrams intravenously. We're not trying to kill the cancer cells; we're trying to keep the body as toxin free as possible. You have to remember when you're doing chemotherapy that all these dead cancer cells have to go somewhere; they go into the bloodstream and ultimately to the kidney, liver, lymph filter.

Keeping the liver as healthy as possible, as clean as possible, is probably the number one thing you can do for a patient with cancer on chemotherapy. And again, when doing chemotherapy, we do vitamin C on the off week.

SS: And how are these patients doing?

MG: They're feeling good and they are confident. When you have a patient who's doing chemotherapy who comes into your office and says, "I feel great," it's an amazing thing. We're not in consultation, unfortunately, with the oncologist, and often the patients have elected not to tell their oncologists that they are working with an integrative doctor who is building up their body simultaneously. I hope this changes in the future.

A lot of oncologists, by the way, especially in the L.A. area, are open to our work and will tell me, "Whatever you're doing, keep doing it." Because basically they're doing their thing, we're doing our thing, the patient's benefiting. The bottom line is everybody wants to help these people. It's just a lack of awareness and education about how to maximize one's health, whether one is on chemo or not.

We measure vitamin D levels, it's a blood test. We like to maximize vitamin D levels with cancer patients in the 70 to 80 range. That usually involves at least 6,000 to 10,000 units of vitamin D every day. We want to stimulate their immune systems.

Mistletoe [Iscador], for example, is a powerful anticancer treatment which builds up your immune system. You know this, of course, Suzanne, because you chose Iscador injections to build up your immune system to prevent a cancer recurrence and you have been cancer-free for the past nine years. It's readily available to all patients with cancer in this country, and I believe it's because of you and all the talking you did about it on television. All a patient's doctor has to do is fax over a request to either Germany or Switzerland. On that request, he must mention the disease and what kind of therapy is being given. Then the manufacturers will send a protocol to the patient of mistletoe and information about how to take it.

There are other ways to build up the immune system: AHCC [a mushroom extract] or MGN-3 [a rice extract]. These activate the natural killer cells, which are key in trying to destroy the cancer cells.

SS: When you get lab numbers back on natural killer [NK] cells, where should they be?

MG: Normally, they should be where you have gotten your levels, around 40. A lot of these NK cell levels you see are 5 or 10 or 11. And vitamin D levels in cancer patients, which we like to see ideally at 70, are usually in the 10 to 20 range. Vitamin D is interesting in that if levels are low, around 10 or 20, they may not have cancer but you know they're sick. D levels are telling you something. German researchers found that zinc supplements interfere with the treatment of cancer.

SS: Why is that?

MG: Zinc activates the cancer process.

SS: Should no one take zinc?

MG: No. People with cancer should not take zinc. Young, healthy people can and should take zinc to help their prostate or to get a healthier testosterone metabolism. Zinc is major—when a couple is trying to get pregnant, it will help increase the motility of the sperm for young men. These are the latest findings presented at A4M last December.

These are the natural treatments we try to give to support and strengthen the body that has cancer. If you're on chemo, we would add melatonin because melatonin potentiates the chemo and helps people sleep. If you don't sleep, nobody gets better, and once you lose the ability to sleep, health deteriorates, but it's important to allow people to sleep naturally. Melatonin does that.

SS: And what about bioidentical hormones relative to cancer?

MG: Bioidentical hormones are key: estrogen, progesterone, testosterone all take away not only symptoms of menopause but also other chemo-induced reactions such as hot flashes that frequently occur. Plus, they have a great mental stimulating effect. They give you your zest for life, and frankly, women look better on bioidentical hormones. When you are taking chemotherapy and you see yourself looking better, it's a huge boost. And if you can stimulate patients' sexual response and help them feel more sexual while being treated for cancer, that's a sign of health. The more you can give people signs that they are healthy, the better their outlook, the better their belief systems, the better the prognosis. So bioidentical hormones are very, very important.

SS: Dr. Gonzalez is very keen on using pancreatic enzymes as part of his protocol for cancer treatment.

MG: Yes, cancer cells have a protective coating, and by giving the patient enzymes, such as Wobenzym, it lets these enzymes attack the cancer cells and take off that protective coating, so that the white blood cells then zoom in and attack the cancer cells.

SS: I know with a cancer patient on Dr. Gonzalez's program they sometimes require 150 or even 300 of these different enzymes daily to do the job. But how many would someone like myself, who is without cancer, take daily?

MG: About fifteen enzymes daily. Five each after a meal for digestion. But when using them to help rid the body of debris of cancer, you always want them on an empty stomach.

SS: Why on an empty stomach if you've got cancer?

MG: We want the enzymes to eat up the cancer debris, kind of like little PacMen that get into the bloodstream. A cancer patient who's doing therapies, whether it be chemotherapy or radiation, has all these dead cells running around in the blood. So getting rid of that debris makes it easier on the liver-lymph detoxification system.

SS: When I'm at your office and when I run into people who are your patients, they just love you. They love your approach to medicine. They love how they feel. It must be rewarding work for you.

MG: Well, I love my patients. They give me purpose. I want to help my patients, and I embrace all challenges.

When I was in emergency medicine I loved the challenge in that it was life or death. You had to work on your instincts. You had to think quickly and decisively. In emergency medicine there's nothing better than saving somebody's life. Sick people are similar; they are huge challenges. It is rewarding to have cancer patients who are receiving chemo and radiation but are feeling well. It's about quality of life before, during, and after treatment, and that's what I try to do with this kind of medicine. Whatever choice they make, it is up to me to honor their belief systems.

This kind of medicine is successful, and as more people realize it is available, they will be willing to take advantage of the breakthroughs being made. They're going to read your book. They're going to read these other doctors in the book and the success stories of their patients.

SS: My choice to go alternative in every facet of my health has been empowering. I feel I am in control of my health and that I can control or manage disease through my understanding of nutrition, detoxification, and supplementation. I've never felt better, and I like working with you as my doctor because of our back-and-forth, the education. You never talk at me; you educate me. It's made me a better patient, and as a result, I take better care of myself. In fact, I honor my health.

MG: You're like the model patient. You're excited, you're interested, you look up things, you e-mail me, you call, you read, you want to know more. You're a unique person. And because you are really into it, that is why you're feeling so great and healthy. In fact, I've never met anybody more into health than you.

SS: When I wake up feeling this great every day and every day is a good one, why wouldn't I do it? And I don't find it difficult; I find it easy. I find the food I eat to be delicious and nutritious. I have no interest in bad food or chemical foods, and I have very little interest in sugar anymore; the cravings are gone. It's just not in my system. And I sleep. I always feel happy and connected. This is the greatest thing I've ever done for myself, and I love having you as my doctor.

I look forward to many more years together. Thank you for all this great information.

MG: My pleasure.

Knock It Out

- Cancer is a disease of the whole body; a tumor is just a symptom of the disease. This means you must treat and support the whole body to beat cancer. We all have cancer cells in our bodies, but you need about a billion cancer cells to get to the lump or bump stage, which is why a tumor takes years to develop. This also means that you have time after being given a diagnosis. It's not necessary to start treatment the next day.
- One of the key elements of healing is to build the patient up first, and then support the patient every day—not only before but also after he or she goes through chemo and radiation. As such, it's essential to find a doctor who honors your belief system and who will support you fully throughout treatment, whatever form it takes.
- When given a cancer diagnosis, a patient needs to eat better, take nutrition seriously, and try to only eat organic foods. Eliminating sources of infection, particularly chronic infection, is also important. The stronger the patient gets, the more likely he or she is to do well with the treatments given, including surgery, chemotherapy, and radiation.
- It is vitally important for cancer patients to limit sugar intake, as cancer cells create energy to grow and spread by fermenting sugar. Cancer patients must also avoid zinc, which activates the cancer process.
- Cancer patients must increase oxygen supply to their cells. Because toxicity gives cancer patients thick blood, garlic, ginkgo, enzymes, and a natural blood thinner called nattokinase can be used to thin the blood, resulting in more nutrients and oxygen getting to the cells. Exercise is crucial. The Budwig diet, which includes a combination of cottage cheese and flaxseed oil, also helps increase oxygen supply to the cells.
- To neutralize and eliminate toxins in the body, the key organs are the liver, kidneys, and lymphatic system. For the liver, take a fresh lemon every morning, cut it in half, squeeze the juice out of both halves, pour it into six to eight ounces of water, and drink it. Consuming vegetables such as carrots, beets, zucchini, squash, and artichokes is also important. To stimulate the lymphatic system, use a trampoline or rebounder, or if you're going to a gym use the elliptical machine, a jump rope, anything that bounces. Deep breathing also helps the lymphatic system.
- To stimulate the immune system, vitamin D levels should be addressed. In addition, mistletoe, otherwise known as Iscador, is a powerful anticancer treatment that builds up the immune system.

Chapter 17

CRISTIANA PAUL, M.S.

We are wiser than we know.

—Ralph Waldo Emerson

Recently I was featured on *The Oprah Winfrey Show*, where I explained my daily regimen of supplementation. Yes, I do take about sixty different supplements daily, as determined by my blood work for deficiencies. I put back what my body needs to keep me at optimum health. I take my vitamins most of the time enthusiastically, thinking about what each supplement is doing to keep me healthy.

Oprah cheerily called me a "wackadoo," and the Internet and talk-show chatter afterward was running over with disbelief at my daily regimen.

But I look around me and it is clear that cancer is an epidemic. People are dropping like flies. So yes, taking these supplements gets a little gaggy at times, but when I am tempted to forgo the day's requirements, I think of the alternatives.

We know that nutrition is key to being healthy. Between organic food, avoiding eating chemicals, and downplaying sugar (which is simply cancer fuel), I believe I can win my own war on cancer.

Cristiana Paul is my nutritionist. In *Breakthrough*, she explained the basics of supplementation for health. For *Knockout*, I asked her to give us information on supplementation that protects and prevents cancer. If this is a possibility, why wouldn't we take these supplements on a daily basis to prevent this dreaded disease?

She is an avid researcher and has a tremendous grasp of nutrition and supplementation. My health has never been better than under her guidance.

You get out of life what you put into it. I desire and treasure good health. It is available to all of us if we make simple changes. The mystery of supplementation is over. Now, through blood work with Designs for Health or Life Extension or certain cutting-edge compounding pharmacies, you can determine your body's exact needs. You put back what is missing. The benefits are vitality, energy, and a strong immune system. These are the tools I believe are necessary for survival in today's world.

SS: Cristiana, I know you do a lot of nutrition research, especially on the effect of nutritional supplements on disease prevention and treatment. Can you explain and summarize for us how the right nutrition can help reduce cancer risk?

CP: The fact is, hundreds of studies come out every day about diet, nutrients, herbal extracts, and their effects on various diseases. [PubMed is an online resource provided by the U.S. National Library of Medicine at the National Institutes of Health.]

SS: On one hand, it's great that there is so much research being done with nutrients and herbs; on the other hand, no wonder not all doctors or nutritionists can keep up with all the information available and the most recent findings. There is quite a bit of contradictory information put out there as well. Which facts do you feel are most important to understand and try to implement every day?

CP: I will take you step by step through the journey of an accidental cancer cell and show you how good nutrition and specific nutrients can intervene at many points in its pathways. They can reduce the chance of it occurring in the first place, or the chances of it surviving, multiplying, and spreading in the body.

SS: I have to ask about this first, though. In the past, vitamin E (alpha-tocopherol) and vitamin A from beta-carotene were considered good antioxidants, and we assumed that taking them would reduce our risk of cancer. But then a few studies showed that supplementing with these caused an increased overall mortality or certain cancers. What do we do with this information? Whom do we believe?

CP: You are right, it's very confusing and sometimes scary. We know and expect to hear that toxins and unhealthy foods may cause cancer, but to hear this about nutritional supplements as well can shake even a nutritionist's core beliefs. The problem is that the media oversimplifies;

they do not tell you which form of vitamin E caused this, that many studies from which they derived these conclusions used the unnatural, synthetic forms of vitamin E. They also did not tell you that there is a big difference between synthetic beta-carotene and mixed natural carotenoids found in fruits and vegetables. We are reminded again and again that we have to pay attention to how things occur in nature and learn from it. Things are much more complex than they appear in the media reports, and you really do not get the whole story because a quick statement is the wrong way to report such study findings.

SS: So did they figure out why beta-carotene supplementation was shown to increase cancer occurrence in that study with smokers?

CP: It was not made clear from that study or any other studies why supplementation with beta-carotene alone did that, but it was interesting that the group that took *both* beta-carotene and vitamin E did not experience the same increased risk of cancer. This aspect of that study gives us a clue that antioxidants work differently if they are given together at the same time. So you see, they left this information out of their media announcements, and people are missing a very important piece of this puzzle. In my opinion, they should have also mentioned findings from other studies showing that antioxidants work better when taken together, not just one of them in huge doses, because natural antioxidants have a way of complementing each other. Antioxidants occur together naturally in foods and evidently there is a good reason for it.

SS: Why was the unnatural, synthetic form of vitamin E used for so long? Even today I see vitamins that have this. Is the natural form that hard to find or that much more expensive?

CP: Initially, I think that it was all that was available. Finally, studies started looking at the effects of the various forms of natural vitamin E and some manufacturers got smarter and started using only the natural form of vitamin E, called mixed tocopherols.

SS: How is this relevant to cancer risk?

CP: Well, it may be relevant in more than one way. For example, one member of the natural vitamin E family that was left out in the synthetic formulation, gamma-tocopherol, happens to be a particularly good protector of DNA, the cell genetic code, and it has additional cardiovascular benefits that alpha-tocopherol does not have. Protecting DNA is an important way to reduce cancer risk. I will explain this in detail later. Not only was gamma-tocopherol left out in the synthetic formulations, but what's worse is that when one takes in large doses of alpha-tocopherol (like 400 IU or more), it is very difficult for the body to absorb the other natural tocopherols that are contained in the diet, because they compete with each other. Alpha-tocopherol acts kind of like a bully pushing around its brothers, the other natural tocopherols, so they have a very hard time getting in the bloodstream, where they are needed. Also, when you supplement exclusively with alpha-tocopherol, you can create a deficiency of other vitamin E forms in the body. This was a very disturbing revelation to me.

SS: So a nutritional supplement can take away your chance of absorbing other nutrients from food if that particular supplement is not balanced as nature would have it. What should we look for on the label of a supplement that contains vitamin E?

CP: Look at the label to see if it contains natural mixed tocopherols. If it has mixed tocotrienols, that is even better; they are another natural form of vitamin E, although not as prevalent in common foods.

SS: Is the tocotrienol form of vitamin E important?

CP: Yes, studies have shown that it can mildly reduce cholesterol synthesis in the body, and there are encouraging studies showing that it can reduce risk of breast, prostate, and colon cancer. It does this by depriving cancer cells of a compound they need for fast proliferation, called mevalonate. This is made in the body on the same pathway where cholesterol is made. By the way, lycopene—found in tomatoes and watermelon—was found to do this, too. Researchers believe that the way lycopene reduces cancer development is by reducing cholesterol and mevalonate availability inside the prostate cells and possibly other cells.

SS: So what should we be careful to avoid on a supplement label?

CP: If the label just says "d-alpha tocopherol" next to the vitamin E entry, it means it is incomplete; it is missing the other tocopherols—beta-, gamma-, delta-tocopherols. This is not good.

Some tricky manufacturers list the majority of vitamin E as d-alpha-tocopherol and then add a very small amount of mixed tocopherols. That to me is purposely deceiving, in order to look good on paper. Do not accept anything other than "mixed tocopherols" as the primary form of vitamin E listed. What is even more disturbing is that whenever they produce synthetic vitamin E, the chemical process automatically creates seven other unnatural vitamin E compounds that are mixed in. And since it is too expensive to separate the artificial ones, they leave them in and call it d,l-alpha-tocopherol. You can recognize this if the label says "d,l-alpha tocopherol." The "d,l" is the clue, but how many people know this? That is only one of the problems with very inexpensive vitamins, and there are lots of them on the market.

SS: What other problems are you referring to? Can these affect cancer risk?

CP: Yes. For example, many nutritional supplements contain artificial dyes. But why put these artificial dyes in our bodies every day? These are also added in foods like puddings, snack bars, fiber supplements, and many packaged foods. That is because they are considered GRAS (generally recognized as safe). For example, the artificial dyes yellow #5 and #6 are still considered safe, but yellow #1, #2, #3, and #4 are now on the list of banned additives, even though they were considered safe in the past. You can read a detailed report on these at www.cspi.com, the website of the Center for Science in the Public Interest.

SS: So the artificial chemicals are considered safe until proven otherwise, or "innocent till proven guilty," while the general population are the guinea pigs on whom we are running experiments to see what happens. I cannot believe we give these chemicals a free pass to be used widely in our food and supplements supply.

CP: A simple look at the history of the GRAS list shows many of these dyes that are now banned due to carcinogenicity or other detrimental health effects were considered safe for a long time.

SS: What about folic acid? I know you told me about this a year ago and I just read in the *Los Angeles Times* health section that there is new awareness from scientists that taking too much folic acid may increase the risk of cancer. They were also emphasizing in the article there are different forms of folate that may have different effects. Can you explain?

CP: Yes, this is a very important public health issue, especially because of the impact of flour fortification with folic acid, and it's finally breaking out in the mainstream media. The article did not explain all the issues well enough, in my opinion, but at least it brought it to everybody's attention.

The issue is that all of a sudden epidemiological studies brought out evidence that too much folic acid may promote the growth of precancerous cells. We also became more aware that there are big differences between synthetic folic acid, which does not occur in nature, and natural folates, found mainly in fruits, vegetables, and liver. Many studies have shown that supplementation with folic acid in people who are deficient can reduce their risk of various cancers. So people figured, "The more the better." Nobody guessed that supplementation with high amounts of folic acid may reach a point of diminishing returns and potentially increase the risk of cancer.

Do not get me wrong—we all still agree that folic acid is important in the right amounts—it varies by individual—to prevent certain birth defects. But that is intended for women of childbearing age. Men and women who cannot conceive may need to keep the folic acid/folate intake at lower levels for optimal health. The problem is that many people may be eating large quantities of fortified-flour products, and so they ingest a proportionally large amount of folic acid they do not really need.

SS: Why do you think that cancer risk increases when there is more folic acid available in the body?

CP: You can think of folic acid like a fertilizer in a garden of cells, which supports the growth of normal cells as well as cancer cells. It actually supports the making of DNA in any new cell.

The problem arises when you throw excess fertilizer in a garden that has weeds, because it may help the weeds grow faster than the plants. It is believed that the downside of excess folic acid may be that it makes it too easy for cancer cells to grow fast, and it makes it that much harder for the immune system to destroy them. Our immune system is like a gardener trying to pluck these cancer weeds out, but it cannot keep up if too much fertilizer is thrown on the garden too frequently.

So folic acid excess does not *cause* cancer per se—it does not start it, for sure—but it may support it to grow faster in a body that has excess folic acid or even other folates around. On the other hand, folic acid deficiency can *cause* cancerous cells to appear, because every new cell formed needs adequate folic acid around it to make its DNA accurate, without errors or mutations.

SS: How much folic acid is too much?

CP: Studies started using larger and larger doses of folic acid, as high as 5 milligrams, with clear benefits for cardiovascular disease. However, recent studies support evidence that daily doses of folic acid above 200 to 400 *micrograms* ingested at any one time may be improperly metabolized and absorbed in the bloodstream, causing people to end up with folic acid in the bloodstream. That is not a natural situation. This does not happen when one takes in natural folates from fruits, vegetables, or supplements that contain the natural forms of folates. So now we need to take another look at which forms of folates one uses and revise the recommended doses. This is especially important because folic acid is used to fortify flour and some people's diets are composed of a large number of those products: cereals, breads, and pasta. Many researchers believe at this time that excess intake of folic acid, specifically in the synthetic form, may increase the risk of polyps and colon cancer, and as I said, other cancers may be stimulated as well.

SS: Can we measure blood levels of folic acid or folate so we can find out what our status is, since this can influence our risk of cancer?

CP: What we should measure, for an adequate estimate of folate status, are the RBC [red blood cell] levels of the natural folate 5-MTHF, which is the preferred natural form of folate that circulates in the blood. This test is available through most common labs. You do not want to be too low or too high in RBC folate, because at both ends the risk of cancer may be increased for different reasons.

As for blood folic acid, we would hope that we have undetectable levels of folic acid in the bloodstream. To ensure that this is the case, it would be good to look for a multivitamin that contains natural folates, but if it contains folic acid, do not take in more than 200 micrograms at a time. As far as foods go, it would be best to get natural folates from fruits and vegetables, not folic acid from refined flour products.

SS: Don't they say not to take folic acid when undergoing chemotherapy?

CP: Yes, for certain chemo agents like methotrexate. It's interesting, because that drug is trying to block the activation of folic acid on the path to making DNA. Cancer cells that multiply fast need DNA, so the drug tries to stop them by cutting off some supplies. What's interesting to me is that some studies have used methotrexate and the natural folate called folinic acid, and they worked great in reducing some side effects of the chemotherapy. Some of them even showed that it made chemotherapy more effective at killing cancer cells.

SS: So copy nature as much as we can in our everyday actions—the way we eat and the way we supplement?

CP: Yes, pay attention to how nature does things, as that is what fits our bodies the best. But sometimes we have to trick nature a bit, too, if we want maximum vitality past our prime reproductive age. We have to supplement with higher doses of nutrients when we need to compensate for some effects of age-related changes, genetics, or environmental challenges. For example, researchers are suggesting we take resveratrol in relatively higher doses than found in any natural food, because we are impressed with its potential benefits for longevity and reducing cancer risk.

SS: How about anticancer foods? We hear that pomegranate juice contains ellagic acid and that red wine contains resveratrol and polyphenols, which have all been shown to reduce cancer risk on top of other health benefits. Should we drink these two every day, and how much?

CP: One thing is for sure: the antioxidants and phytonutrients in pomegranates and grape skins and seeds have been proven to have anti-inflammatory, anticancer, and cardiovascular-protective benefits. However, I am afraid many people will be tempted to just go ahead and drink a lot of both. Let's say, for example, that they drink one or two cups (eight to sixteen fluid ounces) of each every day, which contain about 37 to 72 grams of carbs. That's the same amount of sugar as two to four apples, or two to four slices of bread, or one or two bananas. Well, that is not necessarily good if you already have too much sugar and/or carbohydrates in your diet. On the other hand, everybody needs some specific amount of carbs every day based on their metabolism, so I would say let's get our carbs from the richest sources of antioxidants and anticancer foods. Let's spend our carb allowance really wisely. Same thing with lycopene, which has great data on cancer reduction and is found in tomatoes and watermelon, for example. However, watermelon contains a lot of sugar that is absorbed fast because there is very little fiber in there.

The alcohol from the wine may increase the risk of mouth and throat cancer, and some research suggests that it may increase the risk of breast cancer, but one glass per day may be okay for some people. I know I cannot have a glass every day—my brain just does not function well after that—but I do want the resveratrol, so I take a supplement.

Juices and alcohol may be especially problematic if you have them on an empty stomach. Make sure you have a balanced meal of protein, vegetables, good fats, and moderate amounts of high-quality carbs, and then you may have a little wine and maybe two ounces of pomegranate juice or a slice of watermelon. That way, the alcohol and/or the sugar will be absorbed very slowly through a full stomach, thus causing fewer problems.

SS: How much resveratrol should one take in order to be protected against cancer?

CP: We do not have a clear answer to that from human studies for prevention purposes, although I have heard some cancer studies are going on right now using 1 to 10 grams of it for people with active cancers. Based on the longevity studies, anywhere from 200 to 1,000 milligrams may be very beneficial, yet likely safe. We are making assumptions based on the thousands of studies done so far in vitro, in animals, and a few in humans. Some of us do not want to wait for results from ten- to thirty-year-long human studies. That is always the dilemma.

You should definitely supplement all antioxidants in a balanced way. Just because I take resveratrol, this amazingly powerful antioxidant and genetic modulator, does not mean I will skip the other antioxidants. If a fruit seems great, like pomegranate or grapes, that does not mean we just prioritize that. A mix of them with a large variety of fruits and vegetables will be most protective overall.

SS: So should we also take a pill with extracts of pomegranate, a grape's active components, et cetera, in a supplement to get all the benefits?

CP: That is hard to answer because we never know how the extract was processed and how the supplement was made. If you trust the company that makes it to carefully control everything that goes in it, then you will definitely benefit, but I would do both. I would take some supplements I trust, and then also some of the foods that contain it.

The more I learn, the more I realize how much we do not know about nature's way of interacting with our bodies. I can hardly keep up with all the developments, and I am doing this full-time. ·

Since it's hard to get this variety of beneficial nutrients from a multitude of fruits every day, and they come with added sugar, fruit extract supplements may be a viable alternative. I like Designs for Health Paleo Reds powder because it is an organic blend of eleven antioxidant fruits with additional vegetable extracts, elderberry, and enzymes, with very little sugar. They also produce a matching blend of organic vegetable extracts powder called Paleo Greens. The prefix "Paleo" refers to the Paleolithic nutrition model, which incorporated many fruits and vegetables. They were the only source of carbohydrates that our bodies adapted to when we lived in a natural environment for millions of years.

SS: So how is sugar affecting cancer risk?

CP: The consequence of ingesting a lot of sugar quickly from any starch, high-glycemic-index fruit, or high-sugar liquid, including pomegranate juice or watermelon, is that your blood sugar levels will quickly rise to a point that is damaging to health in general, but most important, it is causing a spike in the hormone insulin. First of all, this sugar is great fuel and stimulus for cancer cells waiting to be fed. High blood sugar is taken in by precancerous cells, which can now multiply faster than they would if less sugar was available. Second, the excess insulin produced by this high-sugar state acts as a stimulating factor that supports cell growth, cell division, and ultimately multiplication of these "bad" cells.

SS: So what you are saying is that pomegranate juice or wine can be a double-edged sword, and if you drink too much of them it may just increase the risk of cancer through their sugar or alcohol content? How much should we have, then, in order to take advantage of its protective effect?

CP: That is the tricky part. It's all about your whole diet, how much you have at any particular meal or snack. The sugar from pomegranate juice is the same as the sugar from any other fruit, table sugar, corn syrup, et cetera. They are all made of two types of molecules: glucose and fructose. This is in addition to the rest of the sugar you get from whatever starch you have in your diet (from bread, cereal, potatoes, et cetera). It's important to pay attention to how much carbohydrate you have at one time, because that determines how high your blood glucose is pushed after that meal. It also matters whether and when you exercise. If you start moving intensely after a high-carb meal, then you can burn them immediately after they are absorbed into your body, and it will not cause much trouble. I say if you overindulge, go for a walk right afterward or go dancing.

All this sugar adds up in your blood, and it does not matter where it is coming from; what matters is the total amount of glucose in the bloodstream at any one time and what your long-term average is. By the way, we can tell what your last three months' average blood glucose is by looking at a blood test called glycated hemoglobin, or HbA1c. Most doctors only test this in diabetics, but some doctors test this in everybody because it is an important marker that needs to be as low as possible in order to reduce the risk of cancer, diabetes, and age-related degenerative diseases, such as cardiovascular diseases.

SS: What about the plastic bottles that the pomegranate juice comes in?

CP: Yes, the plastic bottles are a concern, because they are known to release various chemicals considered hormonelike substances. Also, be aware that most pomegranate juice brands have added sugar, other juices, or artificial flavors.

SS: Reports come out every day on substances, environmental factors, and lifestyle choices that may significantly increase the odds of getting various types of cancers, but you cannot avoid them all. What can we do to compensate for this?

CP: Of course, the media are always capitalizing on the sensational aspect of these news stories. People remember disparate facts and it is virtually impossible for anyone to understand how to sort out this information and what are the most important things to do systematically in their lives to really make a difference, without becoming crazy obsessive at the same time. Let me try to set certain guidelines and a method to this madness.

To understand nutritional interventions for cancer, we have to follow a cancer cell from its accidental birth to its possible growth, multiplication, and spread in the body—to see how many roadblocks we can place in its path with nutrition.

A cancer cell is like a terrorist and thief of health in our bodies, and the immune system is the law enforcement that needs to be efficient at arresting it. Like with any criminal, there are no guarantees that it will be caught, but our chances increase if we put up many roadblocks: if we prevent it from hiding and feeding, from reproducing and multiplying, and if we have a strong and large police force with good weapons that is vigilant twenty-four hours a day. This police force is represented by our immune system cells, and I will review later how nutrition can affect it positively or negatively.

SS: I find it very empowering that what we decide to eat or drink or what we avoid every day will tilt the odds of getting cancer in our favor or our detriment. We cannot control everything perfectly, but at least we know we can follow some useful principles every day without stressing too much about it.

CP: Let me explain things based on a diagram I drew. [See figure 1.] I used to be a software engineer and I have to draw flow charts for myself in order to organize my thoughts, and I find it easier to explain to others this way. I think this diagram will also help readers get the big picture about the most common and typical pathways that cancers start on and how they progress. The good news is that there are so many points where we have the power to change the odds in our favor. That is why I called it "My Power to Change My Cancer Risk" diagram.

I am only noting nine of the most obvious nutritional interventions that are in our power, and I've labeled them A through I. There may be many more ways in which nutrition and nutritional supplements may affect cancer risk, but these are the ones I consider most important and relatively easy to implement.

SS: It is exciting to see at one glance that we can intervene at so many points in the cancer pathway and arrest that accidental cancer cell on its way to causing trouble.

CP: Yes, knowledge is power. I will describe each potential intervention in detail. No one thing will cause or prevent cancer with certainty. There are no guarantees. But we can definitely tilt the odds in our favor,

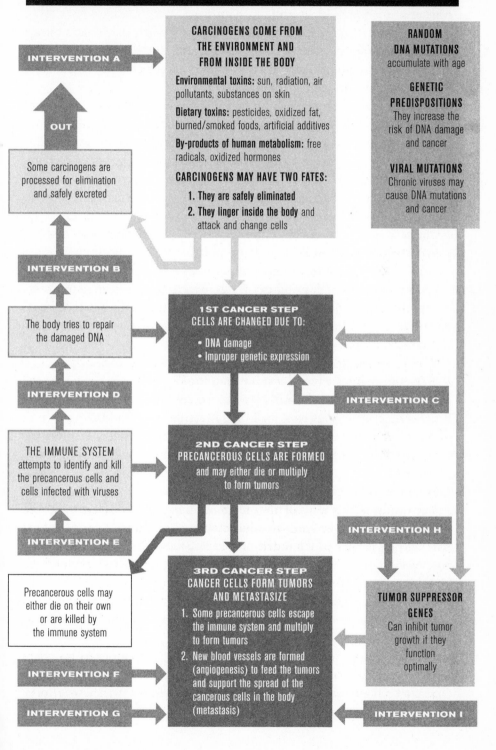

FIGURE 1: MY POWER TO CHANGE MY CANCER RISK
Cancer development steps and nutrition interventions that can reduce cancer risk

INTERVENTION A

CARCINOGENS COME FROM THE ENVIRONMENT AND FROM INSIDE THE BODY

Environmental toxins: sun, radiation, air pollutants, substances on skin

Dietary toxins: pesticides, oxidized fat, burned/smoked foods, artificial additives

By-products of human metabolism: free radicals, oxidized hormones

CARCINOGENS MAY HAVE TWO FATES:

1. They are safely eliminated
2. They linger inside the body and attack and change cells

RANDOM DNA MUTATIONS accumulate with age

GENETIC PREDISPOSITIONS They increase the risk of DNA damage and cancer

VIRAL MUTATIONS Chronic viruses may cause DNA mutations and cancer

OUT

Some carcinogens are processed for elimination and safely excreted

INTERVENTION B

The body tries to repair the damaged DNA

1ST CANCER STEP
CELLS ARE CHANGED DUE TO:

• DNA damage
• Improper genetic expression

INTERVENTION D

INTERVENTION C

THE IMMUNE SYSTEM attempts to identify and kill the precancerous cells and cells infected with viruses

2ND CANCER STEP
PRECANCEROUS CELLS ARE FORMED and may either die or multiply to form tumors

INTERVENTION E

INTERVENTION H

Precancerous cells may either die on their own or are killed by the immune system

3RD CANCER STEP
CANCER CELLS FORM TUMORS AND METASTASIZE

1. Some precancerous cells escape the immune system and multiply to form tumors
2. New blood vessels are formed (angiogenesis) to feed the tumors and support the spread of the cancerous cells in the body (metastasis)

TUMOR SUPPRESSOR GENES
Can inhibit tumor growth if they function optimally

INTERVENTION F

INTERVENTION G

INTERVENTION I

based on all the research we have today and based on our current knowledge of human physiology and biochemistry.

SS: Okay, let's start from the beginning. I see a box that describes carcinogenic substances coming from the environment, but also from inside
our bodies. Please explain. I have always said it's the chemicals, again and
again. Is that the only cause, though?

CP: No, it's not the only cause, but it is certainly the culprit for many
cancers. These odd, artificial, man-made chemicals can be carcinogens,
but chemicals of natural origin can also be a problem, such as aflatoxins
from peanuts, which can cause liver cancer. Obviously, not everybody
who eats peanuts or peanut butter that contains aflatoxin gets liver cancer. This is a good example to show that it takes more than one factor to
lead to full-blown cancer.

I have to say I am not a fan of peanuts because they are a source of oxidized fat, due to the roasting of the polyunsaturated fat they contain,
and this is a source of free radicals that can cause DNA damage.

Peanuts are also high in omega-6 oils, which tend to stimulate excessive proliferation of cancer cells. Keep in mind that omega-3 fats (from
flax, walnuts, and fish oils) have the opposite effect—they reduce cancer
cell proliferation. What matters at the end of the day is your personal
ratio of omega-6 to omega-3.

SS: And there is a blood test for that, too?

CP: Yes, it is called the RBC [red blood cell] fatty acid profile, and it
is performed by various labs, including Metametrix. I find this to be one
of the most important tests that reflect many aspects of health status.

I have to give credit to Barry Sears and his books for enlightening many
people about the impact of these essential fats on the ability of an orga-
nism to function optimally and on the risk of many diseases.

The results of this test tell me a lot about what kind of fats patients eat
(saturated, polyunsaturated, monounsaturated, trans fats), their risk of inflammation, cancer proliferation and angiogenesis (the development of
new blood vessels that feed tumors), vasoconstriction (which leads to
high blood pressure) versus vasodilation (which supports good circulation to all organs), and risk of clotting (through platelet aggregation).

SS: Other than carcinogens, can any other factors give rise to a precancerous cell in the body?

CP: Yes, it's not just chemicals that may do it. As you see in my chart
in the upper right-hand corner box, bad luck (a chance, random genetic
change) or family genetic predisposition could also set the stage for a
precancerous cell to occur, specifically what is called a DNA mutation.

SS: Can you explain the concept of DNA mutation in cells for our readers?

CP: Every cell in our body has a program that tells it what to do, which is called the DNA, or the genetic code. This DNA code is an owner's manual, a set of instructions that guides the cell on when to grow, when to divide and multiply, how to communicate with neighboring cells, how to act as a team member with other cells. This is important because groups of cells form tissues and organs and act like an orchestra. Every cell is also programmed to respond in a very specific way to hormones and other cellular signals that come from the bloodstream or the fluid surrounding them.

All this proper cell behavior can be ruined, however, if the cell DNA code gets changed a bit by a chemical or by free radicals. We call any of these DNA code changes *mutations*, and they cause our cells to have an altered set of instructions, different from the original program we are born with. A cell with mutated DNA acts like a computer that has a bad program or memory problems.

Keep in mind that these mutations can also occur quite frequently by pure chance, when the cells normally divide as part of the process of generating new cells. This is part of the normal process that our tissues, organs, and blood undergo during growth and throughout our lifetime for continuous renewal.

SS: It sounds like our cells can make errors frequently as they continuously divide and turn over.

CP: Yes, the problem is that this process is kind of like making a photocopy of a copy and then making a copy of that copy. So errors just happen, and they accumulate more and more in time; the copies start looking dirtier and fuzzier, they lose their meaning, and start looking nothing like the original. That may be one of the mechanisms behind increased cancer risk with aging. That is why we have to get wiser and wiser about our choices; we just do not get away with "nutritional murder" as we used to when we were younger. Someone said that as we get older we become a less and less perfect copy of our original selves, and there is a lot of truth in that at the cellular and organ level. We can only hope and strive to stay as close to the original as possible by protecting our cells.

SS: So in regard to the random mutations and genetic predisposition factor box in your diagram, is there anything we can do to reduce the impact of those?

CP: Yes. It sounds like bad luck happens, but there are some nutritional interventions that can at least minimize the impact of these potential events, and I marked this as Intervention C in the diagram. What we can do is to make sure we have adequate vitamins such as folate and B_{12} in our diet and/or supplements, because they are necessary for making an accurate new copy of DNA for every new cell. It's like building a puzzle—if you are missing some important pieces, the meaning of the picture being built can change or get lost, which in the case of DNA can end up as different instructions for the cell.

SS: Well, I see this as one more reason why it makes sense to bank our own stem cells.

CP: Yes, that can have major potential in the future, because it saves some of our original cell programs in case technology allows us to reload our cells with "clean" programming. We are like computers that need to be refurbished by reloading with the original disks they came with when we bought them. That is why some parents store cord blood cells from their infants and they may also store the child's stem cells as early as possible after birth.

Also, unfortunately, just like computers, we tend to accumulate viruses and bugs in our cell programs, and the only way we can get rid of these is if the immune system recognizes and kills these infected cells.

So a reload with original DNA programming or any type of DNA correction may be an amazing anticancer, antiaging intervention. In a way, they are doing something similar when they destroy existing marrow cells that generate leukemia cancer cells and reimplant new bone marrow cells that are supposed to generate normal cells.

In the meantime, however, there is a lot we can do to keep our cell programs and minicomputers as clean and unaltered as possible by keeping the chemicals out and the immune system strong.

SS: I know viruses can lead to cancer, but how do they do that?

CP: Viruses that infect humans are known to change the DNA of the cells they infect. This is one reason the hepatitis C virus increases the risk of liver cancer, while HPV [human papilloma virus] increases the risk of cervical or throat cancer. And again, not everybody who is infected with these develops cancer. Some studies have shown that supplementing with vitamin K_2 may protect a liver infected with hepatitis C from developing cancer, while a broccoli extract, called I3C, and adequate folate were shown to reduce the risk of developing cervical or throat cancer in subjects infected with the HPV virus. I will post these studies on my website.

SS: Okay. So one thing is for sure: we need to do everything to avoid letting chemicals into our bodies. What are the most important ones to avoid, and if they do get in, what can we do?

CP: Yes, let's be aware of all detrimental chemicals and avoid them. Some are unavoidable, though, so when they do come in, the second important factor is to support the body's ability to detoxify them, or in other words, facilitate their safe removal.

These are the interventions named A and B in the previously mentioned diagram.

INTERVENTION A:
HOW TO MINIMIZE CARCINOGENIC LOAD IN THE BODY

Avoid getting carcinogens in the body. Avoid as much as possible both environmental and dietary toxins.

Environmental toxins. Sun, radiation (from flying, medical tests, cell phones, computers), air pollutants, substances that contact the skin (toxins found in cosmetics, clothing, or water we shower and bathe in).

Dietary toxins. Pesticides, oxidized fat, burned/smoked foods (especially grilled/burned/smoked meats, roasted coffee, burned toast), artificial additives, colors, sweeteners, emulsifiers, preservatives, contaminants from packaging, cookware (such as Teflon and various toxic metals), serving utensils/dishes/cups. Ceramic cups or plates and crystal glasses may contain and leach lead. I personally switched to all glass mugs and plates.

Avoid producing excessive amounts of carcinogens in the body. Get proper exercise. Excessive aerobic exercise produces free radicals, and studies have clearly shown that this is associated with increased DNA damage. We need to balance our exercise regimen with moderate cardio (not in polluted air), resistance training, and stretching. And then add other beneficial activities such as yoga, tai chi, or martial arts. Exercise should be done in moderation, because the right stimulation is critical for strengthening muscles and bones and joints, while increasing our body's antioxidant defenses.

For women and men. Estrogen (produced in the body or from replacement) that cannot be metabolized properly and excreted may cause DNA damage due to the formation of quinones. Adequate methylating factors (folate, B_{12}, B_6, SAM-e) and cruciferous vegetables and/or supplements that have concentrated extracts of these, such as sulforaphane, DIM, and calcium D-glucarate, help support a safe processing and elimination of estrogen by-products.

For men. Some researchers and doctors believe that testosterone metabolites may need to be adjusted to optimal levels. The conversion of testosterone to estrogen can be reduced by resveratrol, quercetin, chrysin, and adequate zinc status, while the conversion of testosterone to DHT can be reduced by natural compounds such as saw palmetto, GLA, EGCG (from green tea), or plant sterols and, again, adequate zinc status.

INTERVENTION B:
SUPPORT THE BODY'S ABILITY TO
ELIMINATE (DETOX) CARCINOGENS

Have adequate protein throughout the day. It will support the liver's job of processing things that need to be eliminated through the bile and stool (a process called liver detoxification).

Increase fiber. Fiber (both soluble and insoluble) in adequate levels was shown to reduce the risk of colon cancer and hormonally related cancers such as breast and prostate. I think an intake close to 50 grams per day from a combination of soluble and insoluble fiber may offer significant protection. I like Designs for Health Paleo Fiber because it is unique in its composition of twelve different fibers and it is gluten and soy free.

Sweat. Stimulate sweating (sauna, clothing during exercise) because when sweat is excreted, it carries a lot of toxins that have been accumulating in the body, particularly in fat cells.

Drink clean water. Drink plenty of clean water (have it filtered with reliable systems) and not from plastic bottles as much as possible.

Exercise. It will stimulate blood and lymph circulation, as well as sweat production.

SS: In your diagram, the first step in the cancer pathway is described as the process in which some of our normal cells have been changed, due to DNA damage (or DNA mutation) or improper genetic expression. What do you mean by "improper genetic expression," and is there anything we can do to prevent it?

CP: This is another aspect of cell behavior that is influenced by our vitamin status. Each cell has a set of programs with all the instructions it needs in order to function optimally for the specific place it has in the body. Each cell needs to read only certain instructions while other nonrelevant instructions need to be inactivated or "covered up" so they do not confuse the cell about what it needs to do. It's as if you round up a choir and give all the choir members the same book to sing songs from, but you have to specify which songs you want them to sing so that everybody in the choir is on the same page. This makes for harmonious functioning of cells that belong to certain organs with specific tasks. This is implemented in the body with methylating factors provided by vitamins like folate, B_{12}, and B_6 and substances such as choline and SAM-e. This is another way we can ensure that our cells operate properly. When we are deficient in some of these vitamins, however, there is confusion among cells as far as what instructions to follow, and the choir gets out of sync.

SS: How do we know if we have adequate methylating factors?

CP: One way is by checking homocysteine levels, and you may also need to check other measures of adequate folate status such as RBC folate and serum B_{12}, performed by common labs, or urinary markers of folate and B_{12} sufficiency such as urinary organic acids, performed by labs like Metametrix, which specializes in nutrition-related metabolic tests.

SS: Okay, so what happens after the first step in the cancer pathway, with the cells that are now considered precancerous? What are the chances that they will turn into a dangerous cancer?

CP: From this point on, there are factors that may stimulate or reduce the chance of them becoming a tumor, which may or may not spread throughout the body. That is where sugar, insulin, other growth factors, the immune system competence, and other natural compounds can influence their fate. We'll go over them one at a time.

SS: So these cells with bad programming due to mutations do not develop into an unstoppable cancer right away?

CP: Luckily, not always. Here are some good and some bad scenarios that can happen. The body has a system where it checks for errors, and it can do so because we fortunately have two copies of our cell program, kind of like a backup copy of the cell DNA. Believe it or not, the body does a periodic checkup for DNA errors. So sometimes it catches these mutations and it can correct them. However, if a cell divides before the checker comes by for repair, the mutation is passed on to the new cells and is forever unrepairable. Now it has brothers and sisters.

SS: It sounds like there is nothing we can do about this mishap. It's just bad luck?

CP: Actually this is another spot where we have some leverage to influence our chances.

The DNA checkup is more likely to be skipped if cells are growing and dividing really fast, and I mentioned earlier that sugar and insulin are evil supporters in this process. Also, that is not the only way they have detrimental effects on overall cancer risk, as I will describe later. Vitamin D was also shown to be important in supporting this DNA repair process.

SS: Are there any tests that can show us if DNA damage occurs excessively in our bodies, so we can intervene early?

CP: Yes, we can measure urinary DNA damage markers such as 8-OHdG (or 8-hydroxydeoxyguanosine). We can also measure lipid peroxides, which are a marker of oxidized fat and are indicative of an excess of free radicals and the fact that we need more antioxidants. This may be the result of ingesting damaged fats (from fried foods, et cetera) or just too much polyunsaturated fats (such as margarine, sunflower, safflower, soybean, and corn oils) or nuts like roasted sunflower seeds, cashews, peanuts, pine nuts.

SS: So if the DNA mutation can't be detected and corrected, what happens to the cells that have this DNA damage? Are these cells now a real cancer threat?

CP: No, actually this can happen every day with many cells in our bodies, but if we have a powerful immune system, like an army that has an adequate number of soldiers that are equipped with good weapons, these precancerous cells are recognized and killed. For example, the natural killer [NK] cells can recognize cancer cells and kill them. We can actually test patients for NK cell number and activity, to see if their immune system is strong enough and whether we need to work on boosting it. Remember that, as with infections, winning a quick war is about having a strong defense that annihilates the invaders quickly, before they multiply and take over too many local resources. The key is to have a good operating immune system that recognizes these cells as abnormal, almost like foreign invaders. It is critical to kill them before they have a chance to multiply and overwhelm the immune system's ability to eliminate them, just like what happens with tough infections.

SS: What can we do to make sure we have a good operating immune system?

CP: That's what I call Intervention E.

INTERVENTION E:
ENHANCE YOUR IMMUNE SYSTEM

Enhance immune efficiency. Incorporate factors that enhance the immune system's efficiency, such as adequate protein amounts spread evenly throughout the day, vitamins (vitamin C, folate, B_{12}) and minerals (zinc, selenium). Glutamine is fuel for the immune cells; probiotics boost the immune response.

Occasionally get an extra boost. For an extra, occasional immune boost use herbs like echinacea, astralagus, elderberry, andrographis, goldenseal, or various mushroom extracts (maitake, shiitake, reishi, beta-glucan). I have a review of how these work on my website, www.cristianapaul.com, in a paper entitled "Herbal Extracts for Boosting Immunity."

Address what's impairing the system. To keep the immune system from being impaired:
• Reduce stress.
• Do not have excessive amounts of carbs.
• Do not have excessively fatty meals.
• Get adequate sleep.
• Correct depression if possible with lifestyle measures and nutritional interventions.
• Avoid and eliminate toxins (such as mercury or other pollutants).

Know your vitamin K. Vitamin K was shown to be essential in supporting adequate cancer cell killing by the immune system (apoptosis). New research shows evidence we may need at least 1 to 2 milligrams of vitamin K per day for optimal function. One recent study has shown a correlation between prostate cancer risk and vitamin K status; another study supplemented women with vitamin K for bone health and found reduced development of breast cancer.

SS: So the bottom line is that if we have a good immune system, there is a good chance that the mutated cells may be eradicated. Okay, so if the immune system was not able to kill them and mutated cells start multiplying, are there any nutritional interventions that can stop it or slow it down?

CP: That is when things get harder and harder to stop from going down the path of full-blown cancer, but there are many nutritional factors that can slow them down or even cause them to die. In this scenario the cancer cells have a program that instructs them to proliferate fast. In most cases, the new program may direct the cell to not respect or communicate with the neighboring cells. These cancer cells take over the tissue they once belonged to and change it to where the tissue's function is impaired. By the way, here comes the sugar and insulin again, helping these crazy cells to grow and multiply even faster.

Again, the take-home message: keep carbs, sugar, and insulin at moderate/low levels at all times.

And there are quite a few other important physiological/nutritional factors in the body that control the speed of cell division and proliferation, which can rev up or slow down this process of inappropriate cellular growth. I've marked this as Intervention F in the diagram.

INTERVENTION F

Take in adequate omega-3s. Fatty acids and the ratio between omega-6s and omega-3s influence the rate of cell proliferation through hormones called prostaglandins. It's important to take in adequate omega-3 fats from fish oils (also from flax and algae DHA, for vegetarians). Avoid excessive consumption of arachidonic acid from corn-fed animals and their dairy products. Choose instead grass-fed animals and their dairy products as much as possible. Interestingly, cheese from Swiss cows was found to be high in omega-3 fats. This is because those are really "happy cows" grazing in the Swiss Alps only on grass, which is a source of omega-3 fats. Unfortunately, most cows in the United States (except for specific brands) are fed corn, so their meat or dairy products (milk, cheese, yogurt) are high in omega-6 fats.

Keep folate in balance. Excess folic acid or even natural folate may support excess cell proliferation, so it needs to be kept in an optimal middle range, as described earlier, and tested.

Know your IGF-1 levels. Excess IGF-1, a marker of growth hormone, could stimulate excessive cell proliferation. However, adequate growth hormone in the normal reference range may be beneficial because it boosts the immune system.

Keep cholesterol in check. Monitor your cholesterol, as you may need to suppress excess cholesterol production. This is due to the fact that the body makes mevalonate on the same pathway with cholesterol, and they both support cell proliferation. One may need to use tocotrienols, lycopene, and red yeast rice to suppress this pathway if necessary. As I mentioned earlier, there is research showing that these three supplements can reduce prostate cancer risk and development, but they may work the same for many other cancers.

SS: Isn't red yeast rice like a statin?

CP: Yes, it contains molecules similar in function to statins, called monacolins. The similarity is that they all inhibit the enzyme HMG-CoA reductase. But statins and red yeast rice are metabolized a bit differently in the body. One study showed that red yeast rice resulted in ten times lower blood levels of monacolin-K (the statin-like molecule) than an equivalent cholesterol-lowering dose of lovastatin. We could say that red yeast rice is a nicer, gentler statin-like compound, which may have the same cholesterol-lowering effects but with much fewer side effects than the equivalent dose of statin.

In Asia they take grams of red yeast rice in fermented foods, in drinks like rice wine, and in vinegar, and they use it in many foods for color and as a preservative in meats. In the United States, we use nitrates, which are carcinogens, for meat preservation and to retain color.

Red yeast rice is especially useful when all other nutritional and lifestyle interventions did not adjust cholesterol and other blood lipids to optimal levels, ratios, and profiles. Red yeast rice may also be needed when there is a genetic tendency to have high cholesterol. But for cancer, the purpose is not only to lower cholesterol but also to reduce mevalonate, a compound that is made along the same pathway as cholesterol, because both are needed by the cancer cells to thrive. So, in summary, when the enzyme HMG-CoA reductase is inhibited by red yeast rice or a statin, both cholesterol and mevalonate will be reduced at the same time. Many studies have shown that reducing mevalonate availability impairs cancer progression.

SS: Anything else we can do to stop these crazy cancer cells?

CP: Yes, we can take in nutritional factors from foods and/or supplements that can slow down cell proliferation, as well as angiogenesis—the creation of new blood vessels that are brought in to feed the cancerous cells. That is Intervention G.

INTERVENTION G:
SLOWING CANCER CELL PROLIFERATION

Supplement with vitamin D. Vitamin D has been shown to reduce cancer risk and development. It is believed that it does this by reducing excessive cell proliferation. But if supplementing with D, you must also make sure that the body's vitamin K status is adequate, from diet and/or supplements. This is because vitamin D works together with vitamin K as a tag team in distributing calcium to the right places in the body, specifically into the bones and away from arteries or kidneys. When vitamin D levels in the body are increased (through diet, sun, and/or supplements) while vitamin K status is deficient, studies have shown that this situation may lead to increased arterial stiffness and arterial calcification. The bottom line is that vitamin D and vitamin K are a great team in reducing cancer risk and have a multitude of additional health benefits for osteoporosis and heart health.

Know your botanicals. Various botanicals reduce cancer cell proliferation and may actually induce them to die. Here is a list of the ones that I see the most compelling evidence for: resveratrol supplement or a little bit of red wine (not in excess); curcumin as a supplement or from turmeric used in cooking; green tea extract or brewed green tea; broccoli (mature plant and sprouts) as food or as extracts (sulforaphane, DIM); a moderate quantity of grapes (while the skin is most concentrated in the beneficial compounds, the juice is not and it is very high in sugar, so your best bet would be to just eat the skins); grape seed extract; pomegranate extract or juice in moderation; quercetin extract (also found in onions, apples, grapes); CLA (conjugated linoleic acid, as a supplement or found in grass-fed beef and its dairy); luteolin (found in onions, broccoli, carrots, radish, celery, olives); ginger (as extract, supplement, or tea).

Know your natural allies. Here are a few more natural compounds that have been shown to reduce cancer risk through various mechanisms:

- Calcium, to reduce colon cancer risk
- CoQ_{10}, reduce and help with remission of breast cancer
- Perillyl alcohol, found in cherries; similar in structure to limonene (found in citrus peel), and both inhibit cancer
- Garlic, effective against leukemia cells (onions contain anticancer compounds as well)
- Iodine, as a deficiency may have a complex role in the risk of breast and thyroid cancer

CP: This work reaffirms what Hippocrates said twenty-five centuries ago: "Let food be thy medicine and medicine be thy food."

SS: Thank you, Cristiana.

Knock It Out

- Supplement antioxidants in a balanced way. For example, you may take resveratrol, an amazingly powerful antioxidant and genetic modulator, but don't skip the other antioxidants. If a fruit seems great, such as pomegranate or grapes, don't just prioritize that. A mix of antioxidant supplements with a large variety of fruits and vegetables will be most protective against cancer overall.

- Avoid synthetic supplements, as they can block your body from absorbing other nutrients from your diet, and they may not be balanced like natural vitamins and nutrients.
- With supplements that contain vitamin E, look for products that contain natural mixed tocopherols as the primary form of vitamin E listed on the label. If it has mixed tocotrienols, that is even better, as studies have shown promising results that they may reduce the risk of breast, colon, and prostate cancer. Avoid d,l-alpha-tocopherol.
- When choosing a supplement that contains vitamin A, look for mixed carotenoids. A nutritional supplement that contains only beta-carotene as the primary form of vitamin A will cause an imbalance of other natural carotenoids, because they compete for absorption in the body.
- Avoid anything (supplements, processed foods) that contains artificial dyes. Instead, look for products that use natural pigments (e.g., from red grape skin or turmeric) that are also powerful antioxidants.
- While supplementation with folic acid in people who are deficient can reduce the risk of various cancers, there's a big difference between synthetic folic acid and natural folates (found mainly in fruits, vegetables, and liver). Supplementation with high amounts of folic acid may promote growth of precancerous cells. As far as foods go, it would be best to get natural folates from fruits and vegetables, not folic acid from refined flour products.
- Pay attention to how many carbohydrates you consume at one time, as eating too many will increase your blood glucose level. Sugar fuels cancer and precancerous cells and produces excess insulin, which acts as a second stimulating factor for cell growth, cell division, and ultimately multiplication of these "bad" cells. Exercising after a high-carb meal can help you burn the carbs immediately after they are absorbed in your body, so take a walk right after dinner if you've overindulged.
- As people age, cells multiply less accurately. We can protect our cells by making sure we have adequate vitamins such as folate and B_{12} in our diet and/or supplements.

Chapter 18

IF YOU CHOOSE TRADITIONAL TREATMENT, WHAT YOU NEED TO KNOW: AN INTERVIEW WITH BILL FALOON

This isn't mission difficult, it's mission impossible.

–Anthony Hopkins to Tom Cruise, *Mission: Impossible II* (2000)

In doing research for this book, I came across a set of facts that are absolutely earth-shattering. It turns out that what happens in the body in response to surgical removal of the primary tumor is a significant *cause* of metastasis in patients for whom surgery is not curative. In other words, surgery can spread cancer!

The good news is that a wide variety of methods have been identified to protect against surgery-induced recurrence and metastasis. Armed with this knowledge, cancer patients can follow simple steps ahead of time to dramatically improve their odds of a cure.

You would think that cancer surgeons would figure this out themselves. After all, everything I discovered is based on what is already published in the peer-reviewed scientific literature. Sadly, the assembly-line mentality of conventional doctors too often results in these novel methods being overlooked. As I have learned, it is critical that the right choices be made both before and after surgery in order to protect against cancer cells spreading to other parts of the body.

Bill Faloon is the director and cofounder of the Life Extension Foundation. He knows what those choices should be. He is a passionate layperson who fights for what is right, and fights for the truth, sometimes at great personal sacrifice and even danger. His investigations have enabled people to access medical information not available elsewhere through the database supplied by the Life Extension advisory board.

Cancer is a frightening and debilitating diagnosis. For most of us it is our biggest fear. For many people, alternative approaches are just not an option. Mainstream oncologists often offer only one option, and if a patient has not done investigative research on all avenues of healing, then going against orthodox treatments is just too big a leap.

Choice of treatment is very personal and one that I respect. For that reason I have asked Bill Faloon to give me information on how to best utilize *traditional treatment*. How can a person maximize the benefits of chemo and survive harsh chemical poisoning? How can a patient find treatment that fits his particular cancer, rather than the present guessing game? As I have said throughout this book, traditional cancer treatment would no longer be my choice, even though my first time around with breast cancer I did resort to a modified conventional treatment. Although I refused chemotherapy, I did utilize surgery and radiation. But since that time my feelings have changed regarding treatment protocols and now I always choose alternative medicine first as my personal approach to health care. I do acknowledge that pharmaceuticals and Western medicine have their place, particularly where it involves pain, infection, or mental illness. I also realize that when it comes to cancer, many people are not comfortable with alternative choices. I understand and respect any decision a patient chooses to make for themselves regarding their personal health. The purpose of this chapter is to inform you of ways to maximize your success if you do choose to go mainstream.

Some do survive traditional treatment. But building up the body before and during treatment and being sure to work with new advances just makes sense and gives the patient the best shot.

Knowledge is power. Just making the correct choice is no longer enough. Misdiagnosis (such as what I experienced) and medical ignorance are both factors in survival. As patients, we need to be informed and knowledgeable about what is available and what is best for us individually. This interview with Bill Faloon will inform you and enable you to better approach the treatment course you have personally chosen.

Do not allow yourself to give power over your life and health to anyone else. It is always your choice. It is my hope that after reading this book, you come away feeling that you are now an informed patient, and that now you can direct your disease treatment and feel that you have some power over this horrible invader.

Shockingly in many cases mainstream oncologists are overlooking proven methods to better treat their patients. The doctors and scientists at Life Extension offer their subscribers consultations for cancer patients. And this team will introduce you to FDA-approved treatments that are routinely denied to patients because apathetic oncologists seem to prefer to place their patients on highly profitable assembly lines. That is the sad fact. According to Bill Faloon, "The second biggest killer in America is medical ignorance and it is the number one reason people die."

Life Extension has uncovered numerous therapies that can greatly improve a cancer patient's chances of long-term survival or cure. They feel many mainstream oncologists don't even consider the scientifically documented nontoxic approaches to saving their patients' lives, and this is a tragedy. The beginning of this interview discusses a wide range of nontoxic approaches to saving patients' lives and this is critical information if you are choosing traditional "standard of care" treatment. If ever you or a loved one find yourself in the vulnerable position of a cancer diagnosis, you will be helped by knowing this valuable information.

SS: Hello, Bill. Life Extension offers your members a unique consultation service. When a patient calls for information or referrals, what is the first question you ask after they reveal they've been newly diagnosed with cancer?

BF: We ask if they have undergone any conventional treatments, including surgery.

SS: Why is that?

BF: Because cancer patients often call us right before they are about to undergo surgery or some other conventional therapy. We inform them of what we feel are necessary steps to reduce the risk of a recurrence of the primary tumor and the emergence of metastatic disease.

SS: Are you saying there are steps cancer patients can take even before surgery to improve their odds?

BF: Absolutely. The rationale for surgical removal is that you can get rid of the cancer by removing it from the body. This approach does not take into account that after surgery the cancer will frequently metastasize to different organs. Startling scientific findings reveal that cancer surgery can *increase* the risk of metastasis. This flies in the face of conventional medical thinking, but the facts are undeniable.

SS: How does surgery increase metastatic risk?

BF: During the surgical procedure, natural barriers that contain the tumor to a region on the body are breached, enabling cancer cells to escape their original confinement and spread to other parts of the body.

Surgery also induces immune suppression while initiating an inflammatory cascade that provides cancer cells with biological fuel to propagate. Surgery inflicts a wound on the body that requires healing. The body secretes growth factors to facilitate healing. Unfortunately, these same growth factors also stimulate tumor cell growth. Unless the proper steps are taken before surgery, cancer cells can spill into the bloodstream from the surgical margins and establish metastatic colonies in other parts of the body.

SS: What happens after the cancer cells enter the bloodstream?

BF: In some cases, turbulence from the fast-moving blood destroys the cancer cells. Cancer cells must also avoid detection and destruction from immune cells circulating in the bloodstream. This is why it is so important to boost a patient's immune system *before* surgery, so that cancer cells that escape during the surgery are killed by activated immune cells.

SS: What happens if cancer cells are not destroyed?

BF: Rogue cancer cells that survive in the blood can adhere to the lining of the blood vessel and burrow through to invade an organ. These malignant cells can then multiply and become a new metastatic cancer. This is why it is so important to take steps before surgery, so that cancer cells that escape during the surgery are killed by activated immune cells.

SS: How long have scientists known that surgery itself can cause metastasis?

BF: Life Extension uncovered data back in 1985 indicating that surgery increased metastatic risk, and we identified methods to counteract the adverse effects of cancer surgery. Just this year, 2009, in the medical journal *Annals of Surgery*, researchers reported that cancer surgery itself can create an environment in the body that greatly lessens the obstacles to metastasis. Another article in the *British Journal of Cancer* in 2001 stated that "primary tumor removal may result in sudden acceleration of metastatic process." This corroborates observations that relatively soon after surgery, metastatic lesions quickly emerge that were not necessarily evident prior to the surgical procedure.

SS: You are saying these reports indicate that the surgery itself could cause the cancer to spread. So what can those undergoing surgery do to protect themselves against increased risk?

BF: They need to circumvent all the mechanisms that cancer cells utilize to establish metastatic colonies.

SS: Give me an example.

BF: Cancer cells must be able to clump together and form colonies that can expand and grow. It is unlikely that a single cancer cell will form a metastatic tumor, just as one person is unlikely to form a thriving community. Cancer cells use adhesion molecules to facilitate their ability to clump together. Present on the surface of cancer cells, these molecules act like Velcro by allowing freestanding cancer cells to adhere to each other. The adherence of circulating tumor cells to the blood vessel walls is an essential step for the process of metastasis. Cancer surgery increases tumor cell adhesion. In one experiment that mimicked surgical conditions, scientists reported that the binding of cancer cells to the blood vessel walls was increased by 250 percent! Therefore, it is critically important for a person undergoing cancer surgery to take measures that can help to neutralize the surgery-induced increase in cancer cell adhesion. Fortunately, a natural supplement called modified citrus pectin can do just that.

SS: What makes this different from regular citrus pectin?

BF: Citrus pectin—a type of dietary fiber—is not absorbed from the intestine. However, modified citrus pectin has been altered so that it can be absorbed into the blood and exert its anticancer effects.

SS: How does it prevent cancer cell adhesion?

BF: By binding to adhesion molecules on the surface of cancer cells, thereby preventing cancer cells from sticking together and forming a cluster. It also inhibits circulating tumor cells from latching onto the lining of blood vessels. This was demonstrated by an experiment in which modified citrus pectin blocked an adhesion molecule's activity in the lining of blood vessels by an astounding 95 percent. Modified citrus pectin also substantially decreased the adhesion of breast cancer cells to the blood vessel walls.

SS: Does it protect against other kinds of cancer cells?

BF: In a study published in the *Journal of the National Cancer Institute*, a group of mice were given it and then injected with prostate cancer cells. A group of mice not receiving the pectin served as the control group. Lung metastasis was noted in 93 percent of the control group, whereas only 50 percent of the pectin group experienced lung metastasis. Even more noteworthy was the finding that the citrus pectin group had an 89 percent reduction in the size of the metastatic colonies compared with the control group. In a similar experiment, mice injected with melanoma cancer cells experienced a greater than 90 percent reduction in lung metastases compared with the control group.

SS: This is impressive, but I'm sure many will wonder, does this work in humans? Are there human studies?

BF: Human studies have been done on very advanced patients with modest benefits. In one trial, ten men with recurrent prostate cancer received 14.4 grams per day. After one year, a considerable improvement in cancer progression was noted, as determined by a reduction of the rate at which the PSA increased. This was followed by a study in which forty-nine men with advanced prostate cancer were given modified citrus pectin for a four-week cycle. After two cycles of treatment, 21 percent of the men experienced a stabilization of their disease or improved quality of life; 12 percent had stable disease for more than twenty-four weeks. Please remember that these prostate cancer study subjects already suffered from advanced disease. It would appear more logical if these patients had initiated supplementation before surgical procedures to prevent metastatic colonies from being established, as was done in the successful laboratory studies. This is why we at Life Extension try to encourage cancer patients to call us before surgery, so we can suggest supplements like this *before* metastatic colonies have already formed.

SS: What else can cancer patients take to inhibit cancer cell adhesion?

BF: Cimetidine is a drug historically used to alleviate heartburn. Cimetidine also possesses potent anticancer activity. You can purchase this over the counter, and cimetidine inhibits cancer cell adhesion by blocking the expression of an adhesive molecule called E-selectin, which is on the surface of cells lining blood vessels. Cancer cells latch onto E-selectin in order to adhere to the lining of blood vessels. By preventing the expression of E-selectin, cimetidine significantly limits the ability of cancer cell adherence to the blood vessel walls. This effect is analogous to removing the Velcro from the blood vessel walls that would normally enable circulating tumor cells to bind.

SS: How do we know this?

BF: In a study published in the *British Journal of Cancer* in 2002, sixty-four colon cancer patients received standard therapy with or without cimetidine (800 milligrams per day) for one year. The ten-year survival for the cimetidine group was 84.6 percent. This is in stark contrast to the control group, which had a ten-year survival of only 49.8 percent. Remarkably, for those patients with a more aggressive form of colon cancer, the ten-year survival was 85 percent in those treated with cimetidine compared with a dismal 23 percent in the control group. These findings were supported by another study with colorectal cancer patients whereby cimetidine given for just seven days at the time of surgery increased three-year survival from 59 percent to 93 percent! The Life Extension Foundation first recommended cimetidine to cancer patients in 1985. It is absurd to think that virtually no oncologists prescribe it today, despite its efficacy being demonstrated against a wide range of cancers.

SS: What dosages does Life Extension recommend for cimetidine and modified citrus pectin?

BF: The published scientific data provide a compelling case for cancer patients to take, five days prior to surgery, 14 grams of modified citrus pectin and 800 milligrams of cimetidine daily. This combination regimen may be followed for a year or longer to reduce metastatic risk.

SS: What about immune function?

BF: As I mentioned earlier, the surgical procedure suppresses immune function. It is also important for cancer patients to optimize lifelong immune surveillance to reduce the risk of a recurrence, so taking the proper immune-boosting drugs, hormones, and supplements is vitally important.

SS: What types of immune cells are suppressed in cancer patients?

BF: Research has shown that natural killer cells spontaneously recognize and kill a variety of cancer cells. To illustrate the importance of NK cell activity in fighting cancer, a study published in the journal *Breast Cancer Research and Treatment* examined NK cell activity in women shortly after surgery for breast cancer. The researchers reported that low levels of NK cell activity were associated with an increased risk of death from breast cancer. In fact, reduced NK cell activity was a better predictor of survival than the stage of the cancer. In another alarming study, individuals with reduced NK cell activity before surgery for colon cancer had a 350 percent increased risk of metastasis during the following thirty-one months.

SS: Does surgery itself really suppress immunity?

BF: Yes. Numerous studies document that cancer surgery results in a substantial reduction in natural killer cell activity. In an investigation having ominous implications, NK cell activity in women having surgery for breast cancer was reduced by over 50 percent on the first day after surgery. In light of this mounting evidence, a group of researchers stated that even transitory immune dysfunction after surgery may permit cancers to form sizable metastases. This surgically induced NK impairment could not happen at a worse possible time. It is right after surgery that activated immune cells are most needed to fight metastasis.

SS: So what should cancer patients do?

BF: Fortunately, there are nutraceutical and pharmaceutical interventions known to enhance natural killer cell activity in cancer patients. One natural supplement that can increase NK cell activity is called PSK, a specially prepared extract from the mushroom *Coriolus*. PSK has been shown to enhance NK cell activity in multiple studies. PSK's ability to enhance NK cell activity helps to explain why it has been shown to dramatically improve survival in cancer patients. For example, 225 patients with lung cancer received radiation therapy with or without PSK (3 grams per day). For those with more advanced stage III cancers, more than three times as many individuals taking PSK were alive after five years (26 percent), compared with those not taking PSK (8 percent). PSK also more than doubled five-year survival in those individuals with less advanced stage I or II disease (39 percent versus 17 percent).

SS: Does PSK work against other cancers?

BF: Yes. A group of colon cancer patients was randomized to receive standard therapy alone or standard therapy plus PSK, which was taken for two years. The group receiving PSK had an exceptional ten-year survival of 82 percent. Sadly, the group receiving the conventional standard therapy alone had a ten-year survival of only 51 percent. In a similar trial reported in the *British Journal of Cancer* in 2004, colon cancer patients received standard therapy alone or combined with PSK (3 grams per day) for two years. In the group with a more dangerous stage III colon cancer, the five-year survival was 75 percent in the PSK group. This compared with a five-year survival of only 46 percent in the group receiving standard therapy alone. Research has confirmed that PSK also improves survival in cancers of the breast, stomach, esophagus, and uterus/cervix.

SS: What else can help?

BF: Garlic, glutamine, IP6 [inositol hexaphosphate], AHCC [active hexose correlated compound], and lactoferrin all help boost NK activity. One experiment in mice with breast cancer found that glutamine supplementation resulted in a 40 percent decrease in tumor growth paired with a 2.5-fold increase in NK cell activity. Your readers are welcome to receive a free copy of the latest dosing recommendations for these immune-boosting nutrients and drugs by going to your website, www .suzannesomers.com, and clicking on Life Extension.

SS: What about mistletoe extract? I feel that has worked very well for me.

BF: Scientists in Germany explored the effects of mistletoe extract on NK cell activity in sixty-two patients undergoing surgery for colon cancer. The participants were randomized to receive an intravenous infusion of mistletoe extract immediately before they were given general anesthesia, or were given general anesthesia alone. Measurements of NK cell activity were taken before, and twenty-four hours after, surgery. As expected, the group that did not receive mistletoe experienced a 44 percent reduction in NK cell activity twenty-four hours after surgery. The group receiving mistletoe did *not* experience a significant decrease in NK cell activity after surgery. The scientists concluded infusion of mistletoe extracts before surgery can prevent a suppression of NK cell activity in cancer patients.

SS: What about drugs?

BF: Yes. There are drugs proven to work, but most oncologists fail to utilize them properly. Pharmaceuticals used to increase NK cell activity include interferon-alpha and granulocyte-macrophage colony stimulating factor. These drugs are shown to prevent surgery-induced immune suppression when given prior to surgery, yet most oncologists wait until white blood cells drop precipitously before prescribing these immune-boosting drugs. Another immune-boosting drug for cancer patients to consider for preventing or treating metastatic disease is *interleukin-2*. If your readers have any questions about these immune-boosting drugs, they can go to your website, click on Life Extension, and scroll down to a group called International Strategic Cancer Alliance; or call 1-800-327-9009 twenty-four hours a day.

SS: Are cancer vaccines really working?

BF: Yes, they are, and it is too bad the FDA keeps delaying their approval. In a study conducted in 2005, 567 individuals with colon cancer were randomized to receive surgery alone, or surgery combined with vaccines derived from their own cancer cells. The median survival for the cancer vaccine group was over seven years, compared with the median survival of four and a half years for the group receiving surgery alone. The five-year survival was 66.5 percent in the cancer vaccine group, which dwarfed the 45.5 percent five-year survival for the group receiving surgery alone. This glaring difference in five-year survival clearly displays the power of individually tailored cancer vaccines to focus a person's own immunity to target and attack residual metastatic cancer cells. There are vaccines to combat prostate, melanoma, and other cancers, but the FDA mandates that patients fail toxic conventional therapies before being allowed to try these vaccines. At these late stages, when the patient's immune function has been decimated by radiation and chemotherapy, these vaccines do not work nearly as well as they could if given earlier in the treatment process.

SS: I know that the formation of new blood vessels enables cancer cells to rapidly grow. Can you tell my readers more about this and why it's important?

BF: The formation of new blood vessels (angiogenesis) supplying the tumor is a requirement for successful metastasis, since tumors cannot grow beyond the size of a pinhead without expanding their blood supply.

It might be surprising to learn that the presence of the primary tumor serves to inhibit the growth of metastatic cancer elsewhere in the body. The primary tumor produces antiangiogenic factors which restrict the growth of their metastatic offspring. Regrettably, the surgical removal of the primary cancer results in the removal of these antiangiogenic factors, and the growth of metastases is no longer inhibited. That is why it is so important to incorporate antiangiogenesis therapies prior to and immediately after surgery.

After surgery, levels of growth factors that increase angiogenesis are elevated, such as vascular endothelial growth factor [VEGF]. This can result in an increased formation of new blood vessels supplying areas of metastatic cancer, including dormant micrometastatic colonies.

SS: What can be done to suppress VEGF?

BF: Various nutrients have been shown to inhibit VEGF. These include soy isoflavones (genistein), silibinin (a component of milk thistle), green tea (EGCG), and curcumin. In one experiment, EGCG—the active constituent of green tea—was administered to mice with stomach cancer. The results demonstrated that green tea reduced the tumor mass by 60 percent, while also reducing the concentration of blood vessels feeding the tumor by 38 percent. Remarkably, EGCG decreased the expression of VEGF in cancer cells by an astounding 80 percent! The authors of the study concluded that EGCG "is a promising candidate for antiangiogenic treatment of gastric cancer."

SS: Let's talk about curcumin. How does it interfere with angiogenesis?

BF: Researchers at Emory University School of Medicine noted that curcumin is a direct inhibitor of angiogenesis that functions by down-regulating VEGF. The cell adhesion molecules we discussed earlier that facilitate metastasis are up-regulated in active angiogenesis. Curcumin can also block this effect.

SS: Is there a best method for taking these?

BF: Five days prior to surgery, the patient may consider supplementing with standardized green tea extract, curcumin, soy genistein extract, and other nutrients that suppress VEGF—and thus help protect against angiogenesis. Even if a person is fighting cancer that has already metastasized, these same nutrients can help suppress tumor angiogenesis that permits further tumor growth. For the latest dosing recommendations for these nutrients, readers can go to your website and click on Life Extension.

SS: What else can cancer surgery patients do to improve their odds of a cure?

BF: The conventional approach is to use general anesthesia during surgery, followed by intravenous morphine after surgery for pain control. The conventional approach, however, may not be the optimal way to prevent surgery-induced metastasis. The use of morphine directly after surgery poses significant problems. At a time when immune function is already suppressed, morphine further weakens the immune system by diminishing NK cell activity. One study found that morphine increased angiogenesis and stimulated the growth of breast cancer in mice. The researchers concluded that the clinical use of morphine could potentially be harmful in patients with angiogenesis-dependent cancers. Surgical anesthesia has also been shown to weaken NK cell activity.

SS: What should cancer surgery patients ask their doctors to do?

BF: Given the problems associated with morphine and anesthesia, researchers have explored other approaches to surgical anesthesia and pain control. One novel approach is the use of conventional general anesthesia combined with regional anesthesia, which refers to anesthesia that only affects a specific part of the body. The benefits achieved with this approach are twofold: the use of regional anesthesia reduces the amount of general anesthesia required during surgery, as well as decreasing the amount of morphine needed after surgery for pain control.

SS: If their doctors ask, what scientific studies support this?

BF: In one experiment, cancerous mice received surgery with general anesthesia alone or combined with regional anesthesia. The scientists reported that the addition of regional anesthesia to general anesthesia markedly attenuates the promotion of metastasis by surgery. In this study, regional anesthesia reversed 70 percent of the metastasis-promoting effects of surgery caused by general anesthesia alone. Doctors at Pennsylvania State University College of Medicine compared NK cell activity in patients receiving general or regional anesthesia for abdominal surgery. NK cell activity dropped substantially in the general anesthesia group, while NK cell activity was preserved at preoperative levels in the group that received regional anesthesia. In another study, fifty women having breast cancer surgery with general anesthesia combined with regional anesthesia were compared with seventy-nine women who received general anesthesia during their breast cancer surgery followed by morphine for pain control. After a follow-up period of three years, dramatic differences were noted between the two groups. Only 6 percent of patients who received regional anesthesia were diagnosed with liver, lung, or bone metastasis compared with a 24 percent risk of metastatic recurrence in the group that did receive regional anesthesia. Stated differently, women who received regional and general anesthesia had a 75 percent decreased risk for metastatic cancer. Furthermore, the women who did not receive regional anesthesia had almost a sevenfold greater risk of lymph node metastasis compared with the women who received regional anesthesia.

SS: These are startling survival improvements. What about managing chronic pain after surgery?

BF: Our research shows patients requiring morphine for pain control after surgery can consider asking their doctor for a medication called tramadol instead. Unlike morphine, tramadol does not suppress immune function. On the contrary, tramadol has been shown to stimulate NK cell activity. In one experiment, tramadol blocked the formation of lung metastasis induced by surgery in rats. Tramadol also prevented the surgery-induced suppression of NK cell activity.

SS: Are there other methods to reduce the risk of metastasis?

BF: Yes, there are. There is considerable evidence showing that surgeries that are less invasive—and therefore less traumatic—pose less risk of metastasis, compared with more invasive and traumatic surgery. Laparoscopic surgery is one type of minimally invasive surgery, in which operations in the abdomen, pelvis, and other regions are performed through small incisions, as compared to the much larger incisions needed in traditional "open" surgeries.

SS: Again, for a patient's doctor, what human studies are there?

BF: A study published in the *Lancet* compared laparoscopic with open surgery in patients with colon cancer. In contrast to the group receiving traditional open surgery, the laparoscopic surgery group had a 61 percent decreased risk of cancer recurrence coupled with a 62 percent decreased risk of death from colon cancer. A similar study reported a 56 percent decreased risk of death from colon cancer for laparoscopic surgery as compared with traditional open surgery. Minimally invasive surgery has produced substantial improvements in survival for those with lung cancer. Video-assisted thoracic surgery, a minimally invasive surgery, was compared with traditional open surgery. The five-year survival from lung cancer was 97 percent in the video-assisted thoracic surgery group. This greatly contrasts with the 79 percent five-year survival in the open surgery group. Laparoscopic surgery results in faster healing and reduces surgical complications along with pain and discomfort.

SS: You mentioned earlier that the inflammation process caused by surgery facilitates metastasis. How does this happen?

BF: Surgery causes an increased production of inflammatory chemicals, such as interleukin-1 and interleukin-10. These chemicals increase the activity of cyclooxygenase-2 [COX-2], a potent inflammatory enzyme. COX-2 promotes cancer growth and metastasis.

SS: Can you tell us a little more?

BF: An article appearing in the journal *Cancer Research* found levels of COX-2 in pancreatic cancer cells to be sixty times greater than in normal pancreatic cells. Levels of COX-2 were one hundred fifty times higher in cancer cells from individuals with head and neck cancers as compared to healthy volunteers. COX-2 fuels cancer growth by stimulating the formation of new blood vessels feeding the tumor. COX-2 increases cancer cell adhesion to the blood vessel walls. COX-2 also enhances the ability of cancer cells to metastasize, as experiments with mice revealed that colon cancer cells expressing high levels of COX-2 metastasized freely to the liver, while colon cancer cells expressing low levels of COX-2 did not metastasize to the liver.

SS: This is startling information. How long have we known about this?

BF: The Life Extension Foundation incorporated COX-2-inhibiting compounds into its cancer treatment protocols back in 1996, but it was not until much later that cancer researchers began to understand the important role it plays in promoting cancer growth. In a study published in the journal *Clinical Cancer Research* in 2004, 288 individuals undergoing surgery for colon cancer had their tumors examined for the presence of COX-2. The findings were alarming—the group whose cancers tested positive for the presence of COX-2 had a 311 percent greater risk of death compared to the group whose cancers did not express COX-2. A subsequent study in lung cancer patients found that those with high tumor levels of COX-2 had a median survival of only fifteen months, whereas those with low tumor levels of COX-2 had a median survival of forty months.

SS: Walk me through what happens when cancer patients are treated with COX-2 inhibitors.

BF: There are some rather dramatic results against certain cancers. For example, 134 patients with advanced lung cancer were treated with chemotherapy alone or combined with Celebrex (a COX-2 inhibitor). For those individuals with cancers expressing higher amounts of COX-2, treatment with Celebrex resulted in a 66 percent *reduced* risk of death as compared to those who did not receive Celebrex. Treatment with Celebrex also slowed cancer progression in men with recurrent prostate cancer. Perhaps the most impressive display of the antimetastatic effects of COX-2 inhibitor drugs was presented at the annual conference of the American Society of Clinical Oncology in 2008. In this study, the incidence of bone metastases in breast cancer patients who had taken a COX-2 inhibitor for at least six months following the diagnosis of breast cancer was compared to the incidence of bone metastases in breast cancer patients who had not taken a COX-2 inhibitor. Remarkably, those who were treated with a COX-2 inhibitor were 90 percent less likely to develop bone metastases than those who were not treated with a COX-2 inhibitor.

SS: Are there nondrug approaches that have some of the same benefits?

BF: Yes, there are. Nutrients known to inhibit COX-2 include curcumin, resveratrol, vitamin E, soy isoflavones (genistein), green tea (EGCG), quercetin, fish oil, feverfew, and silymarin (from milk thistle). Scientists at Memorial Sloan-Kettering Cancer Center in New York experimentally induced a fourfold increase in COX-2 activity in human breast cells, which was completely prevented by resveratrol. Resveratrol blocked the production of COX-2 within the cell, as well as blocking COX-2 enzyme activity.

SS: With all these choices, how can my readers learn what doses of nutrients and drugs they should take?

BF: As we speak, Suzanne, a dedicated team of clinical oncologists and researchers at the International Strategic Cancer Alliance are preparing a meticulous report on the optimal doses of nutrients and drugs that a cancer patient should consider during the pre- and postoperative period. As with the other information we've discussed, your readers can obtain a free copy of this report by visiting www.suzannesomers.com and clicking on Life Extension.

SS: What about patients whose cancer has already metastasized?

BF: At that point, Suzanne, the patient has to undergo meticulous testing to determine which survival genes in their particular tumor have enabled it to escape eradication by conventional therapy. For example, mutations in one of the genes encoding the ras proteins are associated with up-regulated cell proliferation. These ras mutations are found in an estimated 30 to 40 percent of all human cancers. A mutated ras protein gene behaves like a switch stuck in the "on" position, continuously misinforming the cell, instructing it to divide when the cycle should be turned off. Fortunately, a number of readily available compounds can turn off the cell-proliferating effects of mutated ras oncogenes. Among these are fish oil, garlic, and green tea. The temporary use of high-dose statin drugs can also effectively turn off ras oncogene expression.

SS: How do we know this?

BF: Patients with primary liver cancer were treated with either the standard therapy or a combination of standard therapy and 40 milligrams per day of pravastatin. Median survival increased from nine months among patients treated with only standard therapy to eighteen months when using pravastatin plus standard therapy. When one considers the other integrative therapies available to treat primary liver cancer, the use of compounds that suppress ras oncogene expression offers tremendous potential.

SS: What else can we do to protect ourselves?

BF: As a result of normal aging, the loss of bone mineral density results in the release of a compound that can fuel tumor cell propagation; it's called transforming growth factor. This problem is especially insidious in breast and prostate cancer patients, where tumor cells have a proclivity to invade healthy bones, degrade them, and cause the release of even higher amounts of transforming growth factor. All cancer patients should take extraordinary steps to maintain their bone density, including consuming lots of vitamin D_3, vitamin K_2, and minerals such as boron, magnesium, and calcium. Cancer patients with evidence of circulating tumor cells should also consider an injection of a bisphosphonate drug called Zometa to reduce the ability of tumor cells to bind to bone. Remember, the release of growth factors from bone into the bloodstream can fuel cancer cell growth, so it is important for cancer patients to be especially vigilant in maintaining their bone structure. This is another critical area of cancer treatment so often overlooked by mainstream oncologists.

SS: Wow. There's a lot of incredible information here. Is there anyplace where cancer patients can access your full menu of recommended treatments?

BF: There is, Suzanne. If your readers visit your website and click on Life Extension, they can review an in-depth article we maintain, titled "Cancer Treatment: The Critical Factors." We also maintain at this site our cancer surgery protocol, along with articles that describe the best ways to optimize all cancer treatments.

SS: What about patients with advanced stages of cancer who have failed toxic conventional treatments because they did not know to call Life Extension first?

BF: We have helped quite a few patients drive advanced disease into remission and even attain outright cure.

SS: How have you done that?

BF: Through the International Strategic Cancer Alliance. This group consists of a dedicated team of clinical oncologists and researchers who think way outside the box to deliver evidence-based therapies that are light-years ahead of conventional oncology. Their track record to date is nothing short of earth-shattering. Patients routinely call Life Extension thanking us for referring them to this organization.

SS: What got you so interested in cancer treatment?

BF: Back in the 1970s, I joined a small group of people seeking ways to prevent disease and slow aging. There were only about three hundred of us back then. When our friends or family members were diagnosed with cancer, we reviewed what their oncologists were doing. Some members of the group would then go to a university medical library (this was before the Internet, of course) and see what was being published in the scientific literature. To our astonishment, in each and every case, we would identify therapies that had demonstrated efficacy in published studies but were not being utilized by the treating oncologist. That experience ignited an intense personal interest to educate cancer patients about better ways of treating their disease.

SS: Is that why you cofounded Life Extension?

BF: That is one reason why our nonprofit was formed. Not just for cancer, but for every age-related disorder. We are routinely uncovering scientifically validated methods of preventing and treating diseases that are overlooked by hurried physicians. I have authored hundreds of articles documenting safer and more effective ways of protecting against disease, yet the medical establishment seldom pays attention.

SS: I read your articles every month in *Life Extension* magazine and find them fascinating. I think my readers will be as impressed as I am with the lifesaving information you bring out each month. And I love that you provide free copies, so readers can see for themselves whether they think it's valuable.

BF: Thank you, Suzanne, for enlightening the world to these scientific advances. Since virtually none of what we have just discussed is patented, you won't see these therapies advertised on TV by drug companies, and pharmaceutical reps are not going to promote them to practicing oncologists.

SS: Thank you, Bill. I very much admire the work you are doing.

To learn more about Life Extension, see page 296.

EPILOGUE

As M. Scott Peck so eloquently stated in his book *The Road Less Traveled,* "Life is difficult." It's the wise man who welcomes problems and mistakes, for it is through problems we are able to grow spiritually and emotionally. Problems are our lessons, and in these lessons are always our opportunities.

My nature is to look for the lesson in all negatives, so in reexamining my November experience of being diagnosed by six different doctors with full-body cancer, I had to find the good.

Seeing my death, feeling the pull of thinking I was going to have to leave those I love and cherish most in the world, was excruciatingly painful. I am not a religious person, but in that horrible circumstance I felt the presence of God. I felt a state of grace as comforting, protective, loving arms around me.

I now know what it feels like to be dying. The fact that I didn't die is irrelevant; my cells, my being, had accepted that my life was about to end, and I experienced the valley of fear and a loneliness that can't be explained unless you have been there.

There was a beauty to this experience that changed me forever. I saw my death and got a second chance at life, as if I had been pushed off a building but instead landed on a soft cloud. I was traumatized by the fall but amazed by my good fortune to have been so gently caught.

I chose life. I chose to fight and not give up. I had more to do, and every fiber of my being wanted to stay.

So what was the purpose? Why are we sent these things in life? Where was the good?

And then it came to me so clearly: we could all benefit by this experience. The ray of light, the hope, in that hospital room was the knowledge that I had been compiling information on doctors who were curing cancer. Knowing that these doctors existed and were having success gave me a reason to look forward. I held on to that, and I realized that this is what we all need in our darkest hours: hope and belief that there is a way out.

In this experience I found out who I was. I am a person who loves deeply. I cherish those in my life who love me, and I know that I am deeply loved. Because of this, I feel my life is a success. I now have the chance to apply those feelings and live my life accordingly. It is only about love.

I am not a victim. I used this opportunity to grow spiritually and emotionally. I made it work for me, and so it became my opportunity.

Thankfully, I dodged this bullet, but you, my wonderful readers, might one day be in this same situation. Remember what you have learned from this book: there are doctors who are healing in another way. And maybe, just maybe, if you are ever in this horrible situation, these doctors might give you the hope, comfort, and healing that I was able to garner when I thought my life depended on them.

I cried a lot writing this book. Every patient who told me his or her story brought me to tears. Each doctor moved me deeply with his or her passion, dedication, and courage. I learned a tremendous amount from all these conversations, and now, as a result, I am armed with the knowledge that if I were ever to find myself diagnosed again, I would know what to do; I wouldn't be afraid. I now know that I can manage cancer and that I can possibly be cured of cancer.

In the meantime, I worship the health I am enjoying. I care for my body with all the tenderness and consideration that any precious object would require. I am healthy; it is the greatest gift I have given myself. I now know with certainty what it feels like to think health is gone and life is almost over, and there is nothing more important than health and taking care of this body that houses me.

I hope you have gotten comfort and important knowledge as a result of reading this book. It is an honor to bring this information to you, and I am grateful that I had this experience.

Thank you for spending this time with me, and I am glad to know you are now armed with choices that could save your life.

RESOURCES

Integrative health care practitioners providing support for optimal health, antiaging, and healing from various disease conditions

· ANTIAGING DOCTORS, SPECIALISTS, CLINICS, AND INSTITUTES

The following websites will help you find a doctor in your area:

American Academy of
Anti-Aging Medicine
1510 West Montana St.
Chicago, IL 60614
773-528-4333
www.worldhealth.net

Life Extension Foundation
800-226-2370
www.lef.org/docs

American College for
    Advancement in Medicine (ACAM)
23121 Verdugo Dr., Suite 204
Laguna Hills, CA 92653
800-532-3688

Whenever applicable, the doctors' areas of specialty are specified below. Every effort has been made to ensure the accuracy of each resource listed here. But when making an appointment, be sure to verify the doctor's specialties. "Difficult conditions" means that the doctor is particularly interested in working with patients who have not had success with other conventional treatments for various medical conditions and who are looking for complementary nondrug approaches that minimize the side effects of regular treatment. Their healing approaches look for underlying causes that need to be corrected, and they typically employ a combination of up-to-date conventional, nutritional, and other innovative modalities to treat conditions such as, but not limited to, degenerative diseases (cardiovascular, diabetes, brain conditions such as dementia and Alzheimer's), asthma, infections (such as hepatitis and other viral illnesses), chronic fatigue and fibromyalgia, autoimmune diseases (rheumatoid arthritis, multiple sclerosis, thyroiditis, gastrointestinal problems, lupus), and chronic or mood disorders such as depression and anxiety. Note: BHRT is bioidentical hormone replacement therapy.

Alabama

Marla Wohlman, M.D. (BHRT, antiaging, cosmetic dermatology)
3351 Main St.
Millbrook, AL 36054
866-780-7808
www.drwohlman.com

Arizona

Shaida Sina, N.M.D. (BHRT, integrative medicine)
Gaia Family Medicine
851 South Main St., Suite E
Cottonwood, AZ 86326
928-649-0269
www.gaiamedicine.com

Ty M. Tallman, N.M.D. (medical weight loss [HCG], BHRT—male and female, lipodissolve, natural supplements specialist)
3014 N. Hayden Rd., Suite 122
Scottsdale AZ 85251
480-219-2624
480-802-2474 (fax)
www.giorgii.com
E-mail: info@giorgii.com

Shawn Tassone, M.D., FACOG (BHRT, integrative medicine, ob-gyn)
Kathryn M. Landherr, M.D., F.A.C.O.G.
La Dea Women's Health
7494 N. LaCholla Blvd.
Tucson, AZ 85741
520-544-0906
520-544-5690 (fax)
www.ladeawomenshealth.com

California

David Allen, M.D. (antiaging, BHRT, difficult conditions)
11860 Wilshire Blvd., Suite 200
Los Angeles, CA 90025
310-445-6600
310-445 6601 (fax)
www.davidallenmd.com

Daniel Amen, M.D. (integrative psychiatry, SPECT brain scans)
Amen Clinics
4019 Westerly Pl., Suite 100
Newport Beach, CA 92660
949-266-3700
949-266-3750 (fax)
www.amenclinics.com

Catherine Arvantely, M.D. (BHRT, integrative medicine)
4121 Westerly Pl., Suite 102
Newport Beach, CA 92660
949-660-1399
949-660-1333 (fax)
www.drarvantely.com

Dan Asimus, M.D. (integrative
   psychiatry)
Life Fitness Center
200 E. Del Mar Blvd., Suite 208
Pasadena, CA 91105
626-578-7111
E-mail: lifefitness@earthlink.net

Barbie J. Barrett, M.D. (BHRT,
   antiaging)
1828 El Camino Real, Suite 804
Burlingame, CA 94010
650-552-0395
650-552-0382 (fax)
www.physiciansyouthfulresolutions
   .com

Koren Barrett, N.D. (BHRT,
   integrative medicine, family
   practice)
1831 Orange Ave., Suite A
Costa Mesa, CA 92627
949-743-5770
E-mail: drbarrett@inatural
   medicine.com
www.inaturalmedicine.com

Harvey S. Bartnof, M.D. (antiaging,
   BHRT, integrative medicine)
California Longevity and Vitality
   Medical Institute
450 Sutter St., Suite 2433
San Francisco, CA 94108
415-986-1300
E-mail: DrBartnof@DrBartnof.com
www.longevitymd.net

Arash Bereliani, M.D. (integrative
   cardiology, antiaging medicine)
125 N. Robertson Blvd.
Beverly Hills, CA 90211
310-550-8000
www.optimalvitalemd.com
www.arashbereliani.com

Jennifer Berman, M.D. (sexual health,
   integrative urology, BHRT)
444 North Camden Dr.
Beverly Hills, CA 90210
888-849-9933
www.bermansexualhealth.com

Hyla Cass, M.D. (integrative
   psychiatry, BHRT, antiaging)
Pacific Palisades, CA 90272
Beverly Hills, CA 90211
310-459-9866
310-564-0328 (fax)
www.drcass.com

Phillip Castellano, M.D., ABAAM,
   FAARM (antiaging and
   regenerative medicine)
355 Placentia Ave., Suite 308
Newport Beach, CA 92663
949-574-9492
949-574-4959 (fax)
E-mail: drphilcast@gmail.com
www.drcastellano.net

Yun-Ching Chen, M.D. (integrative
   medicine, BHRT)
720-A Capitola Ave.
Capitola, CA 95010
831-462-6013
www.balancedapproaches.com

Marc Darrow, M.D., J.D. (antiaging,
   BHRT, musculoskeletal care,
   prolotherapy, sports medicine, and
   rehabilitation)
Darrow Wellness Institute
11645 Wilshire Blvd., Suite 120
Los Angeles, CA 90025
310-231-7000
www.drdarrow.com

Howard Elkin, M.D., F.A.C.C.
(cardiology, integrative medicine,
antiaging)
Heartwise Fitness and Longevity
Center
8135 S. Painter, Suite 204
Whittier, CA 90602
562-945-WELL
www.heartwise.com

Ergonique Spa and Anti-Aging Clinic
(antiaging, BHRT)
Alex Martin, M.D.
359 San Miguel Dr., Suite 110
Newport Beach, CA 92660
949-721-8304
949-721-9194
www.ergonique.com

Joe Filbeck, M.D. (BHRT, integrative
medicine)
8929 University Center Ln., Suite 202
San Diego, CA 92122
858-457-5700
www.palmlajolla.com

Drew Francis, L.Ac.,O.M.D. (Oriental
medicine, antiaging, BHRT, difficult
conditions)
Golden Cabinet Medical Healing
Center
2019 Sawtelle Blvd.
West Los Angeles, CA 90025
310-575-5611
310-575-9885 (fax)
www.goldencabinet.com

Michael Galitzer, M.D. (my personal
physician; BHRT, antiaging, integrative medicine, difficult conditions)
12381 Wilshire Blvd., Suite 102
Los Angeles, CA 90025
800-392-2623
www.ahealth.com

Judi Goldstone, M.D. (BHRT,
antiaging, internal medicine)
23823 Hawthorne Blvd.
Torrance, CA 90505
424-247-4962
310-544-4764 (fax)
www.drjudigoldstone.com

Allen Green, M.D. (integrative
medicine, antiaging, BHRT,
difficult conditions)
Center for Optimum Health
11860 Wilshire Blvd., Suite 200
Los Angeles, CA 90025
310-445-6600
310-445 6601 (fax)
www.allengreenmd.com

David L. Greene, M.D. (BHRT,
ob-gyn)
459 W. Line St.
Bishop, CA 93514
760-873-8982

Robert Greene, M.D. (BHRT)
1255 East St., Suite 201
Redding, CA 96001
530-244-9052
www.specialtycare4women.com
www.robertgreenemd.com

Hans Gruenn, M.D. (antiaging,
BHRT, difficult conditions)
Longevity Medical Center
2211 Corinth Ave., Suite 204
Los Angeles, CA 90064
310-966-9194
E-mail: ceo@drgruenn.com
www.drgruenn.com
www.i4sh.com

Prudence Hall, M.D. (antiaging, BHRT, integrative medicine, ob-gyn)
The Hall Center
1148 4th St.
Santa Monica, CA 90403
866-933-HALL (4255)
310-458-0179 (fax)
E-mail: info@thehallcenter.com
www.thehallcenter.com

Karima Hirani, M.D., M.P.H. (BHRT)
9736 Venice Blvd.
Culver City, California 90232
310-559-6634
310-559-6652 (fax)
www.drhirani.com
E-mail: Nicole@drhirani.com

Lisa Hirsch, M.D., FACOG (integrative gynecology/urology, women's wellness, antiaging, difficult conditions)
360 San Miguel, Suite 308
Newport Beach, CA 92660
949-720-0511
949-720-9404 (fax)
www.newportwomenshealthand wellness.com

Andrew H. Jurow, M.D. (BHRT, antiaging, ob-gyn)
1828 El Camino Real, Suite 804
Burlingame, CA 94010
650-552-0395
650-552-0382 (fax)
www.physiciansyouthfulresolutions.com

Vladimir Kaye, M.D., Q.M.E. (integrative medicine, antiaging, musculoskeletal healing)
159 North Raymond Ave.
Fullerton, CA 92831
714-871-2495
714-871-3350 (fax)

Jason Kelberman, D.C. (integrative chiropractic, physical therapy, detox programs, innovative neuropathy healing)
West Side Wellness Center
11645 Wilshire Blvd., Suite 120
Los Angeles, CA 90025
310-231-7000
www.drkelberman.com

Shiva Lalezar, M.D. (antiaging, integrative medicine, BHRT, difficult conditions)
Health and Vitality Center
11600 Wilshire Blvd., Suite 120
Los Angeles, CA 90025
310-477-1166
310-477-9911 (fax)
www.healthandvitalitycenter.com

Candice Lane, M.D.
1250 La Venta Dr., Suite 206
Westlake Village, CA 91361
805-496-7869
877-496-4289
805-496-7879 (fax)

Howard Liebowitz, M.D. (antiaging, BHRT, integrative medicine)
Los Angeles, CA
www.drhowardliebowitz.com

LifeSpan Medicine (integrative medicine, antiaging, BHRT, difficult conditions, highly personalized care)
Christian Renna, M.D.
Robert Maki, N.D.
Dominique Fradin-Read, M.D.
2811 Wilshire Blvd., Suite 610
Santa Monica, CA 90403
310-453-2335
310-453-2337 (fax)
www.lifespanmedicine.com

Cathie Lippman, M.D. (integrative medicine, BHRT)
The Lippman Center for Optimal Wellness
291 S. La Cienega Blvd., Suite 409
Beverly Hills, CA 90211
310-289-8430
310-289-8165 (fax)
www.cathielippmanmd.com

Gary London, M.D. (BHRT, antiaging, ob-gyn)
9201 Sunset Blvd., Suite 902
West Hollywood, CA 90069
310-270-4500
www.garylondonmd.com

Hilda Maldonado, M.D. (BHRT, anti-aging, integrative medicine)
1240 Westlake Blvd., Suite 133
Westlake Village, CA 91361
805-496-6698
805-557-0223 (fax)
www.drhildamaldonado.com

Robert Mathis, M.D. (BHRT, integrative medicine)
9 E. Mission St.
Santa Barbara, CA 93101
805-569-7100
www.baselinehealth.net

Rand McClain, D.O. (antiaging, BHRT, integrative medicine, sports medicine, weight-loss programs)
2701 Ocean Park Blvd., Suite 101
Santa Monica, CA 90405
310-452-3206
310-452-5134 (fax)
15022 Mulberry Dr., Suite B
Whittier, CA 90604
562-906-9700
562-906-9705 (fax)
E-mail: drrandmcclain@drrand mcclain.com
www.focusonlifequality.com

Philip Lee Miller, M.D. (antiaging, BHRT, difficult conditions)
Los Gatos Longevity Institute
15215 National Ave., Suite 103
Los Gatos, CA 95032
408-358-8855
www.antiaging.com

Steven E. Nelson, Pharm.D., Ph.D., N.M.D., Di.Hom. (integrative metabolic medicine)
74-133 El Paseo, Suite 5
Palm Desert, CA 92260
760-776-5001
702-610-3081
760-776-5005 (fax)
E-mail: doc@drstevenelson.com
www.wholehealthamerica.com/dr stevenelson
www.drstevenelson.com

Christine Paoletti, M.D., F.A.C.O.G. (integrative gynecology, BHRT, integrative medicine, women's wellness, difficult conditions)
1304 15th St., Suite 405
Santa Monica, CA 90404
310-319-1819
310-319-1335 (fax)
www.drpaoletti.com

Cristiana Paul, M.S. (preventive and wellness nutrition, difficult conditions)
West Los Angeles, CA 90025
E-mail: info@cristianapaul.com
www.cristianapaul.com

Allen Peters, M.D. (integrative
medicine, BHRT, wellness programs,
antiaging, difficult conditions)
Nourishing Wellness Medical Center
819 N. Harbor Dr., Suite 310
Redondo Beach, CA 90277
310-373-7830
310-373-7840 (fax)
www.nourishingwellness.com

Wendy Miller Rashidi, M.D. (BHRT,
integrative medicine)
Women's View Medical Group
299 West Foothill Blvd.
Upland, CA 91786
909-982-4000
www.womensviewmedical.com

Uzzi Reiss, M.D. (BHRT, integrative
gynecology, women's wellness,
antiaging, difficult conditions)
414 North Camden Dr., Suite 750
Beverly Hills, CA 90210
www.uzzireissmd.com

Ron Rothenberg, M.D., F.A.C.E.P.
(antiaging, BHRT, integrative
medicine)
California HealthSpan Institute
320 Santa Fe Dr., Suite 301
Encinitas, CA 92024
760-635-1996
800-943-3331
www.ehealthspan.com

Gary Ruelas, D.O., Ph.D. (BHRT,
integrative medicine, mental health
support)
Integrative Medical Institute of
Orange County
707 East Chapman Ave.
Orange, CA 92866
714-771-2880
www.integrative-med.org

Joseph Sciabbarrasi, M.D. (BHRT,
antiaging, integrative medicine,
difficult conditions)
2001 S. Barrington Ave., Suite 208
Los Angeles, CA 90025
310-268-8466
310-268-8122 (fax)
www.drjosephmd.com

Priscilla Slagle, M.D. (integrative
medicine/alternative medicine,
BHRT, board certified
psychiatry/neurology)
946 N. Avenida Palos Verdes
Palm Springs, CA 92262
760-322-7797
760-322-7608 (fax)
www.thewayup.com

Allan Sosin, M.D. (integrative medicine,
BHRT, antiaging, difficult conditions)
Institute for Progressive Medicine
4 Hughes, Suite 175
Irvine, CA 92618
949-600-5100
949-600-5101 (fax)
www.iprogressivemed.com

Svetlana R. Stivi, M.D. (BHRT,
integrative medicine, family practice)
New Health Institute
180 Newport Center Dr., Suite 120
Newport Beach, CA 92660
949-644-6969
949-644-6959 (fax)
www.newhealthinstitute.com

Jennifer Sudarsky, M.D. (integrative
medicine, BHRT, family practice,
women's wellness, antiaging,
difficult conditions)
3201 Wilshire Blvd., Suite 211
Santa Monica, CA 90403
310-315-9101
E-mail: jsudarsky@mednet.ucla.edu

Julie Taguchi, M.D. (oncology,
   hematology, internal medicine)
317 West Pueblo St.
Santa Barbara, CA 93105
805-681-7500
E-mail: drtaguchi@thewiley
   protocol.com

Cheryl Thomas, M.D. (integrative
   medicine, family practice)
Total Wellness Medical Corp.
195 S. C St., Suite 100
Tustin, CA 92780
714-669-4700
www.totalwellnessmedical.com

Duncan Turner, M.D. (BHRT, antiaging, ob-gyn)
219 Nogales Ave., Suite A
Santa Barbara, CA 93105
805-682-6340
www.duncanturner.com

Karlis Ullis, M.D. (integrative
   medicine, antiaging, BHRT, sports
   medicine)
2701 Ocean Park Blvd., Suite 101
Santa Monica, CA 90405
310-452-1990
310-452-5134 (fax)
E-mail: kullis@ucla.edu
www.drkarlisullis.com

Cynthia Watson, M.D. (BHRT,
   women's wellness, antiaging,
   integrative medicine, difficult
   conditions, family practice)
Watson Wellness
3201 Wilshire Blvd., Suite 211
Santa Monica, CA 90403
310-315-9101
www.watsonwellness.org

George Weiss, M.D. (BHRT, antiaging,
   weight loss)
WH Longevity Center
300 Carlsbad Blvd., Suite 220
Carlsbad, CA 92008
760-434-5559
760-434-5518 (fax)

Ronald Wempen, M.D.
Health and Energy Medical Clinic, Inc.
14795 Jeffrey Rd., Suite 101
Irvine, CA 92618
949-551-8751
949-551-1272 (fax)
E-mail: lifenergy@cox.net

Julian Whitaker, M.D. (integrative
   medicine, BHRT, antiaging,
   difficult conditions)
Whitaker Wellness Institute Medical
   Clinic
4321 Birch St.
Newport Beach, CA 92660
800-488-1500
www.whitakerwellness.com

COLORADO

James Howton, D.O. (BHRT, antiaging, functional medicine,
   restorative medicine, weight loss)
Radiant Clinic
3553 Clydesdale Pkwy., Suite 210
Loveland, CO 80538
970-278-0900
970-278-4005 (fax)
E-mail: a.howton@radiantclinic
   colorado.com
www.radiantcliniccolorado.com

David Leonardi, M.D. (BHRT,
   integrative medicine)
8400 W. Prentice Ave., Suite 700
Greenwood Village, CO 80111
303-462-5344
www.go2lehi.com

Todd Nelson, N.D., D.Sc. (holistic medicine specializing in clinical nutrition, BHRT)
12600 W. Colfax Ave., Suite A190
Lakewood, CO 80215
303-969-3052
303-969-3049 (fax)
877-DrTodd6
E-mail: info@toddnelsonnd.com
www.toddnelsonnd.com

CONNECTICUT

Peggy Fishman, M.D. (BHRT, integrative medicine)
Institute of Integrative and Age-Management Medicine
267 Westport Rd.
Wilton, CT 06897
203-834-7747
www.iaamed.com

Ilja Hulinsky, M.D., Ph.D. (BHRT, endocrinology, diabetes, metabolism)
755 Campbell Ave.
West Haven, CT 06516

115 Technology Drive
Trumbull, CT 06611
203-374-4490
203-374-0240 (fax)

FLORIDA

Jean Allen, D.O. (integrative medicine, antiaging, family practice)
1502 S. MacDill Ave.
Tampa, FL 33629
813-253-3223
www.southtampamedspa.com

Robert G. Carlson, M.D. (BHRT)
1901 Floyd St., Suite 302
Sarasota, FL 34239
941-955-1815
866-955-1815
www.andlos.com

James Cennamo, D.O. (BHRT, integrative medicine)
2708 E. Oakland Park Blvd.
Fort Lauderdale, FL 33306
954-318-0873

Healthy Choice (ob-gyn)
400 W. Woodward Ave.
Eustis, FL 32727
352-483-3730
352-483-3355 (fax)
www.spencemd.com

Peter Holyk, M.D. (BHRT, integrative medicine)
600 Schumann Dr.
Sebastian, FL 32958
772-388-5554

Beth Moran, A.R.N.P. (BHRT)
Integrated Wellness
4616 Leeta Lane
Sarasota, FL 34234
631-329-7390
631-329-0407 (fax)
www.bethmoran.net

Dr. Jean-Claude Nerette, D.O. (BHRT, antiaging medicine)
2665 Executive Park Dr., Suite 3
Weston, FL 33331
954-384-8989
954-384-8987 (fax)
E-mail: bellissimomedical
spa@gmail.com
www.bellissimomedicalspa.com

Herbert Pardell, D.O. (BHRT, antiaging)
4330 Sheridan St.
Hollywood, FL 33021
954-987-4455

Juan Remos, M.D. (BHRT, antiaging)
The Miami Institute for Age
   Management and Intervention
1441 Brickell Ave., 3rd Floor
Miami, FL 33131
305-624-0009

Herbert Slavin, M.D. (BHRT,
   antiaging, integrative medicine)
7200 W. Commercial Blvd., Suite 210
Lauderhill, FL 33319
954-748-4991
www.drslavin.com

Rudy J. Triana Jr., M.D., F.A.C.S.
   (BHRT, age management)
211 South Ocean Blvd.
Manalapan, FL 33462
800-725-2720
800-298-7012
888-703-6002 (fax)
www.triana-institute.com
www.drjavacoffeecompany.com

Caroline Van Sant-Crowle, M.D.
   (BHRT, antiaging, integrative
   medicine)
2629 McCormick Dr., Suite 102
Clearwater, FL 33759
727-945-9027
www.watershine.biz

Paul Wand, M.D. (BHRT, neuropathy
   treatment)
Neurological Pain Management, Inc.
2855 N. University Dr., Suite 210
Coral Springs, FL 33065
954-340-9772
954-340-9760 (fax)
www.integrativeneurology.com

Genester Wilson-King, M.D.,
   FACOG (weight loss, BHRT, ob-
   gyn, facial rejuvenation)
Hillcrest Aesthetic Institute
130 Hillcrest Ave.
Orlando, FL 32801
407-999-2585
407-999-2628 (fax)

GEORGIA

Donovan Christie, M.D. (BHRT,
   integrative medicine)
2227 Idlewood Rd.
Tucker, GA 30084
678-205-2039
678-205-2040 (fax)
www.anwanwellness.com

Michelle Fischer, M.D. (BHRT,
   integrative medicine)
Anti-Aging and Vitality Center of
   Atlanta
325 Hammond Dr., Suite 204
Sandy Springs, GA 30328
404-255-5583

Milton Fried, M.D. (integrative
   medicine)
4426 Tilly Mill Rd.
Atlanta, GA 30360
770-451-1928

Linda Kelly, M.D. (BHRT, antiaging,
   ob-gyn)
Cobb Longevity and Wellness
4343 Shallowford Rd., Bldg. B, Suite 4
Marietta, GA 30062
770-649-0094
www.cobblongevityandwellness.com

Daniella Paunesky, M.D. (BHRT, antiaging)
11300 Atlantis Pl., Suite A
Alpharetta, GA 30002
770-777-7707
www.atlantaantiaging.com

Elizabeth L. Schultz, D.O. (BHRT, antiaging, ob-gyn)
Network for Optimal Aging and Wellness
1351 Stonebridge Pkwy., Suite 106
Watkinsville, GA 30677
706-769-0720
www.noaw.com

HAWAII

Alan D. Thal, M.D. (integrative medicine)
55-3327 Akoni Pule Hwy.
Hawi, HI 96719
808-889-5556
808-889-5411 (fax)
www.drthal.com

IDAHO

Paul Brillhart, M.D. (integrative medicine, family practice)
1110 E. Polston Ave.
Post Falls, ID 83854
208-773-1311
www.drpaulbrillhart.com

ILLINOIS

Laura Berman, Ph.D. (psychotherapy, sexual health)
Berman Center
211 East Ontario St.
Chicago, IL 60611
800-709-4709
www.bermancenter.com

William Epperly, M.D. (integrative medicine, family practice)
245 S. Gary Ave., Suite 105
Bloomingdale, IL 60108
630-893-9661
www.doctorepperly.com

Geoffrey Jones, M.D. (integrative medicine, BHRT, antiaging, difficult situations)
Jones Institute for Advanced Medicine
120 Oakbrook Center, Suite 308
Oak Brook, IL 60523
630-734-8888
www.jonesinstituteusa.com

Paul Savage, M.D., F.A.C.E.P. (BHRT)
BodyLogicMD
4753 N. Broadway Ave., Suite 101
Chicago, IL 60640
866-535-BLMD (2563)
866-344-2563 (fax)
www.bodylogicmd.com
Other locations (see website), including Chicago, IL; Hartford, CT; Fort Lauderdale, FL; Naples, FL; Jacksonville, FL

INDIANA

Tammy Born, D.O. (integrative medicine, BHRT)
Born Preventive Health Care Clinic
Crossroads Healing Arts
21764 Omega Ct.
Goshen, IN 46528
574-875-4227
www.bornclinic.com

Linda J. Spencer, M.S.N., C.P.N.P.,
F.N.P. (BHRT, family practice)
Complementary Family Medical Care
of Indiana
3850 Shore Dr., Suite 205
Indianapolis, IN 46254
317-298-3850
www.complementaryfamilymedicare
.com

Charles Turner, M.D. (BHRT)
3554 Promenade Pkwy., Suite. H
Lafayette, IN 47909
765-471-1100
www.charlesturnermd.com

George Wolverton, M.D. (BHRT)
647 Eastern Blvd.
Clarksville, IN 47129
812-282-4309
www.21stcenturymed.net

KENTUCKY

Peggy Fishman, M.D. (BHRT,
integrative medicine)
Center for Integrative and Age-
Management Medicine
3703 Taylorsville Rd., Suite 120
Louisville, KY 40220
502-451-7720
502-451-7737 (fax)
www.iaamed.com

Paul Hester, M.D. (BHRT, antiaging,
integrative medicine)
812 East High St.
Lexington, KY 40502
859-266-5483
www.bemedispa.com

Stephen Kiteck, M.D.
600 Bogle St.
Somerset, KY 42503
606-677-0459

MASSACHUSETTS

Barry Elson, M.D. (BHRT, integrative
medicine)
Darren Lynch, M.D.
Liz O'Dair, M.D.
Northampton Wellness Associates
395 Pleasant St.
Northampton, MA 01060
413-584-7787
www.northamptonwellness.com

Todd Lepine, M.D. (integrative
medicine, BHRT)
38 Church St.
Lenox, MA 01240
413-241-7282
www.drlepine.com

MICHIGAN

Tammy Born, D.O. (integrative
medicine, BHRT)
Born Preventive Health Clinic
3700 52nd St. SE
Grand Rapids, MI 49512
616-656-3700
www.bornclinic.com

David Brownstein, M.D. (integrative
medicine, BHRT)
Center for Holistic Medicine
5821 W. Maple Rd., Suite 192
West Bloomfield, MI 48322
248-851-1600
www.drbrownstein.com

Robert DeJonge, D.O. (integrative
medicine, BHRT, antiaging)
350 Northland Dr. NE
Rockford, MI 49341
616-866-4474
www.mannadoc.com

Steven Margolis, M.D.
43956 Mound Rd.
Sterling Heights, MI 48314
586-323-1122

David Nebbeling, D.O. (BHRT,
    integrative medicine)
3918 W. Saint Joseph Hwy.
Lansing, MI 48917
517-323-1833
www.davidnebbelingdo.com

Pamela W. Smith, M.D. (BHRT,
    integrative medicine)
Center for Healthy Living and
    Longevity
63 Kercheval, Suite 14
Grosse Pointe, MI 48236
Other locations in Ann Arbor and
    Rochester
313-884-3288
www.cfhll.com

John O. Wycoff, D.O. (BHRT)
Wycoff Wellness Center
1226 Michigan Ave.
East Lansing, MI 48823
517-333-7270
www.wycoffwellness.com

MINNESOTA

Khalid Mahmud, M.D. (BHRT,
    integrative medicine)
4005 W. 65th St., Suite 212
Edina, MN 55435
952-922-2345
www.idinhealth.com

NEVADA

James W. Forsythe, M.D., H.M.D.
    (homeopathy, integrative
    medicine)
Century Wellness Clinic
521 Hammill Ln.
Reno, NV 89511
775-827-0707
www.drforsythe.com

NEW JERSEY

Vladimir Berkovich, M.D.
Center for Anti-Aging and Integrated
    Medicine
1707 Atlantic Ave., Bldg. B
Manasquan, NJ 08736
732-292-2101

Gary Klingsberg, D.O. (integrative
    medicine, cancer support)
66 North Van Brunt St.
Englewood, NJ 07631
201-503-0007

Allan Magaziner, D.O. (BHRT,
    integrative medicine, antiaging,
    difficult conditions)
Magaziner Center for Wellness
1907 Greentree Rd.
Cherry Hill, NJ 08003
856-424-8222
www.drmagaziner.com

Neil Rosen, D.O. (BHRT, integrative
    medicine, antiaging, difficult
    conditions)
555 Shrewsbury Ave.
Shrewsbury, NJ
732-219-0895
www.doctorneilrosen.com

Judith Volpe, M.D. (BHRT,
  integrative medicine, antiaging,
  difficult conditions)
107 Monmouth Rd.
West Long Branch, NJ 07764
732-542-2638
www.physicians4altmed.com

New York

Scott J. Beres, D.C., C.N.S.
Market Street Chiropractic and
  Nutrition
29 E. Market St., Suite 101
Corning, NY 14830
607-936-4141
607-936-4144

Kenneth Bock, M.D. (BHRT,
  integrative medicine, antiaging,
  difficult conditions)
Steven Bock, M.D.
Michael Compain, M.D.
The Rhinebeck Health Center
108 Montgomery St.
Rhinebeck, NY 12572
845-876-7082
www.rhinebeckhealth.com

Kenneth Bock, M.D.
Steven Bock, M.D.
The Center for Progressive Medicine
Pinnacle Place, Suite 224
10 McKown Rd.
Albany, NY 12203
518-435-0082
www.rhinebeckhealth.com

Eric Braverman, M.D. (integrative
  medicine, antiaging, BHRT)
PATH Medical
304 Park Ave. South, 6th floor
New York, NY 10010
212-213-6155
212-889-5204 (fax)
E-mail: pathmedical@aol.com
www.pathmed.com

Ronald Hoffman, M.D. (integrative
  medicine, difficult conditions)
The Hoffman Center
40 E. 30th Street
New York, NY 10016
212-779-1744
www.drhoffman.com

Alexander N. Kulick, M.D.
625 Madison Ave.
New York, NY 10022
212-838-8265
www.ostrow.medem.com

Richard Linchitz, M.D. (integrative
  medicine, BHRT, difficult
  conditions)
Linchitz Medical Wellness
70 Glen St., Suite 240
Glen Cove, NY 11542
516-759-4200
www.linchitzwellness.com

Ron Livesey, M.D. (integrative
  medicine, BHRT)
PhysioAge Medical Group
30 Central Park South
New York, NY 10019
877-888-3210
www.physioage.com

Beth Moran, A.R.N.P. (BHRT)
Integrated Wellness
26 King St.
East Hampton, NY 11937
631-329-7390
631-329-0407 (fax)
www.bethmoran.net

Jeffrey A. Morrison, M.D., C.N.S.
  (integrative medicine, BHRT,
  difficult conditions)
103 Fifth Ave., 6th floor
New York, NY 10003
212-989-9828
212-989-9827 (fax)
E-mail: drmorrison@themorrison
  center.com
www.themorrisoncenter.com

John Salerno, M.D. (integrative
  medicine, BHRT, family practice)
14 W. 49th St., Suite 1401
New York, NY 10020
212-582-1700
www.salernocenter.com

Michael Schachter, M.D. (integrative
  medicine, BHRT, difficult
  conditions)
2 Executive Blvd., Suite 202
Suffern, NY 10901
845-368-4700
www.mbschachter.com

Judith Volpe, M.D. (BHRT,
  integrative medicine, antiaging,
  difficult conditions)
250 W. 49th St., Suite 503
New York, NY 10019
212-545-9730

NORTH CAROLINA

R. Ernest Cohn, M.D., N.D. (BHRT,
  integrative medicine, difficult
  conditions)
Robert G. Apgar, M.D.
Holistic Medical Clinic of the
  Carolinas
308 East Main St.
Wilkesboro, NC 28697
336-667-6464
336-667-4488 (fax)
E-mail: info@holisticmedclinic.com
www.holisticmedclinic.com

Neal Speight, M.D. (integrative
  medicine, difficult conditions)
1258 Mann Dr., Suite 100
Matthews, NC 28105
704-847-2022
www.drnealshousecall.com

OHIO

James Frackelton, M.D. (BHRT,
  integrative medicine, antiaging)
24700 Center Ridge Rd.
Westlake, OH 44145
440-835-0104
www.prevmedgroup.com

Felicitas Juguilon, M.D. (BHRT,
  integrative medicine, antiaging)
Anti-Aging and Vitality Center of
  Cleveland
6000 Lombardo Center Dr., Suite 150
Seven Hills, OH 44131
216-573-5600
www.antiagingandvitality.com

Thomas Violand, D.O. (BHRT)
1790 Town Parks Blvd.
Uniontown, OH 44685
330-563-4424

OREGON

Nisha Jackson, Ph.D., M.S.,
    W.H.C.N.P., H.H.P.
3156 State St.
Medford, OR 97504
877-ASK-NISH
541-772-WELL
541-773-1113 (fax)
E-mail: asknish@ventanawellness.com
www.ventanawellness.com
www.justasknish.com

Daniel Laury, MD (BHRT)
786 State St.
Medford, OR 97504
541-773-5500

PENNSYLVANIA

Adrian J. Hohenwarterm, N.D. (also
    compounds hormones)
Family Practice and Alternative
    Medicine
745 S. Grant St.
Palmyra, PA 17078
717-832-5993

Ruth Jones, D.O.
342 S. Richard
Bedford, PA 15522
814-623-8414

Conrad Maulfair, D.O. (family
    medicine, integrative medicine)
403 North Main St.
Topton, PA 19562
610-682-2104
www.drmaulfair.com

Ralph Miranda, M.D. (integrative
    medicine)
Holistic Health Center
196 Old Route 30
Greensburg, PA 15601
724-838-7632
www.ralphmiranda.com

SOUTH CAROLINA

Mickey Barber, M.D. (BHRT, age
    management)
Cenegenics Carolinas
211 King St., Suite 310
Charleston, SC 29401
843-724-7272
843-577-8482 (fax)
E-mail: mbarber@
    cenegenics-carolinas.com
www.cenegenics-carolinas.com

TENNESSEE

Marc Houston, M.D. (integrative
    medicine, progressive cardiology,
    antiaging, BHRT)
Hypertension Institute
4230 Harding Rd., Suite 400
Nashville, TN 37205
615-297-2700
615-467-0365

L. Morgan Williams, M.D.
321 Billingsly Ct., Suite 20
Franklin, TN 37067
615-771-8832

TEXAS

Barry Beaty, D.O. (BHRT)
North Texas Institute for Healing and
    Wellness
4455 Camp Bowie Blvd., Suite 211
Fort Worth, TX
817-737-6464
www.northtexashealing.com

Sakina Davis, M.D. (antiaging, BHRT, family practice)
Woodlands Wellness and Cosmetic Center
9595 Six Pines Dr., Suite 6250
The Woodlands, TX 77380
281-362-0014
281-466-8044 (fax)
www.woodlandswellness.com

Linda Ho, M.D. (BHRT, ob-gyn)
Anti-Aging and Vitality Center of Dallas
6101 Chapel Hill Blvd.
Plano, TX 75093
972-312-8881

Steven Hotze, M.D. (BHRT, integrative medicine)
Hotze Health and Wellness Center
20214 Braidview Dr., Suite 215
Katy, TX 77450
877-698-8698
281-698-8698
www.hotzehwc.com
www.drhotze.com

LifeSpan Medicine (integrative medicine, antiaging, preventive medicine, BHRT, difficult conditions)
Christian Renna, M.D.
David Lancaster, D.O.
2706 Fairmount St.
Dallas, TX 75201
214-303-1888
214-303-1550 (fax)
www.lifespanmedicine.com

Alice Pangle, D.O. (general primary care, bariatrics, endocrinology)
South Plains Bariatric Clinic
3303 University Ave.
Lubbock, TX 79411
806-795-6466
800-772-6466
www.southplainsbariatrics.com

Jose Reyes, M.D. (BHRT)
12730 IH 10 W., Suite 306
San Antonio, TX 78256
210-694-5800
www.800-menopause.com

John Sessions, D.O. (family practice, preventive medicine)
1609 S. Margaret Ave.
Kirbyville, TX 75956
409-423-2166
409-423-5496

UTAH

Rachel Burnett, N.D., L.Ac. (antiaging, BHRT, naturopathy)
Utah Natural Medicine
242 South 400 East, Suite A
Salt Lake City, UT 84111
801-363-8824
www.utahnaturalmedicine.com

Gordon Reynolds, M.D. (BHRT, antiaging)
Green Valley Spa
1871 W. Canyon View
St. George, UT 84770
435-628-8060
www.greenvalleyspa.com

Simmon Wilcox, M.D. (BHRT)
1999 W. Canyon View Dr.
St. George, UT 84770
435-619-1577
972-947-3958 (fax)

VIRGINIA

Dima Ali, M.D. (aesthetic and anti-
    aging medicine)
1801 Robert Fulton Dr., Suite 540
Reston, VA 20191
703-787-9866
703-787-9861 (fax)
E-mail: dr.dima@wellmedica.com
www.wellmedica.com
www.cosminology.com

George Guess, M.D., D.Ht.
    (homeopathic medicine)
233 Hydraulic Ridge Rd., Suite 101
Charlottesville, VA 22901
434-295-0362
434-295-0798 (fax)
www.drgeorgeguess.com

Jennifer Krup, M.D. (BHRT)
2232 Virginia Beach Blvd., Suite 104
Virginia Beach, VA 23454
757-306-4300
757-306-1460 (fax)
E-mail: doctor@rejuvinage.com
www.rejuvinage.com
www.thehormonereplacementcenter
    .com

Lynese L. Lawson, D.O. (BHRT,
    antiaging/functional medicine)
8300 Greensboro Dr., Suite 800
McLean, VA 22102
703-822-5003
703-621-7157 (fax)
E-mail: info@proactivewellness.com
www.proactivewellness.com

WASHINGTON

Jonathan V. Wright, M.D. (BHRT,
    antiaging, preventive medicine,
    integrative medicine, difficult
    conditions)
Tahoma Clinic
801 S.W. 16th St., Suite 121
Renton, WA 98057
425-264-0059
425-264-0071 (fax)
www.tahomaclinic.com

WISCONSIN

Steven Meress, M.D. (BHRT,
    integrative medicine)
180 Knights Way
Fond du Lac, WI 54935
920-922-5433
www.foxvalleywellness.com

BRITISH COLUMBIA

Corrine Dawson, N.D. (BHRT,
    naturopathic physician)
Integrated Health Clinic
202-23242 Mavis Ave.
Fort Langley, BC V1M 2R4
604-888-8325
www.integratedhealthclinic.com

Nishi Dhawan, M.D., C.C.F.P. (BHRT,
    integrative medicine)
Bal Pawa, M.D.
Westcoast Women's Clinic
1003 West King Edward Ave.
Vancouver, BC V6H 1Z3
604-738-9601
604-738-9605 (fax)
www.westcoastwomensclinic.com

Karla Dionne, M.D. (BHRT, antiaging,
   weight loss)
EnerChanges Clinic
M11-601 West Broadway
Vancouver, BC V5Z 4C2
604-681-8380
604-681-7003 (fax)
www.enerchanges.com

Brian Martin, B.Sc., N.D. (BHRT,
   antiaging, weight loss)
Karla Dionne, M.D.
EnerChanges Clinic
Canada's 1st Medically Supervised
   Anti-Aging and Weight-Loss Clinic
M11-601 West Broadway
Vancouver, BC V5Z 4C2
604-681-8380
604-681-7003 (fax)
www.enerchanges.com

ONTARIO

Metalife BioMedical Clinic
The International Center for
   Metabolic Testing (ICMT)
NutriChem
1303 Richmond Rd.
Ottawa, ON K2B 7Y4
613-820-4200
613-829-2226 (fax)
www.nutrichem.com

Alvin Pettle, M.D., F.R.C.S. (BHRT,
   women's health)
The Ruth Pettle Wellness Center
3910 Bathurst St., Suite 207
Toronto, ON M3H 3N8
416-633-4101
416-633-3400 (fax)
www.drpettle.com

Maria Schleifer, M.D.
H.O.P.E. Clinic of Integrative
   Medicine
4195 Dundas St. West
Toronto, ON M8X 1Y4
416-236-8788

Natasha Turner, N.D.
The 3-Step Clear Medicine Lifestyle
   System—An integrated medicine
   program focused on hormonal
   health
123 Dupont St.
Toronto, ON, M5R 1V4
416-579-9105
647-349-3009 (fax)
E-mail: clinic@clearmedicine.com
www.clearmedicine.com

BELGIUM

Thierry Hertoghe, M.D. (BHRT,
   antiaging)
7–9 Avenue Van Bever
B-1180 Brussels, Belgium
3227366868
3227325743 (fax)
E-mail: secretariathertoghe@
   hotmail.com (for appointments)
www.hertoghe.eu

BAHAMAS

Norman R. Gay, M.D. (antiaging,
   BHRT, integrative medicine)
Bahamas Anti-Aging Medical
   Institute
West Bay St.
P. O. Box N3222
Nassau, Bahamas
242-328-4100
242-328-4104
E-mail: drnormangay@yahoo.com
www.bahamaslllt.com

NEW TECHNOLOGIES

All three of these companies can be contacted by direct links on my website, www.suzannesomers.com.

David Schmidt
LifeWave
1020 Prospect St., Suite 200
La Jolla, CA 92037
858-459-9876
866-420-6288
www.suzannesomers.com (click on
  LifeWave)

Robin Smith, M.D., M.B.A.
NeoStem, Inc.
420 Lexington Ave., Suite 450
New York, NY 10170
212-584-4180
646-514-7787 (fax)
www.suzannesomers.com (click on
  NeoStem)

Ondamed
www.suzannesomers.com (click on
  Ondamed)

MASTER HERBALIST

Paul Schulick
New Chapter
99 Main St.
Brattleboro, VT 05301
802-257-9345
www.newchapter.info

OTHER HELPFUL WEBSITES

Dr. Russell L. Blaylock
Advanced Nutritional Concepts, LLC
www.russellblaylockmd.com
www.newportnutritionals.com
Blaylock Wellness Report,
  www.blaylockreport.com

Julie Carmen
www.JulieCarmenYoga.com
www.yogatalks.com

Suzanne Somers
www.suzannesomers.com

Don Tolman
www.dontolmaninternational.com

TESTING HORMONE LEVELS

Aeron LifeCycles
1933 Davis St., Suite 310
San Leandro, CA 94577
800-631-7900
www.aeron.com

Life Extension Foundation
Fort Lauderdale, FL
888-884-3666
www.lef.org/goodhealth

Sabre Sciences, Inc.
2233 Faraday Ave., Suite K
Carlsbad, CA 92008
www.sabresciences.com

TESTING FOR NUTRITIONAL DEFICIENCIES

Doctor's Data
3755 Illinois Ave.
St. Charles, IL 60174-2420
800-323-2784 (USA, Canada)
· 0871-218-0052 (United Kingdom)
E-mail: inquiries@doctorsdata.com
www.doctorsdata.com

Genova Diagnostics
63 Zillicoa St.
Asheville, NC 28801
800-522-4762
www.gdx.net

Metametrix Clinical Laboratories
4855 Peachtree Industrial Blvd.
Norcross, GA 30092
770-446-5483
www.metametrix.com

Cristiana Paul, M.S.
Los Angeles, CA
E-mail: cristiana@cristianapaul.com
www.cristianapaul.com

CHEMOSENSITIVITY TESTING

Biofocus Institute for Laboratory
  Medicine
Dr. med Dipl. Chem. Doris Bachg
Dr. med Uwe Haselhorst
Berghauser Str. 295
45659 Recklinghausen, Germany
Contact: Dr. Lothar Prix
+49 2361-3000-130
+49 2361-3000-169 (fax)
E-mail: prix@biofocus.de

Research Genetic Cancer Centre
  (R.G.C.C.)
P.O. 53070
Florina, Greece
+30-24630-42264
+30-24630-42265 (fax)
E-mail: jpapasot@doctors.org.uk

NONSURGICAL FACIAL REJUVENATION

Dr. Peter Hanson
Cherry Creek Center for Healing and
  Pain Relief
3300 East First Ave., Suite 600
Denver, CO 80206
303-733-2521
www.peterhansonmd.com

COMPOUNDING PHARMACIES BY STATE

These websites list compounding pharmacies by state:

http://www.angelfire.com/fl/endohystnhrt/pharmacy.html

Professional Compounding Center of America (PCCA)

www.pccarx.com

For a referral to the closest compounding pharmacy in your area:

International Academy of Compounding Pharmacists
P.O. Box 1365
Sugar Land, TX 77478
800-927-4227
www.iacprx.org

ARIZONA

Women's International Pharmacy
12012 N. 111th Ave.
Youngtown, AZ 85363
800-279-5708
www.womensinternational.com

CALIFORNIA

The Compounding Pharmacy of
  Beverly Hills
9629 West Olympic Blvd.
Beverly Hills, CA 90212
310-284-8675
888-799-0212
www.compounding-expert.com

Dr. Eleanor Kong, Pharm.D.
3435 Ocean Park Blvd., Suite 105B
Santa Monica, CA 90403
310-393-2755
E-mail: eleanor155@aol.com

Leiter's Rx Pharmacy
1700 Park Ave, Suite 30
San Jose, CA 95126
800-292-6773
408-292-6772
408-288-8252 (fax)

Medical Center Pharmacy
Redondo Beach, CA
Pharmacist: Nilesh Bhakta
310-540-3312

San Diego Compounding Pharmacy
Jerry Greene, R.Ph., F.A.C.A.
5395 Ruffin Rd., Suite 104
San Diego, CA 92123
858-277-8884
866-413-2673
858-277-8889 (fax)
E-mail: sdcprx@gmail.com

Santa Ana Tustin Pharmacy
801 North Tustin Ave.
Santa Ana, CA 92705
714-547-3949

Steven's Pharmacy
1525 Mesa Verde Dr. East
Costa Mesa, CA 92626
800-352-3784
www.stevensrx.com

Town Center Drugs and
    Compounding Pharmacy
72624-A El Paseo
Palm Desert, CA 92260
760-341-3984
877-340-5922

COLORADO

College Pharmacy
3505 Austin Bluffs Pkwy., Suite 101
Colorado Springs, CO 80918
800-888-9358
719-262-0022
800-556-5893 (fax)
719-262-0035 (fax)

FLORIDA

The Compounding Shop
4000 Park St. North
St. Petersburg, FL 33709
727-381-9799
866-792-6731
727-347-2050 (fax)
www.gotocompoundingshop.com

MARYLAND

Village Green Apothecary
Paul Garcia, marketing director
5415 W. Cedar Lane
Bethesda, MD 20814
301-530-0800
240-644-1362 (fax)
www.myvillagegreen.com

NEVADA

Kronos Pharmacy (formerly Medical
    Center Pharmacy)
3675 South Rainbow Blvd.
Las Vegas, NV 89103
800-723-7455

NEW JERSEY

Pharmacy Creations
Compounding and Nutritional Pharmacy
Bernard Covalesky Jr., R.Ph., M.S.
540 Route 10 West
Randolph, NJ 07869
973-328-8756
973-328-8731 (fax)
www.pharmacycreations.com

OHIO

The Medicine Shoppe Pharmacy
649 West High St.
Piqua, OH 45356
937-773-1778
888-723-5344
www.hormoneconnection.biz

PENNSYLVANIA

Hazle Compounding
7 N. Wyoming St.
Hazleton, PA 18201
570-454-2958
800-213-0592
800-400-8764 (fax)
E-mail: info@hazlecompounding.com
www.hazlecompounding.com

TENNESSEE

Solutions Pharmacy
4632 Hwy. 58 North
Chattanooga, TN 37416
423-894-3222
800-523-1486
www.solutions-pharmacy.com

TEXAS

Apotheca Compounding Pharmacy
Pharmacist/owner: Mike Anderson,
  R.Ph.
14603 Huebner Rd., Suite 2602
San Antonio, TX 78230
210-226-1112
210-226-1119 (fax)

ApotheCure, Inc.
4001 McEwen Rd., Suite 100
Dallas, TX 75244
972-960-6601
800-969-6601
www.apothecure.com

VERMONT

Custom Prescription Shoppe
Scott W. Brown, P.D.
42 Timber Lane
South Burlington, VT 05403
800-928-1488
802-864-0812
E-mail: scott@customrxshop.com

VIRGINIA

Leesburg Pharmacy
Jay Gill, Pharm.D.
36-C Catoctin Circle
Leesburg, VA 20175
703-737-3305

WISCONSIN

Health Pharmacies
2809 Fish Hatchery Rd., Suite 103
Madison, WI 53713
800-373-6704

ONTARIO

NutriChem Pharmacy
1303 Richmond Rd.
Ottawa, ON K2B 7Y4
613-820-4200
613-829-2226 (fax)
www.nutrichem.com

Trutina Pharmacy
201 Wilson St. East
Ancaster, ON L9G 2B8
866-418-9303
905-304-9300

York Downs Pharmacy
3910 Bathurst St.
Toronto, ON M3H 5Z3
416-633-2244
800-564-5020
416-633-3400 (fax)
www.yorkdownsrx.com

NATURAL BEAUTY PRODUCTS AVAILABLE AT SUZANNESOMERS.COM

I am always looking for ways to reduce my exposure to chemicals and preservatives; this philosophy also applies to my line of skin care products. SUZANNE Beauty products include natural botanical extracts and fragrances, healing enzymes, essential oils, skin-nurturing antioxidants, even organic fruits and vegetables. As this line expands, I will continue to utilize all the newest scientific developments to keep my products as pure and clean as possible while incorporating the most effective antiaging ingredients.

Product List

SPA MASKS

Botanical Spa—Apple Pectin Mask

BASIC SKIN CARE

Hydrating Therapy—Gentle Exfoliating Cleanser

Hydrating Therapy—Soothing Aloe Vera Toner

Balancing Therapy—Clarifying Cleanser

Balancing Therapy—Healing Enzyme Toner

Balancing Therapy—Daily Moisturizer

Anti-Aging Therapy—Night Repair Cream

Anti-Aging Therapy—Intensive Eye Cream

Anti-Aging Therapy—Hydra Lift Serum PM Treatment

Fresh Face Gentle Cleansing Gel

Hydra Lift & Soft as Silk Firming Set

BODY CARE

Fit to Be Tight Firming Body Treatment—AM with Natural Tint and PM

Ginger Mango Body Glow and Body Butter

Lemongrass Jasmine Body Glow and Body Butter

Rosemary Lavender Body Glow and Body Butter

COSMETICS

Spray-on Makeup—Professional Foundation

Spray-on Primer—Perfecting Base

PERSONAL CARE

SomerSmile Get White Tooth Whitening System

SomerSmile Stay White Daily Whitening System

LifeWave Nanopatches

Life Extension for blood testing

NeoStem for stem cell collection information

FaceMaster, www.suzannesomers.com

EXERCISE PRODUCTS

ThighMaster
www.thighmaster.com

EZ Gym
www.ezgym.com

LIFE EXTENSION FOUNDATION

Founded in 1980, the Life Extension Foundation is a nonprofit organization dedicated to discovering innovative approaches to prevent and treat diseases like cancer.

Since its inception Life Extension has introduced evidence-based therapies that are often decades ahead of conventional medicine. These scientific advances are chronicled in *Life Extension* magazine, read by over 300,000 people each month.

The Life Extension Foundation supports a large cancer research program and utilizes its scientific findings to educate cancer patients about novel methods to help eradicate their disease. Unlike today's cancer bureaucracy that too often stifles innovation, Life Extension quickly moves discoveries out of the laboratory to patients in need.

Forward-thinking oncologists and cancer patients join the Life Extension Foundation to obtain the latest information about novel diagnostic procedures and nontoxic treatments that are too often overlooked by the medical mainstream.

Foundation members have free seven-day-a-week phone and e-mail access to knowledgeable health advisors, some with specialized expertise in complementary approaches to cancer treatment.

Life Extension also maintains an enormous library of meticulously referenced protocols that provide unique insight into an array of natural methods to combat specific forms of cancer, such as pancreatic, breast, prostate, colon, lung, and others. Some of the recommendations made in Life Extension's protocols, such as using agents that inhibit the cyclooxygenase-2 and 5-lipoxygenase enzymes, have demonstrated survival improvements in clinical studies. Yet hurried oncologists too often fail to prescribe these safe adjuvant approaches, even though the evidence supporting efficacy appears in their own medical journals.

You learned in the preface of this book about an over-the-counter drug called cimetidine that dramatically reduces the recurrence of colon cancer. It was Life Extension that first recommended cimetidine to cancer patients back in 1985, yet few oncologists prescribe it even today. Discovering these bits of lifesaving information alone justifies cancer patients becoming Foundation members.

It costs $75 to join the Life Extension Foundation, and the benefits are too numerous to describe. New members, for instance, receive a 1,600-page reference book called *Disease Prevention and Treatment* that provides invaluable health information published by the Foundation over the past three decades. Each month, members are updated about new medical technologies in *Life Extension* magazine. To become a member, call 888-884-3666 or log on to www.lef.org/goodhealth.

INTEGRATIVE HEALTH CARE PRACTITIONERS PROVIDING SUPPORT FOR CANCER PREVENTION DURING CANCER TREATMENT AND/OR REMISSION

The health care practitioners featured in this section may be medical doctors (M.D.'s) or osteopaths (D.O.'s, similar to M.D.'s but with additional training), licensed acupuncturists (L.Ac.'s), and/or nutritionists. They employ comprehensive modalities to improve human physiology in order to support a patient's health and ability to heal from cancer, as well as reduce risk of cancer recurrence and overall cancer risk.

Priya Advani, L.Ac.
1526 14th St., Suite 101
Santa Monica, CA 90404
310-463-8323
E-mail: contact@PriyaAdvani.com
www.PriyaAdvani.com

She is a licensed acupuncturist located in Santa Monica. With cancer patients, she uses energy healing and acupuncture and herbal formulas, especially for patients going through chemotherapy treatments. She also works with meditation/visualization, qi gong, and nutrition to bring patients' bodies back into balance.

David Allen, M.D.
11860 Wilshire Blvd., Suite 200
Los Angeles, CA 90025
310-445-6600
310-445 6601 (fax)
www.davidallenmd.com

Dr. Allen offers an integrative approach to health. By combining the best of traditional Western medicine, preventative medicine, and the mind-body connection, the totality of the patient is evaluated and treated. Dr. Allen offers nutritional support during and after cancer treatment, as well as cancer prevention.

Koren Barrett, N.D.
1831 Orange Ave., Suite A
Costa Mesa, CA 92627
949-743-5770
E-mail: drbarrett@inatural
  medicine.com
www.inaturalmedicine.com

Provides complementary care for patients who wish to prevent, currently have, or are interested in avoiding a recurrence of breast cancer. Also screens for nutritional deficiencies (such as vitamin D), excess insulin, and inflammation, all associated with cancer, and makes specific supplement recommendations based upon laboratory testing to assist patients' immune systems.

Roger Billica, M.D.
William Billica, M.D.
Mark Hoenig, M.D.
TriLife Health, PC
2362 E. Prospect Rd., Suite A
Fort Collins, CO 80525
970-495-0999
970-495-1016 (fax)
www.trilifehealth.com

TriLife Health, PC, is an integrative clinic of licensed M.D.'s that offers a wide range of supportive and adjunctive therapies to patients who are dealing with cancer. They do not claim to cure cancer; instead they offer support, such as IV vitamin C and other IVs, hyperbaric oxygen, frequency-specific microcurrent, ultraviolet blood illumination, metabolic typing for pH balancing, massage, FIR sauna, and nutritional therapies for detoxification and functional support.

Russell Blaylock, M.D.
www.russellblaylockmd.com
www.newportnutritionals.com

Stanislaw R. Burzynski, M.D., Ph.D.
Burzynski Clinic
9432 Old Katy Rd., Suite 200
Houston, TX 77055
713-335-5697
713-935-0649 (fax)
www.burzynskiclinic.com

Hyla Cass, M.D.
Pacific Palisades CA 90272
Beverly Hills, CA 90211
310-459-9866
310-564-0328 (fax)
www.drcass.com

In over twenty-five years of clinical practice, Dr. Cass has combined the best of modern medicine with natural methods, given with care and compassion. For cancer treatment support and prevention, she uses specific metabolic lab testing, and treats at the deepest level with specific diet, nutrition, and mind-body support. She has created innovative nutritional formulas that are used by other physicians in their practices. Free health e-newsletter: www.cassmd.com/newsletterenroll .html.

Nalini Chilkov, O.M.D.
530 Wilshire Blvd., Suite 206
Santa Monica, CA 90401
310-395-4133
310-451-3975 (fax)
www.nalinichilkov.com

Dr. Chilkov is known for her compassion and clinical excellence. She draws upon over twenty-five years of experience, combining advanced training in both modern health sciences and traditional Oriental medicine to provide truly integrative and highly individualized care. Integrative cancer care/prevention/support/recovery, acupuncture, herbal medicine, clinical nutrition, dietary therapies for prevention of cancer due to family history or toxic exposures; supportive integrative care related to surgery, radiation, and chemotherapy and their side effects; assistance making health care choices; preventing recurrence; restoring lifelong health and wellness after treatment. Phone consultations available.

Marc Darrow, M.D., J.D.
Darrow Wellness Institute
11645 Wilshire Blvd., Suite 120
Los Angeles, CA 90025
310-231-7000
www.drdarrow.com

Dr. Darrow was trained by his grandfather (born in the late 1800s) in natural healing. He is an author and assistant professor of medicine at the UCLA School of Medicine, where he teaches complementary and alternative medicine to residents. In his practice Dr. Darrow strives to move beyond the patient diagnosis and to awaken in him or her "healing consciousness." His complementary approach with cancer patients is to strengthen the immune system with natural supplements, balance the hormones, and use nutrition that will not support cancerous growth. His nutrition program favors a Paleolithic diet to lower sugar and insulin and reduce the body's inflammation. For the musculoskeletal pain that accompanies cancer, Dr. Darrow focuses on the healing technique prolotherapy.

Martin Dayton, M.D., D.O.
Dayton Medical Center
18600 Collins Av.
Sunny Isles Beach, FL 33160
305-931-8484
305-936-1849 (fax)
www.daytonmedical.com

Jeanne Drisko, M.D.
University of Kansas Medical Center
3801 Rainbow Blvd.
Kansas City, KS 66160
913-588-5000
Linus Pauling, Ph.D., discovered that vitamin C had a negative effect upon cancer. This was taken up by Dr. Hugh Riordan, who had extensive experience in the use of high-dose vitamin C in the treatment of all cancer. Jeanne Drisko, M.D., took over Dr. Riordan's outreach and is now at the University of Kansas Medical Center using high-dose vitamin C. High doses of vitamin C administered intravenously converts vitamin C into a pro-oxidant, not an antioxidant, and this pro-oxidant activity is particularly useful at treating cancer.

Kelly Marie Fitzpatrick, B.S.N.,
    M.P.S., N.D.
1695 Jefferson St.
Eugene, OR 97402
541-344-9658
After sixteen years as a registered nurse, ten years as a naturopathic physician, and a diagnosis and treatment of stage III endometrial cancer, she is a firm believer in the benefits of having a fully integrated medical plan in the treatment of cancer. During the office visit, each patient has an individualized treatment plan utilizing nutrition, botanicals, homeopathy, physical medicine, IV therapy, and lifestyle management to improve the prognosis of the cancer diagnosis; reduce side effects of surgery, chemotherapy, and radiation; and reduce recurrence. Many insurances cover naturopathic physician services. Long-distance treatment is available.

James W. Forsythe, M.D., H.M.D.
Century Wellness Clinic
521 Hammill Ln.
Reno, NV 89511
775-827-0707
www.drforsythe.com

Drew Francis, O.M.D., L.Ac.
Golden Cabinet Medical Healing
    Center
2019 Sawtelle Blvd.
Los Angeles, CA 90025
310-575-5611
www.goldencabinet.com

Dr. Drew Francis, O.M.D., L.Ac., has over twenty-five years of experience integrating both Eastern and Western medicines to provide the most advanced integrative supportive care. His clinical strengths include state-of-the-art gene testing that reveals each individual's unique liver detoxification enzymes. Nutritional testing reveals vitamin, mineral, amino acid, essential fatty acid, and antioxidant status; markers of metabolism efficiency; as well as DNA damage; oxidized fats; and toxic elements load. He offers supportive care for any degenerative disease or cancer with his expertise in managing side effects, reducing the risk of recurrence, and establishing lifelong knowledge of how to cultivate radiant health through personally empowering each patient.

Sonja N. Fung, N.D.
Live Well Clinic
78-370 Hwy. 111, Suite 100
La Quinta, CA 92253
760-771-5970
760-771-5982 (fax)
www.livewellclinic.org

Dr. Sonja Fung, N.D., is a board-certified family practice naturopathic doctor and one of the medical directors at Live Well Clinic in La Quinta, California. Along with integrative cancer care, Dr. Fung provides intravenous nutritional therapy, prolotherapy, and bio-identical hormone balancing.

Robert J. Gilbard, M.D., Medical
    Director
Ray Hammon, D.C., D.N.B.H.E.,
    N.M.D., Clinic Director
Alternative and Traditional Medical
    Center
5429 Lakeview Pkwy.
Rowlett, TX 75088
972-463-1744
972-463-8243 (fax)
www.atmctx.com

They've been working with a geneticist and cancer researcher from Greece for over five years now with several hundred cancer cases. Use of a simple peripheral blood test provides them with a wealth of information about an individual's cancer and how to better customize a complete approach to their treatment. They are able to test the chemosensitivity and resistivity of over forty-four chemo drugs, and also an additional fifty-plus nutritional products, which helps them to support each patient individually.

Burton Goldberg
309 Paradise Dr.
Tiburon, CA 94920
415-435-8222
E-mail: burton@burtongoldberg.com

Steve Gomberg, L.Ac., C.C.N., R.H.
    (A.H.G.)
Eastern Center for Complementary
    Medicine
5910 Monterey Rd.
Los Angeles, CA 90042
323-551-5962
www.herbalroom.com

Steve Gomberg is a practitioner of acupuncture, clinical nutrition, and botanical medicine, specializing in the herbal and nutritional management and treatment of cancer and chronic degenerative diseases. A proponent of a multidisciplinary approach to healing, Steve works very closely with both M.D.'s and other health care practitioners in a fully integrative way to maximize the potential for successful therapeutic outcomes. In cancer management, his emphasis is on evidence-based botanical medicine and nutritional interventions. He has published in peer-reviewed publications on the use of botanicals in breast cancer management.

Nicholas Gonzalez, M.D.
36A E. 36th St., Suite 204
New York, NY 10016
212-213-3337
212-213-3414 (fax)
www.dr-gonzalez.com

Allen Green, M.D.
Center for Optimum Health
11860 Wilshire Blvd., Suite 200
Los Angeles, CA 90025
310-445-6600
310-445 6601 (fax)
www.allengreenmd.com
Allen Green, M.D., is a board-certified family physician with over twenty years of experience practicing integrative medicine. He believes that cancers arise from the immune system's failure to destroy cancer cells before they cause disease; therefore, he emphasizes nutritional and natural therapies for strengthening and balancing immune function. Patients receive various immuno-restorative therapies including intravenous vitamins and minerals, herbs, detoxification programs, and alkalinizing diet plans. Testing for nutritional deficiencies, hormone imbalances, hidden infections, and heavy metal toxicity is provided in the search for the underlying causes of weakened immunity. Patients undergoing conventional treatments are offered therapies to minimize side effects and even enhance treatment benefits.

Payam Hakimi, M.D.
144 S. Beverly Dr., Suite 602
Beverly Hills, CA 90212
310-247-9997
www.bodyofharmony.com
A board-certified family physician, Dr. Payam Hakimi has had diverse medical training and has combined Western medicine with specialized alternative medical modalities to create an integrative and comprehensive medical practice. He believes health is a dynamic process in which energetic, hormonal-chemical, physical, emotional-mental, and spiritual aspects converge to produce balance and harmony. Dr. Hakimi uses osteopathic treatments, homeopathic medicine, and supplements to help with symptoms of cancer and the side effects of treatments.

Steve Haltiwanger, M.D., C.C.N.
LifeWave
1020 S. Prospect, Suite 200
La Jolla CA 92037
858-459-9876

Mary Hardy, M.D.
Simms/Mann-UCLA Center for Integrative Oncology
200 UCLA Medical Plaza, Suite 502
Los Angeles, CA 90095
310-794-6644
www.simmsmanncenter.ucla.edu

Mary Hardy, M.D., offers counseling and education to answer questions about nutrition, dietary supplements, and complementary medicine before, during, and after conventional cancer treatment. These one-and-a-half-hour private sessions help patients develop strategies to optimize wellness, select appropriate nutritional/dietary supplements/herbs, choose other CAM treatments, and manage conventional treatment side effects. She is well versed in both conventional and complementary treatments to help decrease toxicity from conventional treatment while adding the best of CAM to maximize wellness. This comprehensive assessment takes into consideration your medical history, nutrition, CAM practices, mind-body strategies, spiritual practices, and goals.

Lisa Hirsch, M.D.
Newport Women's Health & Wellness
360 San Miguel, Suite 308
Newport Beach, CA 92660
949-720-0511
949-720-9404 (fax)
www.newportwomenshealthand
  wellness.com

Dr. Hirsch specializes in natural hormone replacement and balance, based on the latest published research and her twenty-plus years of clinical practice and study. She works in close collaboration with a cutting-edge oncologist to assess individual genetic risk through testing of genetic markers and genetic counseling. Each patient receives individualized nutritional assessments based on testing of specific nutritional deficiencies, markers of nutritional imbalances, DNA damage, toxic metal load, and gastrointestinal infections. Dr. Hirsch's goal is to provide preventive health awareness and education that will promote total wellness and longevity and reduce risk of cancer.

Janet Hranicky, Ph.D.
The American Health Institute, Inc.
12381 Wilshire Blvd.
Los Angeles, CA 90025
310-207-3314
800-392-2623
310-207-3342 (fax)
E-mail: jhranicky@ahealth.com,
  customerservice@ahealth.com
www.hranickypsychooncology.com
www.ahealth.com

The Hranicky Psycho-Oncology Program is a one- to three-week intensive patient program for people with cancer that combines the latest advances both from the field of psychoneuroimmunology and bioenergetic regeneration medicine. It is held throughout the year on specific dates at the Hippocrates Health Institute West at Serra Retreat Center in Malibu, California. The program has been designed to empower people with cancer to use the power of their minds and emotional states to successfully maximize their recovery potential, and is ideal for use in conjunction with both standard medical treatment and alternative therapeutic approaches. Dr. Hranicky also incorporates her exciting clinical research in the fields of psychoneuroimmunology, epigenetics, and cancer into a prevention (antiaging and longevity) model.

Institute for Progressive Medicine
4 Hughes, Suite 175
Irvine, CA 92618
949-600-5100
949-600-5101 (fax)
www.iprogressivemed.com

The Institute for Progressive Medicine combines traditional and alternative approaches. Their staff includes board-certified medical doctors, naturopaths, and registered nurses with many years of experience treating all types of chronic and acute conditions. Unique treatment options include high-dose intravenous vitamins, minerals, and antioxidants for a wide variety of medical conditions, including cancer, heart disease, diabetes, neurological conditions, detoxification, infertility, and bacterial and viral infections. IV therapies are also excellent for pre- and postoperative support. Patients often experience symptoms of lesser duration and intensity when treated with IV therapy. For more information and to read patient success stories, please visit their website.

Geoffrey Jones, M.D.
Jones Institute for Advanced Medicine
120 Oakbrook Center, Suite 308
Oak Brook, IL 60523
630-734-8888
www.jonesinstituteusa.com

Dr. Jones's program stimulates the body's natural ability to repair. He helps correct hormonal deficiencies (using bioidentical hormones), improves gastrointestinal health, strengthens nutrition through an individualized diet and supplement plan, improves sleep quality, increases the body's ability to handle stress, and strengthens the im-

mune system. Patients notice more energy, greater ability to handle stress, easier weight loss, and a sharper mind.

Aaron E. Katz, M.D.
Columbia University Medical Center
Center for Holistic Urology
New York, NY 10032
212-305-0114

Dr. Katz is founder and director of the Center for Holistic Urology (established 1998) at Columbia University Medical Center (CUMC), where he also serves as vice chairman of urology. The center performs consultations and research and conducts clinical trials that investigate the role of natural therapies within urology. Dr. Katz has an office at CUMC as well as an East Side office in midtown Manhattan for consultations. Medicare and several commercial insurances are accepted.

Carolyn Katzin
866-471-0529
www.carolynkatzin.com
www.cancernutrition.com

Carolyn Katzin is a certified nutrition specialist with over twenty years of experience in clinical nutrition, with an emphasis on optimizing health and wellness. Carolyn provides integrative oncology nutrition counseling to cancer patients and their families at Beverly Hills Cancer Center, Premiere Oncology in Santa Monica, and Eisenhower's Lucy Curci Cancer Center in Rancho Mirage. She has published a nutrition handbook including recipes and specific drug-nutrient interactions, available from her website www.cancernutrition.com as well as other bookstores. She is an internationally acclaimed public speaker on the topic of nutrition and cancer.

Shiva Lalezar, M.D., D.O.
Health and Vitality Center
11600 Wilshire Blvd., Suite 120
Los Angeles, CA 90025
310-477-1166
310-477-9911 (fax)
www.healthandvitalitycenter.com

Dr. Shiva Lalezar is a holistic physician who supports her patients with nutrients to boost their immune system and reduce their risk of cancer by detoxification in conjunction with other therapies. Dr. Lalezar uses high-dose vitamin C infusion protocols and a variety of other nutrients to optimize health. Special dietary counseling is provided with a focus on alkalizing the blood and balancing body function. A multitude of techniques are used to reduce side effects of chemotherapy and enhance the outcome as well as improve patients' quality of life.

Howard Liebowitz, M.D.
Los Angeles, CA
www.drhowardliebowitz.com

Dr. Liebowitz believes that inflammation is the fundamental cause of virtually all disease, especially cancer. His approach to illness concentrates on modalities that reduce or eliminate inflammation in the body. By integrating nutritional support, the use of nutraceuticals, natural bioidentical hormone balancing, detoxification, and the mind-body connection, he decreases inflammation. As a result, the overburdened immune system is allowed to recover, helping to protect against cancer reoccurrence. With a balanced, healthful diet free of high-glycemic-index foods and toxic substances, along with the power of the mind, the natural healing energy of the body can be enlisted to return to optimum health and life.

Anja Lindblad, N.D.
1756 Lacassie Ave., Suite 102
Walnut Creek, CA 94596
925-939-0300
925-939-3181 (fax)
E-mail: manager@dranja.com
www.dranja.com

As a licensed naturopathic doctor, Dr. Anja Lindblad works with cancer patients alongside their oncologists as an adjunctive care specialist. Using the principles found in naturopathic medicine, she addresses each cancer patient as a unique individual, not as their diagnosis. Analysis of a patient's case typically includes a variety of tests, including nutrient, hormonal, and pathology testing. Therapies used in treatment may include diet and lifestyle changes, botanical medicines, and nutritional supplements, as well as other therapeutics deemed necessary for each individual case.

Rand McClain, D.O.
2701 Ocean Park Blvd., Suite 101
Santa Monica, CA 90405
310-452-3206
310-452-5134 (fax)

15022 Mulberry Dr., Suite B
Whittier, CA 90604
562-906-9700
562-906-9705 (fax)
E-mail: drrandmcclain@drrand
   mcclain.com
www.focusonlifequality.com

Cancer may arise from a multifaceted breakdown in the body's protective mechanisms. Dr. McClain recommends health optimization through the use of nutrition designed specifically for the individual. Movement (exercise) is an essential component of the definition of life itself and of any of his protocols. He provides hormonal replacement with bioidentical hormones for men and women in a form and quantity optimized for each individual's goals, while reducing cancer risk by optimizing their metabolism in the body.

Andreas Moritz
Ener-Chi Wellness Center
9 Night Hawk Way
Landrum, SC 29356
864-895-6285
864-895-2422 (fax)
www.ener-chi.com

Ralph Moss, Ph.D.
814-466-6514
www.ralphmoss.com

Steven E. Nelson, Pharm.D., Ph.D., N.M.D., Di.Hom.
74-133 El Paseo, Suite 5
Palm Desert, CA 92260
760-776-5001
702-610-3081
760-776-5005 (fax)
E-mail: doc@drstevenelson.com
www.wholehealthamerica.com/ drstevenelson
www.drstevenelson.com

Nourishing Wellness Medical Center
819 N. Harbor Dr., Suite 310
Redondo Beach, CA 90277
310-373-7830
310-373-7840 (fax)
www.nourishingwellness.com

They are a passionate doctor/dietitian/chef team who believe that food is the best medicine to change an underlying cause of cancer and create a favorable outcome in treatment. They assess and strengthen immunity through cutting-edge, science-based laboratory/ medical tests, antioxidant scans, nutritional assessment, and a personalized food and supplement program. Nutrient-dense foods can be delivered to your home. They will work in tandem with the patient's extended care team.

Nicole Ortiz, N.D.
Live Well Clinic
78-370 Hwy. 111, Suite 100
La Quinta, CA 92253
760-771-5970
760-771-5982 (fax)
E-mail: info@livewellclinic.org
www.livewellclinic.org

Dr. Nicole Ortiz, N.D., received her doctoral degree in naturopathic medicine with honors in research from the National College of Natural Medicine. She is one of the medical directors at Live Well Clinic in La Quinta, California, providing comprehensive and compassionate care in women's health from puberty through fertility, menopause, and beyond. Dr. Ortiz trained under the nation's leading naturopathic doctors in the areas of women's health, integrative cancer care, graceful aging, and regenerative medicine. She received additional training in prolotherapy, IV nutritional therapy, bioidentical hormone replacement, nasospecific technique, and personal fitness.

Christine Paoletti, M.A., M.D.,
F.A.C.O.G.
1304 15th Street, Suite 405
Santa Monica, CA 90404
310-319-1819
310-319-1335 (fax)
E-mail: info@drpaoletti.com
www.drpaoletti.com

Dr. Paoletti specializes in women's general health, with a special interest in bioidentical hormone replacement. She communicates with other experts in the fields of women's hormones, oncology, and immunology, and uses the information to formulate and individualize the treatment that she dispenses. Dr. Paoletti places an emphasis on regular and complete screening for colon, breast, thyroid, and all gynecological cancers with each major visit. She screens for nutritional, digestive, and immunological deficiencies and, among other things, provides risk assessments for all of the major health risks that women face as well as recent information about their behavioral and nutritional prevention.

Christian Renna, D.O.
Dominique Fradin-Read, M.D.
Robert Maki, N.D.
LifeSpan Medicine
2811 Wilshire Blvd., Suite 610
Santa Monica, CA 90403
310-453-2335
310-453-2337 (fax)
www.lifespanmedicine.com

Christian Renna, D.O.
David Lancaster, D.O.
LifeSpan Medicine
2706 Fairmount St.
Dallas, TX 75201
214-303-1888
214-303-1550 (fax)
www.lifespanmedicine.com

For over twenty-five years, Lifespan Medicine has offered a comprehensive, integrative approach to cancer recovery. They perform in-depth evaluations and comprehensive laboratory panels on each individual. This approach allows them to investigate the underlying cause of the disease, the problems created by treatment, and the persisting factors that increase the risk of recurrence or a new cancer. They emphasize restoring normal detoxification processes, repair of tissue, and recovering healthy immune function through diet, supplementation, IV therapies, and hormone balancing.

Emmey Ripoll, M.D.
Rocky Mountain Center for
Advanced Medicine
3434 47th St., Suite 101
Boulder, CO 80301
303-565-3889
303-444-0838 (fax)
www. rmcam.com

Dr. Emmey Ripoll is board-certified in urology/holistic medicine with a fellowship in urologic oncology. She has a diverse practice, specializing in oncology and antiaging medicine using both Western and complementary approaches. She believes each person can find the health within, and utilizes a range of therapies to discover this optimal state: hormone replacement, IV treatments, acupuncture, herbs, homeopathy, and nutritional and lifestyle modification.

Mark Rosenberg, M.D.
2512 N. Federal Hwy., Suite 105
Delray Beach, FL 33483
561-272-1956
www.alternativecancersolution.com
www.antiagemed.com

Martin Rossman, M.D.
Collaborative Medicine Center
1341 S. Eliseo Dr., Suite 350
Greenbrae, CA 94904
415-925-8600
E-mail: mrmd555@aol.com

The Collaborative Medicine Center provides expert physiological and psychological support for cancer patients going through chemotherapy, radiation therapy, and surgery. They utilize nutrition, mind-body medicine, and Chinese medicine to support each patient individually and work closely with them and their oncologists to get the best outcomes possible.

David Schmidt
LifeWave LLC
1020 S. Prospect, Suite 200
La Jolla, CA 92037
858-459-9876
E-mail: knockout@lifewave.com
www.suzannesomers.com

LifeWave technology is a new method for dramatically elevating your body's master antioxidant glutathione without having to take pills or injections. As a comparison, a glutathione pill will increase your antioxidant levels by about 14 percent in thirty days. With LifeWave your glutathione antioxidant levels increase on average to more than 300 percent in only one day, giving you better protection from the harmful effects of environmental toxins and aging. How is this possible? The scientific principle is very similar to how sunlight causes your body to make biochemicals, such as vitamin D and melanin. Instead of having one ingest a pill, LifeWave uses a nontransdermal patch that you apply to the body on specific acupuncture points, gently stimulating those points all day.

Joseph Sciabbarrasi, M.D.
2001 S. Barrington Ave., Suite 208
Los Angeles, CA 90025
310-268-8466
310-268-8122 (fax)
www.drjosephmd.com

Their approach to cancer patients is built upon customized, individualized care utilizing state-of-the-art testing and treatment. Most patients they treat are receiving conventional therapy. They offer hope, reassurance, and a full array of immune-enhancing therapies and highly specialized labs to guide individualized treatment, including intravenous vitamin C to achieve optimal blood levels, natural immune cell stimulants supported by university-based clinical trials, nutritional consultation, tailored supplements based upon individual testing, bioidentical hormone replacement therapy in specific cases, heavy metal testing and chelation therapy, acupuncture for energy and immune health, and deep tissue bodywork.

Stephen T. Sinatra, M.D., F.A.C.C.,
F.A.C.N., C.N.S., C.B.T.
c/o Optimum Health Building
257 East Center St.
Manchester, CT 06040
860-645-0288
860-643-2531 (fax)
www.heartmdinstitute.com

Robin Smith, M.D., M.B.A.
NeoStem, Inc.
420 Lexington Ave., Suite 450
New York, NY 10170
212-584-4180
646-514-7787 (fax)
www.neostem.com
www.suzannesomers.com (click on
NeoStem)
   Dr. Robin L. Smith is chief executive officer of NeoStem, Inc. (AMEX:NBS), an adult stem cell collection processing and long-term storage company focused on enabling people to donate and store their own stem cells when they are young and healthy for their personal use in times of future medical need. Additionally the company is focused on advancing stem cell–based therapies. Dr. Smith also serves on the board of trustees of the NYU Medical Center and is chairman of the board of directors for the NYU Hospital for Joint Diseases and the Stem for Life Foundation.

Jennifer Sudarsky, M.D.
3201 Wilshire Blvd., Suite 211
Santa Monica, CA 90403
310-315-9101
310-829-9860 (fax)
E-mail: jsudarsky@mednet.ucla.edu
www.LAvitamindoc.com
   In her integrative approach to medicine, Dr. Jennifer Sudarsky helps patients achieve optimal overall health by addressing primary care needs as well as more specialized issues like immune strengthening and hormone balancing. She also collaborates with patients who wish to explore alternative therapies, including nutritional supplementation and intravenous vitamins and herbal remedies. A graceful and intuitive healer, Dr. Sudarsky has her own history of autoimmune dysfunction, which has given her a broader understanding of patients' needs when struggling with these concerns. A member of the clinical faculty at UCLA, Dr. Sudarsky is also a diplomate of both the American Board of Family Medicine and the American Board of Holistic Medicine.

Tahoma Clinic
801 SW 16th St., Suite 121
Renton, WA 98055
425-264-0059
425-264-0071 (fax)
   The staff includes Jonathan V. Wright, M.D. (medical director); Olivia Franks, N.D.; Lauren Russel, N.D.; Wendy Ellis, N.D.; Christa Hinchcliffe, N.D. (thermography, BHRT for women, hormone balancing for younger women—not menopausal, headaches, thyroid balancing, osteoporosis, malabsorption, toxic metal detoxification, digestive issues, food sensitivity—including gluten sensitivity, fatigue, and many other health concerns for women, ADD/ADHD, children, young adults with various health issues, and male patients); Davis Lamson, N.D. (hepatitis C, liver disorders, autoimmune disorders, cancer support therapies, food sensitivities, especially gluten, gut reconditioning, chelation for toxic heavy

metals, therapies for arterial calcification).

Karlis Ullis, M.D.
2701 Ocean Park Blvd., Suite 101
Santa Monica, CA 90405
310-452-1990
310-452-5134 (fax)
E-mail: kullis@ucla.edu
www.drkarlisullis.com

Karlis Ullis, M.D., is a board-certified physician and was a UCLA faculty member for thirty years. Dr. Ullis carefully balances hormones along with metabolic factors, specific diets, nutrients, deep tissue therapies (Rolfing, Heller, Neuromuscular-NMT), and exercise programs for specific conditions, including health recovery after cancer and further cancer risk reduction. Dr. Ullis's programs include metabolic rate studies, anabolic lifestyle protocols to prevent muscle loss (sarcopenia) and regain muscle and bone strength, and optimal health and vitality to achieve reduced biological aging. Dr. Ullis also treats men who have been cured of prostate cancer with testosterone, if indicated.

Cynthia M. Watson, M.D.
3201 Wilshire Blvd., Suite 211
Santa Monica, CA 90403
310-315-9101
310-829-9860 (fax)
www.watsonwellness.org

Cynthia M. Watson, M.D., is board-certified in family medicine and has a thriving integrative medicine practice in Santa Monica, California, handling all areas of primary care. Dr. Watson is known for incorporating conventional medicine with herbal medicine, homeopathy, and nutrition. In her medical practice she specializes in women's health, bioidentical hormones, antiaging medicine, and intravenous vitamin therapy. Dr. Watson works with various detoxification programs tailored to each patient's individual needs, including chemicals, mold, and heavy metals. She also has assisted many patients in recovering from cancer and the side effects of chemotherapy and radiation with nutritional therapy.

Julian Whitaker, M.D.
Whitaker Wellness Institute Medical
  Clinic
4321 Birch St.
Newport Beach, CA 92660
800-488-1500
www.whitakerwellness.com

Since 1979, the Whitaker Wellness Institute has treated more than 45,000 patients with diabetes, heart disease, cancer, and other serious conditions. The clinic's six physicians, scores of health care professionals, and numerous therapeutic modalities make it one of the country's largest and most comprehensive complementary medicine clinics. Therapies offered for the treatment of cancer include Dr. Stanislaw Burzynski's treatment protocols, IV vitamin C, low-dose naltrexone, hyperbaric oxygen therapy, and targeted nutritional supplementation.

Jonathan Wright, M.D.
Tahoma Clinic
801 S.W. 16th St., Suite 121
Renton, WA 98055
425-264-0059
425-264-0071 (fax)
www.tahomaclinic.com
See Tahoma Clinic, page 308.

HEALTH CARE ATTORNEY

Richard A. Jaffe
Phoenix Tower
3200 Southwest Freeway, Suite 3200
Houston, TX 77027
713-626-3550
713-626-9420 (fax)
E-mail: rickjaffeesq@aol.com
www.richardjaffe.com

Richard Jaffe is a health care litigator and counselor specializing in cutting-edge medical technologies and representing alternative and integrative health care practitioners in criminal, civil, and administrative cases. He also acts as counsel to a number of complementary health groups and trade organizations. His recently published book, *Galileo's Lawyer,* describes the struggles among medical mavericks, the government, and the church of medical orthodoxy.

BOOKS BY OR ABOUT
<u>KNOCKOUT</u> DOCTORS

Balch, Phyllis A. *Prescription for Nutritional Healing*, 4th ed. Penguin Group (USA), 2006.

Blaylock, Russell. *Health and Nutrition Secrets*. Health Press, 2006.

———. *Natural Strategies for Cancer Patients*. Twin Streams Books/ Kensington Publishing, 2003.

———. *Excitotoxins: The Taste That Kills*. Health Press, 1997.

Campbell, T. Colin, and Thomas M. Campbell. *The China Study: The Most Comprehensive Study of Nutrition Ever Conducted and the Startling Implications for Diet, Weight Loss and Long-Term Health*. BenBella Books, 2006.

Cham, Bill. *The Eggplant Cancer Cure: A Treatment for Skin Cancer and New Hope for Other Cancers from Nature's Pharmacy*. Smart Publications, 2008.

Critser, Greg. *Generation Rx: How Prescription Drugs Are Altering American Lives, Minds, and Bodies*. Houghton Mifflin Harcourt, 2005.

Dayton, Martin. *The Case for Intravenous EDTA Chelation Therapy*. Self-published, 1995.

Elias, Thomas. *The Burzynski Breakthrough: The Century's Most Promising Treatment . . . and the Government's Campaign to Squelch It*. General Publishing Group, 1997.

Fox, Cynthia. *Cell of Cells: The Global Race to Capture and Control the Stem Cell*. W. W. Norton, 2007.

Galitzer, Michael. *Clinical Bioenergetics* [pamphlet]. Apex Energetics, 1994.

Geller, Alan. *Scary Diagnosis*. Three Rings Publishing, 2007.

Goldberg, Burton. *Women's Health: Alternative Medicine Definitive Guides.* Future Medicine Publishing, Inc., 1998.

Goldberg, Burton, John W. Anderson, and Larry Trivieri. *Alternative Medicine: The Definitive Guide.* 2nd ed. Celestial Arts, 2004.

Goldberg, Burton, and the Burton Goldberg Group. *Alternative Medicine: The Definitive Guide to Cancer.* Future Medicine Publishing, 1997.

Goldberg, Burton, W. Lee Cowden, and Ferre Akbarpour. *Longevity.* AlternativeMedicine.com, 2000.

Goldberg, Burton, W. John Diamond, and W. Lee Cowden. *An Alternative Medicine Definitive Guide to Cancer.* Future Medicine Publishing, Inc., 1997.

Goldberg, Burton, and the Editors of *Alternative Medicine Digest. Alternative Medicine Guide to Heart Disease.* Future Medicine Publishing, 1998.

Goldberg, Burton, and Jay Gordon. *Natural Medicine Chest and Home Remedies.* Future Medicine Publishing, 1994.

Goldberg, Burton, Jesse Hanley, Mari Florence, and Kerry Hughes. *Women: Everything You Need to Know: How Proven and Natural Therapies Can Help You.* Future Medicine Publishing, 1998.

Goldberg, Burton, Konrad Kail, and Bobbi Lawrence. *Allergy Free: An Alternative Medicine Definitive Guide.* AlternativeMedicine.com, 2000.

Goldberg, Burton, Lita Lee, Lisa Turner, and Richard Leviton. *The Enzyme Cure: An Alternative Medicine Guide.* Future Medicine Publishing, 1998.

Goldberg, Burton, Robert D. Milne, and Blake More. *Alternative Medicine Definitive Guide to Headaches.* Future Medicine Publishing, 1997.

Goldberg, Burton, William H. Philpott, and Dwight K. Kalita. *Magnet Therapy: An Alternative Medicine Definitive Guide.* Alternative Medicine.com, 2000.

Goldberg, Burton, Herbert Ross, and Keri Brenner. *Sleep Disorders: An Alternative Medicine Definitive Guide.* AlternativeMedicine.com, 2000.

Goldberg, Burton, James Strohecker, and Leon Chaitow. *You Don't Have to Die: Unraveling the AIDS Myth.* Future Medicine Publishing, 1994.

Goldberg, Burton, and Larry Trivieri Jr. *Chronic Fatigue, Fibromyalgia and Lyme Disease.* AlternativeMedicine.com, 2004.

Goldberg, Burton, Eugene Zampieron, and Ellen Kamhi. *Arthritis: An Alternative Medicine Definitive Guide.* AlternativeMedicine.com, 1999.

Hagen, Bruce C. *How to Live to Be 100 in Spite of Your Doctor.* Hagen Publishing, 2006.

Haltiwanger, Steve. *Winning in the New World: With Help From the Power of Anti-aging Peptides and Hormones.* Intec Publishing, 2002.

Hauser, Ross A., and Marion A. Hauser. *Treating Cancer with Insulin Potentiation Therapy.* Beulah Land Press, 2002.

Hertoghe, Thierry, and Jules-Jacques Nabet. *The Hormone Solution: Stay Younger Longer with Natural Hormone and Nutrition Therapies.* Three Rivers Press, 2002.

Horwitz, Len, with contributions by Steve Haltiwanger. *DNA: Pirates of the Sacred Spiral.* Tetrahedron Publishing, 2004.

Hotze, Steven F., and Kelly Griffin. *Hormones, Health, and Happiness: A Natural Medical Formula for Rediscovering Youth.* Forrest Publishing, 2005.

Jaffe, Richard A. *Galileo's Lawyer: Courtroom Battles in Alternative Health, Complementary Medicine and Experimental Treatments.* Thumbs Up Press, 2008.

Mahmud, Khalid. *Keeping aBreast: Ways to Prevent Breast Cancer.* Strategic Book Publishing, 2008.

McLeod, Donald M., and Philip A. White. *Doctors' Secrets: The Road to Longevity.* McLeod and White, 2001.

Mercola, Joseph, and Kendra Pearsall. *Take Control of Your Health.* Mercola.com, 2007.

Miller, Philip Lee, and Monica Reinagel. *The Life Extension Revolution: The New Science of Growing Older Without Aging.* Bantam, 2005.

Morgentaler, Abraham. *Testosterone for Life: Recharge Your Vitality, Sex Drive, Muscle Mass, and Overall Health.* McGraw-Hill, 2008.

Moritz, Andreas. *The Amazing Liver and Gallbladder Flush.* Ener-Chi Wellness Press, 2006.

———. *Cancer Is Not a Disease—It's a Survival Mechanism.* Ener-Chi.com, 2008.

———. *Diabetes—No More!.* Ener-Chi.com, 2006.

———. *Ending the AIDS Myth.* Ener-Chi.com, 2006.

———. *It's Time to Come Alive.* Ener-Chi Wellness Press, 2005.

———. *Lifting the Veil of Duality: Your Guide to Living Without Judgment.* Ener-Chi.com, 2005.

———. *Timeless Secrets of Health and Rejuvenation,* new ed. Ener-Chi Wellness Press, 2005.

Moritz, Andreas, and John Hornecker. *Simple Steps to Total Health.* Ener-Chi.com, 2006.

Moss, Ralph W. *Alternative Medicine Online: A Guide to Natural Remedies on the Internet.* Equinox Press, 1997.

————. *Antioxidants Against Cancer.* Equinox Press, 2000.

————. *The Cancer Industry, New Updated Edition.* Equinox Press, 1996.

————. *Cancer Therapy: The Independent Consumer's Guide to Non-Toxic Treatment and Prevention.* Equinox Press, 1992.

————. *Herbs Against Cancer.* Equinox Press, 1998.

————. *Questioning Chemotherapy.* Equinox Press, 1995.

Moss, Ralph W., and Josef Beuth. *Complementary Oncology: Adjunctive Methods in the Treatment of Cancer.* Thieme Publishing, 2005.

Moss, Ralph W., and Theron G. Randolph. *An Alternative Approach to Allergies: The New Field of Clinical Ecology Unravels the Environmental Causes of Mental and Physical Ills.* Harper Perennial, 1989.

Moynihan, Ray, and Alan Cassels. *Selling Sickness: How the World's Biggest Pharmaceutical Companies Are Turning Us All into Patients.* Nation Books, 2006.

Murphy, Christine. *Iscador: Mistletoe in Cancer Therapy.* Lantern Books, 2001.

Owens, Paula. *The Power of 4: Your Ultimate Guide Guaranteed to Change Your Body and Transform Your Life.* NetSource Distribution, 2008.

Plasker, Eric. *The 100 Year Lifestyle: Dr. Plasker's Breakthrough Solution for Living Your Best Life—Every Day of Your Life!* Adams Media, 2007.

Rothenberg, Ron, Kathleen Becker, and Kris Hart. *Forever Ageless, Advanced Edition.* California HealthSpan Institute, 2007.

Rowe, John Wallis, and Robert L. Kahn. *Successful Aging.* Dell, 1999.

Segala, Melanie. *Disease Prevention and Treatment,* 4th ed. Life Extension Publications, 2003.

Servan-Schreiber, David. *Anticancer: A New Way of Life.* Viking, 2008.

Simoncini, Tullio. *Cancer Is a Fungus.* Edizon, 2007.

Sinatra, Stephen. *A Cardiologist's Guide to Optimum Health.* Lincoln-Bradley Publishing Group, 1996.

————. *CoenzymeQ10 and the Heart.* Keats Publishing, 1999.

————. *The CoenzymeQ$_{10}$ Phenomenon.* Keats Publishing, 1998.

————. *Heartbreak and Heart Disease: A Mind/Body Prescription for Healing the Heart.* Keats Publishing, 1999.

————. *Lose to Win: A Cardiologist's Guide to Weight Loss and Nutritional Healing.* Lincoln-Bradley Publishing Group, 1992.

————. *Lower Your Blood Pressure in Eight Weeks: A Revolutionary Program for a Longer, Healthier Life.* Ballantine Books, 2003.

———. *Optimum Health: A Natural Lifesaving Prescription for Your Body and Mind.* Bantam Books, 1997.

———. *The Sinatra Solution: Metabolic Cardiology.* Basic Health, 2008.

———. *The Sinatra Solution: New Hope for Preventing and Treating Heart Disease.* Basic Health, 2005.

Sinatra, Stephen, and Connie Bennett. *Sugar Shock! How Sweets and Simple Carbs Can Derail Your Life—and How You Can Get Back on Track.* Berkley Trade, 2006.

Sinatra, Stephen, and Jim Punkre. *The Fast Food Diet.* John Wiley and Sons, 2006.

Sinatra, Stephen, and James Roberts. *Reverse Heart Disease Now.* John Wiley and Sons, 2007.

Sinatra, Stephen, Graham Simpson, and Jorge Suarez-Menendez. *Spa Medicine: Your Getaway to the Ageless Zone.* Basic Health Publications, 2004.

Sinatra, Stephen, and Jan Sinatra. *L-Carnitine and the Heart.* Keats Publishing, 1999.

Sinatra, Stephen, Jan Sinatra, and Roberta Jo Lieberman. *Heart Sense for Women: Your Plan for Natural Prevention and Treatment.* Plume, 2000.

Small, Gary, and Gigi Vorgan. *The Longevity Bible: 8 Essential Strategies for Keeping Your Mind Sharp and Your Body Young.* Hyperion, 2007.

Sutherland, Caroline. *The Body Knows . . . How to Stay Young: Healthy-Aging Secrets from a Medical Intuitive.* Hay House, 2008.

Thompson, Robert, and Kathleen Barnes. *The Calcium Lie: What Your Doctor Doesn't Know Could Kill You.* In Truth Press, 2008.

Wallach, Joel D., and Ma Lan. *Dead Doctors Don't Lie.* Legacy Communications, 1999.

Watson, Brenda. *The HOPE Formula: The Ultimate Health Secret.* Renew Life Press, 2007.

Wright, Jonathan V. *Book of Nutritional Therapy: Real-Life Lessons in Medicine Without Drugs.* Rodale Press, 1979.

———. *Dr. Wright's Guide to Healing with Nutrition.* Rodale Press, 1984.

———. *Maximize Your Vitality and Potency for Men Over 40.* Smart Publications, 1999.

Wright, Jonathan V., et al. *The Natural Pharmacy: Complete A–Z Reference to Natural Treatments for Common Health Conditions.* Three Rivers Press, 1999.

Wright, Jonathan V., and Alan R. Gaby. *Natural Medicine, Optimal Wellness.* Vital Health Publishing, 2006.

Wright, Jonathan V., and Lane Lenard. *D-Mannose and Bladder Infection: The Natural Alternative to Antibiotics.* Dragon Art, 2001.

———. *Why Stomach Acid Is Good for You.* M. Evans, 2001.

———. *Xylitol: Dental and Upper Respiratory Health.* Dragon Art, 2003.

Wright, Jonathan V., and John Morgenthaler. *Natural Hormone Replacement for Women Over 45.* Smart Publications, 1997.

Wright, Jonathan V., and John Neustadt. *Thriving Through Dialysis.* Dragon Art, 2005.

INDEX

Abraham, Dr. Guy, 197
Adriamycin, 47, 48, 103
Aflatoxins, 73–74, 175, 240
Aging, 75
    antiaging doctors, specialists,
        clinics, and institutes, 271–289
    cancer and, 153–155
    genetics and, 154, 241
    glutathione and, 174, 176
AHCC (active hexose correlated
    compound), 259
Ali, Dr. Majid, 121
Alkalinazation, 104–105, 125
Allergies, 166
Alternative medicine
    conventional medicine's attitude
        toward, 216–217
    future prospects, 54–55, 129–130,
        221–222
    Goldberg's involvement with,
        163–164

pharmaceutical industry and, 106
    See also Integrative medicine;
        Prevention of cancer;
        Treatment of cancer
Alzheimer's disease, 63, 158
American Cancer Society, 45, 46
Amines, 175
Amino acids, 63–64
Aminocare supplements, 68, 77
Androstenediol, 193
Anesthesia use during surgery,
    261–263
Angiogenesis, 260–261
Antibiotics in food, 167
Antineoplaston replacement therapy,
    21, 59, 61
    administration of medications, 70
    animal testing for, 63
    brain cancer and, 67, 70, 81–83
    breast cancer and, 66, 71, 85–86
    chemistry of peptides, 63–64

Antineoplaston replacement therapy
    (continued)
  chemotherapy used with, 67
  curing of cancer with, 70–71,
      78
  deficiency of peptides in people
      with cancer, 61–62, 63, 68
  duration of treatment, 70
  efficacy of, 66, 67, 70–71
  genetics of, 65–67, 68
  information processing and,
      64
  killing of cancer cells, 65
  liver cancer and, 71, 72, 74
  lymphoma and, 78–81
  medulloblastoma and, 83–84
  melanoma and, 71
  pancreatic cancer and, 71, 72
  patient testimonials about,
      78–86
  for post-chemotherapy patients,
      69–70
  supplementation and, 74–77
Antioxidants, 174–175, 178, 230
  resveratrol, 234–236
Apoptosis, 49
Armstrong, Lance, 95
Aromatase, 161
Arrogance of doctors, 13
Arthritis, 175
Ashkenazi Jews, 66
Aspartame, 98
Astrocytoma, 67
Asyrus devices, 171
Ativan, 7
Autologus vaccines, 171
Autonomic nervous system, 99–101,
      104–105
Avastin, 51, 65

Belief in healing, 106–107, 201–204,
      205–206, 213–214, 220–221
  BHRT and, 139
Beta-carotene, 229–230
BHRT. *See* Bioidentical hormone
      replacement therapy
Bioenergetic therapy, 204, 207
BioFocus blood test, 171
Bioidentical hormone replacement
      therapy (BHRT), 25
  belief in healing and, 139
  bone loss and, 139–140
  breast cancer and, 134–139, 141,
      185–187, 188
  cancer from using bioidenticals,
      196
  compounding pharmacies and,
      140
  cream form of hormones used in,
      184–185
  DHEA hormone, 183–184
  estrogens, 185–187, 188–192, 196
  5-alpha-reductase, 193–194
  Knock It Out recommendations,
      199
  medical education and, 192
  misunderstandings about,
      141–142
  pharmaceutical industry/FDA
      policy on, 186, 189–191
  progesterone, 196
  testosterone, 193, 194–196
Biopsies, 11, 12, 105
Birth control pills, 28–29, 101–102
Blaylock, Dr. Russell, 24–25, 101
  background of, 147–148
  interview with, 148–162
Blood thinning, 215
Bone loss, 139–140

Bowel movements, 223
Brain cancer
  antineoplaston replacement
    therapy and, 67, 70, 81–83
  Avastin and, 51
  cell phone use and, 101
  vitamin D3 and, 154–155
Brassica vegetables, 188
Braverman, Dr. Albert, 20
Breast cancer
  antineoplaston replacement
    therapy and, 66, 71, 85–86
  BHRT and, 134–139, 141,
    185–187, 188
  birth control pills and, 102
  chemotherapy and, 158, 159
  childhood abuse and, 187
  COX-2 inhibitors and, 264–265
  environmental toxins and,
    167–168
  enzyme therapy and, 115–116,
    117–118, 119–120
  estrogen and, 185–187, 188
  fibrocystic disease and, 152,
    187
  homeopathic therapy and, 125,
    130–131
  internal conflict and, 209–210
  iodine intake and, 187–188
  mammograms and, 149–152
  MRI scans for, 152
  overdiagnosis of, 149, 158
  preventive strategies, 137
  root canals and, 218
  Somers's experience with, 28, 29,
    181, 186–187
  soy consumption and, 161
  supplementation and, 152–153,
    159
    synthetic hormone replacement
      and, 182
    transforming growth factor and,
      266
Breast Cancer Action, 51
Brenner, Barbara, 51
Budwig diet, 215–216
Burzynski, Dr. Stanislaw, xvi, 20, 30,
    53–54, 103, 137, 181, 198
  background of, 59–61
  interview with, 61–78
  legal actions against, 21–23
  patient testimonials about, 78–86

Calcium, 101
Campaign financing, 167
Cancer
  adhesion by cancer cells,
    255–258
  aging and, 153–155
  anaerobic metabolism of cancer
    cells, 183, 215
  angiogenesis and, 260–261
  BHRT as source of, 196
  chemical carcinogenesis, 178
  DNA mutation and, 240–242,
    244–246
  energy metabolism of cancer cells,
    125–126, 176
  environmental toxins and, 41–42,
    164–166, 167–168, 176–177,
    240
  folic acid and, 153, 232–234
  grief and, 206–207
  infections and, 218–219
  inflammation as cause of, 153,
    154, 155, 263–265
  internal conflict and, 209–210
  iron intake and, 159–160

Cancer *(continued)*
  precancerous cells' transformation
    to cancer cells, 245–247
  proliferation of cancer cells,
    247–250
  stem cells and, 214
  sugar intake and, 155–156, 215,
    236–237
  supplementation and the
    increased risk for cancer,
    229–230, 232–234
  surgery-induced recurrence and
    metastasis, 252, 254–255
  viruses and, 242
  vitamin E and, 229–230
  See also Prevention of cancer;
    Treatment of cancer; *specific
    forms of cancer*
Cancer vaccines, 260
Carbohydrate intake, 237
CAT scans, 4, 5–6
Cavalieri, Dr. Ercole, 189
Celebrex, 264
Cell phones, electromagnetic
    radiation from, 97, 101, 206
Center for Science in the Public
    Interest, 232
Cervical cancer, 242
Cham, Dr. Bill, 197
Chemical carcinogenesis, 178
Chemosensitivity testing, 29, 31, 38,
    127–128
  medical community's rejection of,
    48–49
Chemotherapy
  antineoplaston replacement
    therapy used with, 67
  approval process for new drugs,
    51–52
  breast cancer and, 158, 159
  doctors' refusal of chemotherapy
    for themselves, 50
  economics of, 49–50, 51, 52–53
  folic acid intake and, 234
  homeopathic therapy used with,
    125, 126
  individualized approach to, 47,
    49–50, 53
  ineffective drugs, 48, 103, 128
  ineffectiveness for major cancer
    killers, 95–96
  integrative medicine and, 214,
    223–224
  low-dose chemotherapy, 169
  medical education and, 71–72,
    96
  multidrug resistance and, 157,
    159
  nutrition and, 169
  patients' faith in, 97
  placebo function for terminal
    patients, 52
  racket of, 31–32
  "response" of tumors to, 97
  side effects of, 127, 158–159
  success issue, 51, 158–159
  survival rates of patients, 123–124
  testicular cancer and, 95
  See also specific drugs
Chemotherapy concession, 52
Childhood abuse, 187
Chinese aspirin, 125
Chlebowski, Dr., 137
Cholesterol, 231, 248, 249
Cigarette smoke, 220
Cimetidine, 257–258
Citrus pectin, 256–258
Coffee consumption, 92–93

Coffee enemas, 89, 92–93
Colonics, 223
Colorectal cancer, 52, 100
  cancer vaccines and, 260
  cimetidine therapy and, 257–258
  COX-2 inhibitors and, 264
  enzyme therapy and, 115–116
  mistletoe extract and, 259–260
  PSK mushroom extract and, 259
Compounding pharmacies, 140
  state-by-state listing of, 292–294
Computers, electromagnetic
    radiation from, 97
COMT enzyme, 190
Congress, U.S., 22
Conventional cancer therapy
  anesthesia use during surgery,
    261–263
  "big business" dimension of, 29
  biopsies, 11, 12, 105
  cancer vaccines and, 260
  cure for cancer as threat to, 60–
    61, 157–158
  evidence-based medicine and,
    161–162
  faulty paradigm of, xv–xvi, 60
  immune system and, 258–260,
    262, 263
  inflammation and, 263–265
  mammograms, 149–152
  morphine use after surgery,
    262–263
  overdiagnosis of cancer, 149, 158
  palliation and, 148
  precautions patients can take to
    increase likelihood of success,
    254–267
  radiation therapy, 50, 151
  "standard of care" protocol, 38

  surgery, 252, 254–255, 258,
    261–263
  See also Chemotherapy;
    Integrative medicine
Coumadin, 10
Crying, 209
Curcumin (turmeric), 68–69, 76,
    157, 261
Curry lines, 219
Cyclooxygenase-2 (COX-2) enzyme,
    264–265

Day, Philip, 87
Dayton, Dr. Marty, 169
Dendritic cell therapy, 168–169
Depression, 140, 166
Devito, Esther, 113–114
DHEA hormone, 183–184
Diabetes, 102
Diamond, Jared, 40
Dihydrotestosterone (DHT), 193
DIM supplement, 188
DNA. See Genetics
D'Orisio, Lolli, 85–86
Drug approval process, 51–52
Drug companies. See Pharmaceutical
    industry
Drug development process, 44
Dyes, artificial, 232

Einstein, Albert, 1
Electromagnetic contamination, 97,
    101, 206
Ellagic acid, 234
Emerson, Ralph Waldo, 228
Energy patches, 173, 178–179
Environmental toxins, 41–42,
    164–166, 167–168, 176–177,
    240

Enzyme therapy, 88, 225
  autonomic nervous system and,
    99–101, 104–105
  breast cancer and, 115–116,
    117–118, 119–120
  colorectal cancer and, 115–116
  cost of, 89–90
  curing of cancer with, 94–95, 102
  detoxification component, 89–90,
    92–93
  dietary component, 89, 100–101
  efficacy of, 90
  enzyme supplementation
    component, 89
  liver cancer and, 116–117
  lung cancer and, 115–116
  lymphoma and, 111–114
  management of cancer as chronic
    disease, 102–103
  myeloma and, 101
  ovarian cancer and, 109–111
  pancreatic cancer and, 90–91, 94,
    108–109, 118–119
  patient program design, 91
  patients beyond the help of,
    90–91
  patient testimonials about,
    108–120
Eosinophils, 36–37
E-selection molecule, 257
Estrogens, 185–187, 188–192, 196
Evidence-based medicine, 161–162

Faloon, Bill, xvii, 26, 29, 252–253
  interview with, 254–267
Fatty liver disease, 103–104
Fawcett, Farrah, xx, 29
Fenn, Forrest, 36, 145
Fibrocystic disease, 152, 187

FIGHT program, 218–220
5-alpha-reductase, 193–194
Flick, Wanda, 117–118
Folic acid, 153, 232–234, 248
Food and Drug Administration
  (FDA), 29, 61
  approval process for new drugs,
    51–52
  BHRT and, 186, 189–191
  Burzynski and, 21, 22
  cancer vaccines and, 260
  pharmaceutical industry and, 32,
    45, 46–47
  scientific legitimacy, loss of, 32
Food intolerances, 166–167
Foods to eat and to avoid, 159–161
Forsythe, Dr. James, 20, 23–24, 198
  interview with, 121–130
  legal actions against, 24
  patient testimonials about,
    130–133
Forsythe Immune Therapy (FIT),
  125
Free radicals, 154, 155, 174–175,
  240, 241
Fruit extracts, 236
Fungal infections, 37

Gadsden, Henry, 40
Galileo, xv
Galitzer, Dr. Michael, 25, 36
  interview with, 212–226
Gandhi, M. K., 221
Garlic, 259
Gemzar, 51, 96–97
Genetically modified foods (GMO),
  167
Genetics
  aging and, 154, 241

of antineoplaston replacement
therapy, 65–67, 68
belief in healing and, 201–202
DNA mutation, 240–242, 244–
246
human genome, 75
hypermethylated genes, 137
of liver cancer, 75
mammograms and, 150
prevention of cancer and, 68–69,
75–77
supplementation and, 68–69,
241–242
vitamin E and, 230–231
Genistein, 76, 261
Geopathic stress, 219
Gettino, Jenny and Sophia, 81–83
Glutamates, 160
Glutamine, 259
Glutathione, 36, 154, 173
prevention of cancer and,
174–176, 177–178
treatment of cancer and,
179–180
Glycated hemoglobin test, 237
Glyco-benzaldehyde, 125
Gold, Dr. Joseph, 170
Goldberg, Burton, 25, 31, 217
background of, 163–164
interview with, 164–172
Gonzalez, Dr. Nicholas, 20, 23, 30,
47, 53–54, 170, 225
background of, 87–88
interview with, 88–107
patient testimonials about,
108–120
Gordon, Dr. Gary, 218
Granulocyte-macrophage colony
stimulating factor, 260

Green tea, 68, 261
Grief, 206–207

Halsted, Dr. William, xvi
Haltiwanger, Dr. Steve, 179
Hancock, Sharon, 130–131
Hands-on approach to medicine,
204–205
Harrowsmith, Marilyn, 132–133
Healing, normal patterns of,
208–209
Heart disease, 204, 209
Heparin, 7
Hepatitis B, 72–74
Hepatitis C, 242
Herceptin, 48
Higher source, connecting with,
221
HIV/AIDS, 73, 122
Homeopathic therapy, 122–123
advanced cancer patients and,
127
breast cancer and, 125, 130–131
chemotherapy used with, 125,
126
efficacy of, 126
individualized approaches to, 126
lung cancer and, 132–133
management of cancer as chronic
disease, 127
patients beyond the help of, 127
patient testimonials about,
130–133
prostate cancer and, 125,
131–132
supplementation used in,
124–126, 128–129
Hormones
balance of, 28

Hormones (continued)
    FIGHT program and, 219–220
    in food, 167
'   prevention of cancer and, 77–78
    synthetic hormone replacement,
        182
    See also Bioidentical hormone
        replacement therapy
Hospital stays, dangers of, 32–33
HPV (human papilloma virus), 242
Hydrazine sulfate therapy, 170–171
Hydroxyestrogens, 188–189
Hypermethylated genes, 137
Hyperthermia therapy, 171, 217
Hysterectomies, 192

Immune system, 64–65, 166,
        174–175, 233, 238
    conventional cancer therapy and,
        258–260, 262, 263
    mistletoe extract and, 224,
        259–260
    PSK mushroom extract and,
        258–259
    supplementation for
        enhancement of, 246–247
Immune therapies, 168–169
Indole-3 carbinol (I3C), 188
Infections, 218–219
Inflammation as cause of cancer,
        153, 154, 155, 263–265
Information processing, 64
Insulin, 63–64, 125
Insulin potentiation therapy, 169–
        170
Integrative medicine, 123, 169, 171,
        213
    chemotherapy and, 214, 223–224
    listing of practitioners, 297–309

Interferon-alpha, 260
Interleukin-2, 260
Internal conflict, 209–210
International Strategic Cancer
        Alliance, 265, 266–267
Iodine intake, 187–188, 197
Iodolipids, 187
IP6 (inositol hexaphosphate), 259
Iron intake, 159–160
Iscador, 171, 224
Issels, Dr., 217, 218

Jaffe, Richard, 21–22
Johnson, David, 118–119

Kelley, Dr. William Donald, 88, 89,
        93–94, 95, 100, 102, 105,
        106–107
Kennedy, John F., 1
Kidney cancer, 214
King, Martin Luther, Jr., 57
Kunnari, Mary Ann and Dustin,
        21–22, 83–84

Lactoferrin, 259
Laetrile, 30, 45–46
Laparoscopic surgery, 263
Lemon, Dr. Henry, 185, 189
Leukemia, 30, 242
    radiation therapy and, 151
Levaquin, 7
Life Extension Foundation, 32, 252,
        254, 258, 264, 267, 295–296
Lipoic acid, 124
Lipton, Bruce, 201
Liver, fatty infiltration of, 103–104
Liver cancer, 240, 242
    antineoplaston replacement
        therapy and, 71, 72, 74

enzyme therapy and, 116–117
epidemic of, 72–74
genetics of, 75
radiation therapy and, 151
ras oncogene expression and, 266
Liver flushes, 92
Lowen, Alexander, 204
Lung cancer, 72
COX-2 inhibitors and, 264
enzyme therapy and, 115–116
grief and, 206–207
homeopathic therapy and,
132–133
PSK mushroom extract and, 259
video-assisted thoracic surgery
and, 263
Lycopene, 231, 235
Lymphatic system, stimulation of,
222–223
Lymphoma, 30
antineoplaston replacement
therapy and, 78–81
enzyme therapy and, 111–114

Magnesium, 101
Malaria, 184
Mammograms, 149–152
Management of cancer as chronic
disease, 102–103, 127
Manganese, 161
Manilow, Barry, 11
Marquee professors, 53
Mathé, Georges, 34
Mayo Clinic, 95
McCoy, Joy Lee, 111–113
McQueen, Steve, 93
Meat consumption, 159–160, 218
Medical education, 31
BHRT and, 192

chemotherapy and, 71–72, 96
pharmaceutical industry and, 156
problems of, 156
Medicalization of daily life, 40–41
Meditation, 221
Medulloblastoma, 83–84
Melanoma, 71
Melatonin, 154, 196, 225
Menopause, 75
Merck company, 40
Mercury intake, 175, 220
Methotrexate, 234
Methylating factors, 245
Methylcobalamin, 192
Methylfolate, 192
Mevalonate, 231, 249
Mind-body connection, 204
Mistletoe extract, 171, 224, 259–260
Monacolins, 249
Morgentaler, Abraham, 78
Moritz, Andreas, 145, 181, 200
Morphine use after surgery, 262–263
Moss, Ralph, 20, 30
interview with, 43–55
Moyers, Bill, 154
MRI scans, 152
MSG, 41, 155
Multidrug resistance, 157, 159
Munoz, Dr., 168–169
Myeloma
enzyme therapy and, 101
Poly-MVA therapy and, 170
radiation therapy and, 151
"My Power to Change My Cancer
Risk" diagram, 238–250

Nagourney, Dr. Robert, 31, 49, 128
National Cancer Institute, 45, 46, 48
Nattokinase, 10, 215

Natural killer [NK] cells, 224, 246, 258–260, 262, 263
Nitrates, 249
Normal patterns of healing, 208–209
Nutrition
    chemotherapy and, 169
    foods to eat and to avoid, 159–161
    as foundation of good health, 105
    Paleolithic nutrition model, 236
    vegetarian diet, 218
    See also Supplementation

Obesity, 41
Oliver, Miles, 131–132
Omega-3 oils, 41–42, 155, 240, 248
Omega-6 oils, 41–42, 155, 160, 240
Ondamed machine, 171
Osteoporosis, 188, 189
Ovarian cancer, 109–111
Oxidative therapies, 125

Paleolithic nutrition model, 236
Palladium, 124
Palliation, 148
Pancreatic cancer, 30
    antineoplaston replacement therapy and, 71, 72
    enzyme therapy and, 90–91, 94, 108–109, 118–119
    estrogen and, 190
Panzem, 189–191
Paracelsus, 202
Parkinson's disease, 175
Patient advocacy groups, 51
Paul, Cristiana, 26
    background of, 228–229
    interview with, 229–250

Pauling, Dr. Linus, 19
Pawpaw, 124, 126
Peanuts, 240
Peck, M. Scott, 269
Peptides. *See* Antineoplaston replacement therapy
Perl, Fritz, 204
Pharmaceutical industry, 29
    alternative medicine and, 106
    BHRT and, 186, 189–191
    chemotherapy racket and, 31–32
    drug development process, 44
    FDA and, 32, 45, 46–47
    medical education and, 156
    patient advocacy groups and, 51
Phosfood, 92
Plastic bottles, 237
Poly-MVA therapy, 124, 126, 170
Pomegranate juice, 234–235, 236–237
Pregnancy, 151, 185
Premarin, 136–137
Prevention of cancer
    breast cancer, 137
    energy patches and, 178–179
    FIGHT program, 218–220
    foods to eat and to avoid, 159–161
    genetics of, 68–69, 75–77
    glutathione and, 174–176, 177–178
    hormones and, 77–78
    iodine and, 187–188, 197
    Knock It Out recommendations, 142–143, 162, 180, 199, 211, 227, 250–251
    political obstacles to, 167–168

stem cells and, 172, 242
toxicity reduction, 222–223
See also Bioidentical hormone replacement therapy; Supplementation
Progesterone, 196
Propecia, 193
Proscar, 193
Prostate cancer
citrus pectin supplementation and, 256–257
COX-2 inhibitors and, 264
dendritic cell therapy and, 168–169
estrogen and, 188
5-alpha-reductase and, 193–194
homeopathic therapy and, 125, 131–132
overdiagnosis of, 149, 158
testosterone and, 77–78
transforming growth factor and, 266
Proteins, 63–64
Provera, 136–137
PSK mushroom extract, 258–259
Psychotherapy, 204, 207, 208–209

Radiation therapy, 50, 151
Ras proteins, 265–266
Rau, Dr., 218
RBC (red blood cell) fatty acid profile, 240
Rectal cancer. *See* Colorectal cancer
Red yeast rice, 248, 249
Reeve, Dana, 207
Resveratrol, 234–236
Root canals, 218
Royal jelly, 77

S-adenosyl methionine (SAM-e), 192
Salicinium, 125, 126
Sanchez, Dr. Albert, 124
Saul, Stephanie, 40
Savino, Raphaela, 109–111
Saw palmetto, 194
Schmidt, David, 25
background of, 173–174
interview with, 174–180
Schopenhauer, Arthur, 60
Schuman frequency, 219
Sears, Barry, 240
Secondhand cigarette smoke, 220
Shilts, Randy, 122
Siegel, Bernie, 207
Siegel, Mary Jo, 78–81
Silibinin, 261
Sinatra, Dr. Stephen, 25, 170, 220
background of, 200–201
interview with, 201–210
Skin cancer, 197
melanoma, 71
Slamon, Dr. Dennis, 48
Sloan-Kettering Cancer Center, 43, 45
Smith, Dr. Robin, 172
Soda pop, 98
Somers, Suzanne
breast cancer experience, 28, 29, 181, 186–187
cancer misdiagnosis experience, 3–17, 33, 34–37, 202–203, 205, 207
Sontag, Susan, 28
Soy consumption, 160–161
Soy isoflavones, 261
Spontaneous remissions, 217–218
Statins, 249

Stem cells, 214
  banking one's own stem cells,
    172, 242
Steroids, 13
Stress, 99, 190–191, 204
Sugar intake, 98, 103–104, 155–156,
    171–172, 215, 236–237
Supplementation, 228–229
  antineoplaston replacement
    therapy and, 74–77
  breast cancer and, 152–153, 159
  cancer cell proliferation, control
    of, 248–250
  cancer risk increased by, 229–230,
    232–234
  citrus pectin, 256–258
  dyes in supplements, 232
  to eliminate (detox) carcinogens,
    244
  folic acid, 232–234
  fruit extracts, 236
  genetics and, 68–69, 241–242
  homeopathic therapy and,
    124–126, 128–129
  for immune system enhancement,
    246–247
  information sources on, 229
  iodine, 187–188
  to minimize carcinogenic load in
    the body, 243–244
  mistletoe extract, 259–260
  multidrug resistance and, 157
  "My Power to Change My Cancer
    Risk" diagram, 238–250
  as natural approach to cancer,
    156–157
  PSK mushroom extract, 258–259
  resveratrol, 234–236
  vitamin E, 229–231

Surgery, 252, 254–255, 258,
    261–263

Taguchi, Dr. Julie, 25, 182
  interview with, 134–142
Tamoxifen, 159
Taxol, 103
Testicular cancer, 30, 95
Testosterone
  BHRT and, 193, 194–196
  prostate cancer and, 77–78
Texas Medical Board, 21
Thermograms, 152
Throat cancer, 242
Tocopherols, 230–231
Tonsillectomies, 218–219
Toxicity reduction, 222–223
Traditional cancer treatment. See
    Conventional cancer therapy
Tramadol, 263
Transforming growth factor, 266
Treatment of cancer
  belief in healing and, 106–107,
    201–204, 205–206, 213–214,
    220–221
  blood thinning and, 215
  Budwig diet and, 215–216
  conventional approaches to (See
    Conventional cancer therapy)
  dendritic cell therapy, 168–169
  glutathione therapy, 179–180
  hydrazine sulfate therapy,
    170–171
  hyperthermia therapy, 171, 217
  immune therapies, 168–169
  management of cancer as chronic
    disease, 102–103, 127
  Poly-MVA therapy, 124, 126, 170
  questions to ask your doctor, xvii

spontaneous remissions and, 217–218

whole body approach to, 212–213

zinc intake and, 224–225

See also Antineoplaston replacement therapy; Enzyme therapy; Homeopathic therapy

Turmeric. *See* Curcumin

2-methoxyestradiol, 189–192

Ungar, George, 63

Uterine cancer, 159

Vaccines, 153, 171, 260

Valley fever (coccidiomycosis), 10, 14, 35–37

Van Stratten, Arlene, 108–109

Vascular endothelial growth factor (VEGF), 261

Video-assisted thoracic surgery, 263

Viruses, 64, 242

Vitamin A, 229–230

Vitamin B$_{12}$, 192

Vitamin C, 36, 223

Vitamin D, 224, 249–250

Vitamin D$_3$, 154–155

Vitamin E, 229–231

Vitamin K, 247

Vitamin K$_2$, 242

Warburg, Otto, 215

Water intake, 104, 160, 177, 222

Watermelon, 235

Weight gain, 138

Weisenthal, Dr. Larry, 31, 48–49, 128

Whitaker, Dr. Julian, xv–xviii, 22–23, 60

Wine, 160, 234–235, 236–237

Winfrey, Oprah, 228

Women's Health Initiative, 182

Wright, Dr. Jonathan, 5, 14–15, 16, 25

interview with, 183–199

Wurtman, Richard, 98

Wycoff-Fields, Carol, 119–120

Yoffee, David, 116–117

Young, Hester, 115–116

Zinc intake, 194–195, 224–225

Zometa, 266